Women's Health in Clinical Practice

Current Clinical Practice

Neil S. Skolnik, MD • Series Editor

Targeted Cancer Therapy, edited by *Razelle Kurzrock and Maurie Markman,* 2008

Essential Infectious Disease Topics for Primary Care, edited by *Neil S. Skolnik and Ross H. Albert,* 2008

Anxiety Disorders: *A Pocket Guide for Primary Care,* edited by *John R. Vanin and James D. Helsley,* 2008

Practical Evaluation and Management Coding: *A Four-Step Guide for Physicians and Coders,* by *Christopher L. Taylor,* 2008

Women's Health in Clinical Practice: *A Handbook for Primary Care,* edited by *Amy Lynn Clouse and Katherine Sherif,* 2008

Primary Care Sleep Medicine: *A Practical Guide,* edited by *J. F. Pagel and S. R. Pandi-Perumal,* 2008

Essential Practice Guidelines in Primary Care, edited by *Neil S. Skolnik,* 2007

Sexually Transmitted Diseases: *A Practical Guide for Primary Care,* edited by *Anita Nelson and JoAnn Woodward,* 2007

Allergic Diseases: *Diagnosis and Treatment, Third Edition,* edited by *Phil Lieberman and John A. Anderson,* 2007

Headache and Chronic Pain Syndromes: *The Case-Based Guide to Targeted Assessment and Treatment, Dawn A. Marcus,* 2007

Bone Densitometry in Growing Patients: *Guidelines for Clinical Practice,* edited by *Aenor J. Sawyer, Laura K. Bachrach, and Ellen B. Fung,* 2007

The Handbook of Contraception: *A Guide for Practical Management,* edited by *Donna Shoupe and Siri L. Kjos,* 2006

Obstetrics in Family Medicine: *A Practical Guide, Paul Lyons,* 2006

Psychiatric Disorders in Pregnancy and the Postpartum: *Principles and Treatment,* edited by *Victoria Hendrick,* 2006

Disorders of the Respiratory Tract: *Common Challenges in Primary Care,* edited by *Matthew L. Mintz,* 2006

Cardiology in Family Practice: *A Practical Guide, Steven M. Hollenberg and Tracy Walker,* 2006

Bronchial Asthma: *A Guide for Practical Understanding and Treatment, Fifth Edition,* edited by *M. Eric Gershwin and Timothy E. Albertson,* 2006

Dermatology Skills for Primary Care: *An Illustrated Guide, Daniel J. Trozak, Dan J. Tennenhouse, and John J. Russell,* 2006

Thyroid Disease: *A Case-Based and Practical Guide for Primary Care, Emanuel O. Brams,* 2005

Type 2 Diabetes, Pre-Diabetes, and the Metabolic Syndrome: *The Primary Care Guide to Diagnosis and Management, Ronald A. Codario,* 2005

Chronic Pain: *A Primary Care Guide to Practical Management, Dawn A. Marcus,* 2005

Bone Densitometry in Clinical Practice: *Application and Interpretation, Second Edition, Sydney Lou Bonnick,* 2004

Cancer Screening: *A Practical Guide for Physicians,* edited by *Khalid Aziz and George Y. Wu,* 2001

Hypertension Medicine, edited by *Michael A. Weber,* 2001

Allergic Diseases: *Diagnosis and Treatment, Second Edition,* edited by *Phil Lieberman and John A. Anderson,* 2000

Parkinson's Disease and Movement Disorders: *Diagnosis and Treatment Guidelines for the Practicing Physician,* edited by *Charles H. Adler and J. Eric Ahlskog,* 2000

Women's Health in Clinical Practice

A Handbook for Primary Care

Edited by

Amy L. Clouse, MD

Family Medicine Residency Program
Abington Memorial Hospital
Abington, PA

Katherine Sherif, MD

Department of Medicine
Drexel University College of Medicine
Philadelphia, PA

Humana Press

999 Riverview Drive, Suite 208
Totowa, New Jersey 07512
www.humanapress.com

This publication is printed on acid-free paper. ∞

ANSI Z39.48-1984 (American National Standards Institute) Permanence of Paper for Printed Library Materials.

Cover design by Karen Schulz

Production Editor: Christina Thomas

For additional copies, pricing for bulk purchases, and/or information about other Humana titles, contact Humana at the above address or at any of the following numbers: Tel.: 973-256-1699; Fax: 973-256-8314; E-mail: orders@humanapr.com, or visit our Website: http://humanapress.com

ISBN 978-1-61737-683-2

Printed in the United States of America. 10 9 8 7 6 5 4 3 2 1
eISBN: 978-1-59745-469-8

Library of Congress Cataloging-in-Publication Data
Women's health in clinical practice: a handbook for primary care / edited by Katherine Sherif, Amy L. Clouse.
p. ; cm. – (Current Clinical Practice)

1. Women's health services. 2. Women–Health and hygiene. 3. Primary care (Medicine)
I. Sherif, Katherine. II. Clouse, Amy L. III. Series.
[DNLM: 1. Women's Health. 2. Primary Health Care. WA 309 W8722 2007]
RA564.85.W6683 2007
362.1082--dc22
2007004640

Series Editor's Introduction

As most young clinicians loosely observe, until some extraordinary attention is paid to the significant differences in health needs, interventions, and outcomes that occur between men and women, neither gender will receive optimal health care. That the needs of men and women differ has been clearly delineated over the last two decades. Whether it is as simple as the different benefit/risk ratios incurred by men and women in the prescription of aspirin for the prevention of cardiovascular disease, the increasing proportion of women affected by hypertension, or the differences in screening protocols and outcomes for sexually transmitted diseases such as Chlamydia, the continued examination, delineation, and communication of the importance of appropriate approaches to gender-based risk assessment and treatment have become more and more apparent. Drs. Clouse and Sherif add to the existent literature on the subject by putting often difficult to find information in one easy-to-read, well-organized textbook that can be embraced and used by primary care physicians in their practices.

For this they deserve our thanks.

Neil Skolnik, M.D.
Professor of Family and Community Medicine
Temple University School of Medicine
Associate Director of the Family Medicine Residency Program
Abington Memorial Hospital

Preface

Traditionally, women's health has been synonymous with obstetrics and gynecology. With the exception of Family Medicine physicians who are trained in obstetric and gynecologic issues, most primary care physicians have received little training in reproductive health issues even though they care for women and girls. Furthermore, the concept of women's health has evolved beyond the reproductive organs. There has been growing recognition that sex differences do exist between the organ systems of women and men. Research about male and female physiologic differences has bolstered the growing body of knowledge about sex differences.

This text is intended to present the most recent changes in this current research and provide the user with an easily accessible reference to common women's health issues. The topics in this text range from health problems that largely affect only women, like cervical cancer and breast disease, to health problems that present differently in women than in men, such as cardiovascular disease and diabetes. Chapters on polycystic ovary syndrome and oral health issues address health problems that bring together multiple organ systems including reproductive, cardiovascular and dental health. There are also useful chapters not typically found in primary care texts like eating disorders, interpersonal violence and sexual health.

Women's Health: A Handbook for Primary Care is succinct and well organized. It contains easily understood, practical information for the most common health problems seen in women. Each of the 17 chapters, meticulously researched and referenced, has been written by experts in their respective fields. *Women's Health* is a valuable text for anyone who practices primary care medicine.

Amy L. Clouse, MD
Katherine Sherif, MD

Contents

Color Plate

The following color illustrations are printed in the insert.

Contributors

DEIRDRE ANGLIN, MD, MPH • *Department of Emergency Medicine, Keck School of Medicine, University of Southern California, Los Angeles, CA*

LYNDA M. BASCELLI, MD • *West Jersey-Memorial Family Practice Residency at Virtua, Voorhees, NJ*

TAMARA G. BAVENDAM, MD • *Pfizer Pharmaceuticals, Exton, PA*

DEBORAH M. BETHARDS, MD • *Division of Gastroenterology, Milton S. Hershey Medical Center, Hershey, PA*

BRENDA BUTLER, MD • *Department of Psychiatry, Drexel University College of Medicine, Philadelphia, PA*

AMY L. CLOUSE, MD • *Family Medicine Residency Program, Abington Memorial Hospital, Abington, PA*

RONALD CODARIO, MD • *Department of Medicine, University of Pennsylvania and Jefferson Medical College, Thomas Jefferson University, Philadelphia, PA*

HARRIS B. COHEN, MD • *Hatboro Medical Associates, Hatboro PA*

DEBORAH EHRENTHAL, MD • *Department of Obstetrics and Gynecology, Christiana Care Health System, Wilmington, DE*

M. HAMED FAROOQI, MD • FACE *Joslin Diabetes Center, Mease Countryside Hospital, Safety Harbor, FL*

SUSANNE K. GIORGIO, RDH • *Private Practice, Elkins Park, PA*

JOAN I. GLUCH, PhD • *Division of Pediatric and Community Oral Health, University of Pennsylvania School of Dental Medicine, Philadelphia, PA*

SERGE JABBOUR, MD • *Division of Endocrinology, Diabetes & Metabolic Diseases, Department of Medicine, Jefferson Medical College, Thomas Jefferson University, Philadelphia, PA*

LORI JARDINES, MD • *Department of Surgery, Albert Einstein Medical Center, Philadelphia, PA*

SUSAN MATHER, MD • *Wyeth Pharmaceuticals, Jefferson Medical College, Thomas Jefferson University, Philadelphia, PA*

SHAHAB MINASSIAN, MD • *Department of Obstetrics & Gynecology, Drexel University College of Medicine, Philadelphia, PA*

LAURA MINSK, DMD • *Department of Periodontics, University of Pennsylvania School of Dental Medicine, Philadelphia, PA*

CONNIE MITCHELL, MD • *Consultant, Health and Forensic Care of Intimate Partner Violence, Los Angeles, CA*

JANICE E. NEVIN, MD, MPH • *Department of Family and Community Medicine, Christiana Care Health System,Wilmington, DE*

Ann Ouyang, MD • *Division of Gastroenterology and Hepatology, Department of Medicine, Milton S. Hershey Medical Center, Hershey, PA*

Harriette M. Scarpero, MD • *Department of Urologic Surgery, Vanderbilt University, Nashville, TN*

Katherine Sherif, MD • *Department of Medicine, Drexel University College of Medicine, Philadelphia, PA*

Barbara Steinberg, DDS • *Department of Surgery, Drexel University College of Medicine, Philadelphia, PA*

Leonore Tiefer, PhD • *Department of Psychiatry, NYU School of Medicine, New York, NY*

Colleen Veloski, MD • *Division of Endocrinology and Metabolism, Temple University School of Medicine, Philadelphia, PA*

1 Contraception

Lynda M. Bascelli, MD

CONTENTS

During a busy morning office session, three women inquire about contraception, each with different goals and concerns. The first, 30 years old and married, has two young children. She and her husband think that they do not want more children, but not so certainly that they desire "permanent" birth control. She is looking for contraception that is safe, convenient, and reversible. The second woman, in her early 20s, is single and in a monogamous relationship. She has no children, but wants to have children someday. She also seeks a contraceptive method that is convenient and safe, but with the added benefit of protection against sexually transmitted infections. She suffers from dysmenorrhea. The third woman, in her late 30s and married, has firmly decided with her partner that they do not want any children. She is looking for a highly effective method to prevent pregnancy.

From: *Current Clinical Practice: Women's Health in Clinical Practice*
Edited by: Clouse and Sherif © Humana Press Inc., Totowa, NJ

INTRODUCTION

Assisting women as they decide which contraceptive method to use is an increasingly complex task because many new products have been introduced in the last decade. Novel options include oral contraceptives with novel hormones (Yasmin®) or novel regimens (Seasonale®), a levonorgestrel-releasing intrauterine device (Mirena®), a transdermal combination hormonal patch (Ortho-Evra®), and a transvaginal combination hormonal ring (NuvaRing®). A new permanent method of sterilization (Essure®) is available. Emergency contraception is available in both combination hormonal regimens (Yuzpe regimen) and progestin-only regimens (Plan B®).

These new approaches to contraception join the list of older methods, not only augmenting available options but also expanding the range of factors that differentiate these methods—factors that women now can consider when making their selection. As suggested by the examples above, different women have different goals and concerns, which typically address a method's:

1. Effectiveness, both with perfect and typical use of the method.
2. Safety (likelihood of personal harm).
3. Convenience (ease of use).
4. Reversibility (likelihood of and/or length of time to return to fertility on cessation of method).
5. Ancillary benefits (desirable side effects).
6. Acceptability (risk of undesirable side effects and whether the mechanism of action conforms to a woman's religious or other beliefs).
7. Cost.

To be most successful, a method first must be compatible with a woman's preferences and priorities, and second must be used consistently and correctly in the context of her lifestyle. A clinician can be most helpful to a woman seeking contraception by not only knowing what methods are available, but also how to help a woman decide what method will best fit into her life. Accordingly, this chapter focuses on newer technologies available for contraception, and reviews older methods, organizing the discussion of each approach to consider each of the major considerations of effectiveness, safety, convenience, reversibility, ancillary benefits, acceptability, and cost.

Before we begin, let us briefly review the definition and measure of effectiveness. In reports of contraceptive effectiveness, a group of sexually active women who use the method of contraception are observed for the first year of use of the method to determine what percentage of these women become pregnant (in other words, the failure rate of the method). This failure rate is reported for both perfect use (which is defined as consistent and correct use of the method) and typical use (defined as use of the method that is not always consistent or not always correct). This proportion is then compared with the established 85% of sexually active women who typically become pregnant each year if they are using no form of birth control. In this chapter, all information regarding effectiveness is based on the data reported in *Contraceptive Technology*, which is the gold-standard source in this field *(1)*. Finally, all data regarding cost is based on the 2005 summary published online by *Consumer Reports (2)*.

ORAL CONTRACEPTIVES

The combination oral contraceptive (which contains both estrogen and progesterone) is historically important: hundreds of millions of women have used the multitude of formulations collectively known as "the pill" as a means to prevent pregnancy since it was first introduced in the 1960s. Furthermore, the newer formulations available today are ensuring that oral contraceptives remain a popular, effective, and safe method of birth control.

- Effectiveness: Women who use combination oral contraceptives perfectly (that is, take the pill at the same time every day) have a 0.3% chance of becoming pregnant; more typical use of the pill (including missing doses or not taking the pill at the same time every day) can result in an 8% chance of becoming pregnant. There is insufficient data from randomized controlled trials to distinguish any difference in effectiveness between oral contraceptives containing 20 μg ethinyl estradiol and those containing greater than 20 μg *(3)*. In women with a body mass index greater than 27, the oral contraceptive may be less effective *(4)*.
- Safety: Among women who do not smoke, the oral contraceptive pill has an established safety record. Smoking, however, especially in women older than the age of 35 years, increases the risk of thrombosis, stroke, and myocardial infarction. Lower doses of ethinyl estradiol in oral contraceptives are thought to account for a lower risk of venous thromboembolism, but the type of progestin may also be responsible for the cardiovascular risk associated with oral contraceptives *(5)*. Although controversial, the data regarding breast cancer risk in the users of oral contraceptives seems to indicate no additional risk than in nonusers: a recent case–control study demonstrated that the incidence of breast cancer is the same among women aged 35 to 64 years who have never taken the pill, who used to take the pill, and who currently take the pill *(6)*. The use of the combination oral contraceptive is not recommended in women who have a history of thrombosis or cardiovascular disease, liver disease, hypertension, breast cancer, unexplained vaginal bleeding, or migraine headaches with focal neurological symptoms *(5)*.
- Convenience: The oral contraceptive pill must be taken daily for 21 days of each 28-day cycle; most pill packs dispense a 7-day placebo course to help maintain a daily routine. Seasonale® is an extended-cycle oral contraceptive that may be beneficial to those women with menstrual-related disorders

such as dysmenorrhea, because it allows for only four withdrawal bleeds each year by using 84, instead of 21, hormone-containing pills per cycle.

- Reversibility: Fertility returns immediately on discontinuation of the oral contraceptive.
- Ancillary Benefits: Benefits of the combined oral contraceptive include protection against endometrial and ovarian cancer, treatment of dysmenorrhea and treatment of acne. Drospirinone, a new progestin (Yasmin®) related to spironolactone, is antiandrogenic, antimineralocorticoid, and associated with less weight gain and more improvement in acne compared with other oral contraceptives. Seasonale® (ethinyl estradiol/levonorgestrel) reduces dysmenorrhea by reducing the number of cycles. Standard contraceptive pills used continuously for 3 months and skipping the placebo week will also reduce the number of menstrual cycles to four per year. There are no advantages of multiphasic contraceptive pills, which vary estrogen or progestin doses, over monophasic pills.
- Acceptability: The oral contraceptive pill works by preventing ovulation; its mechanism of action may also include thickening the cervical mucous, which inhibits sperm motility, and inducing endometrial changes that prevent implantation. Contraceptive pills may be associated with nausea, breast tenderness, mood changes, and headache, all of which stop on cessation of therapy. Breastfeeding women should not use combination oral contraceptives because they may decrease milk production; the evidence for this, however, is not overwhelming *(7)*. Women who are taking oral contraceptives with low-dose (20 μg) ethinyl estradiol experience more irregular bleeding than women who take higher doses of estrogen *(3)*, but this side effect could potentially be attributed to the type of progestin in the pill as well. There is some evidence that oral contraceptive pills containing 20 μg of ethinyl estradiol may have adverse effects on bone mineral density in young women *(8)*. Oral contraceptives provide no protection against sexually transmitted infections.
- Cost: The average cost per month of contraception is approx $30, but ranges between $20 and $50. A 3-month course of Seasonale is $115, but this 84-day regimen can be duplicated by using the active pills of monthly contraceptive pills continuously.

PROGESTIN-ONLY ORAL CONTRACEPTIVE

The progestin-only "mini-pill" is used in the same way as the combination oral contraceptive pills, but has the benefit of being appropriate in breastfeeding. Progestin-only pills are also safe in women in whom estrogen is contraindicated, such as smokers older than age 35 years, and women with a history of venous thromboembolism, hypertension, cardiovascular disease, or stroke. The progestin-only pill is taken every day with no hormone-free withdrawal period to ensure that ovulation is suppressed by a consistent level of hormone. However, it is more likely to be associated with irregular bleeding and amenorrhea. To ensure effectiveness, the mini-pill must be taken at nearly the exact same time every day to provide a failure rate of 0.3% with perfect use and 8% with more typical use. The mini-pill costs between $30 and $50 per month.

TRANSDERMAL HORMONAL CONTRACEPTIVE PATCH

Approved by the Food and Drug Administration (FDA) in 2001, the combined hormonal contraceptive patch (Ortho-Evra®) provides an average daily dose of 20 μg of ethinyl estradiol and 0.15 mg of norelgestromin via transdermal delivery. Overall similar to the oral contraceptive pill in terms of mechanism of action, efficacy, safety, and side effects, the patch differs chiefly with regard to convenience.

- Effectiveness: Ortho-Evra® is equally efficacious in preventing pregnancy as the combination oral contraceptive pill, with a failure rate of 0.3% with perfect use and 8% with typical use. It may not be as effective in preventing pregnancy in women who weigh more than 90 kg *(9)*.
- Safety: Similar to the contraceptive pill, the patch is associated with an increased rate of venous thromboembolism, stroke, and myocardial infarction, especially in women older than age 35 years or women who smoke. Women with a history of venous thromboembolism or cardiovascular disease, or a history of hypertension, liver disease, unexplained vaginal bleeding, or smokers older than age 35 years should not use the transdermal patch. In late 2005, the FDA updated labeling for Ortho-Evra® to include a bolded warning that users are exposed to 60% more total estrogen in their blood than if they were taking a combination birth control pill containing 35 μg of estrogen. However, it is still not known whether this extra estrogen exposure results in an increase in thromboembolic events *(10)*.
- Convenience: The patch is applied once a week to the upper torso, arm, abdomen, or buttocks. Each patch is worn for 1 week and removed before applying the next patch, with one patch-free week after 3 weeks of use to allow for a withdrawal bleed. The patch is beige in color, and can be seen on the skin if not placed in an area covered by clothing. Women's self-reported compliance is better with the patch than with the pill *(11)*.
- Reversibility: As with the combination oral contraceptive pill, fertility is restored once the patch is discontinued.
- Ancillary Benefits: Similar to the pill, the patch provides protection against ovarian and endometrial cancer.
- Acceptability: The patch prevents pregnancy chiefly by preventing ovulation. As with the oral contraceptive pill, its mechanism of action may also involve changes in the cervical mucous and changes in the endometrium to hinder sperm motility and implantation, respectively. The patch may cause dysmenorrhea and breast tenderness more often then the pill; the patch may also result in increased spotting, but this usually resolves after two cycles of use. The most

common adverse reaction resulting in patch discontinuation is local skin reactions. The patch provides no protection against sexually transmitted infections.

- Cost: The cost is approx $39 per month, roughly the same as a 1-month supply of oral contraceptive pills.

TRANSVAGINAL CONTRACEPTIVE

The NuvaRing®, available in the United States since 2002, is a soft, flexible ring that is placed into the vagina by the user, where it remains in place for 3 weeks and is removed for 1 week to allow for a withdrawal bleed before it is replaced by a new ring for the next cycle. It requires no fitting, and delivers a dose of 15 μg of ethinyl estradiol and 0.12 mg of etonogestrel daily while in place.

- Effectiveness: The ring has the same failure rate as the oral contraceptive: 0.3% with perfect use and 8% with typical use.
- Safety: The ring has the same hormone-associated risks as the oral contraceptive pill of venous thromboembolism, stroke, and myocardial infarction. The same women who should not use combination hormonal contraception—smokers older than 35 years, women with a history of venous thromboembolism or cardiovascular disease, and women with liver disease, hypertension, breast cancer, or unexplained vaginal bleeding should not use the transvaginal ring.
- Convenience: The transvaginal ring offers the convenience of administration every 3 weeks as opposed to daily pill usage or weekly transdermal patch usage. If the ring falls out or is removed for more than 3 hours, it can be replaced, but back-up contraception (a barrier method) should be used for the next 7 days.
- Reversibility: Fertility is restored on discontinuation of the transvaginal ring.
- Ancillary Benefits: The transvaginal ring offers menstrual cycle control and the same benefits of the combination oral contraceptive in terms of protection against endometrial and ovarian cancer, with an overall lower dose of hormones.
- Acceptability: The transvaginal ring works by preventing ovulation. In addition, its mechanism of action may include alteration of the cervical mucous to create an environment that impairs sperm motility and it may cause changes in the endometrium that inhibit implantation. As with the pill, ring use can lead to headache, nausea, and breast discomfort; additionally, local reactions to the ring may include vaginal discomfort and discharge. A woman needs to be comfortable inserting and removing the ring herself for this method of birth control to be acceptable to her. The transvaginal ring provides no protection against sexually transmitted infections.
- Cost: Similar to the transdermal patch, the transvaginal ring costs roughly the same as a 1-month supply of oral contraceptives, approx $37 per month.

INJECTABLE CONTRACEPTION

Medroxyprogesterone acetate (DMPA, specifically Depo-Provera®) is a progestin-only injectable contraceptive administered once every 3 months.

- Effectiveness: DMPA provides highly effective contraception with a failure rate of 0.3% if used perfectly and 3% with typical use.
- Safety: DMPA, unlike combination hormonal-based methods of birth control, is not associated with an increased risk of thrombosis. DMPA has been associated with decreases in bone-mineral density; a recent study suggested that the loss in bone density is reversed after discontinuation of DMPA *(12)*. DMPA has also been associated with increases in low-density lipoprotein and total cholesterol and a decrease in high-density lipoprotein.
- Convenience: With no need to take a daily pill, DMPA does require a woman to make an office visit every 3 months to receive the injection.
- Reversibility: Fertility is delayed 6 to 12 months after discontinuation of DPMA, and may be delayed longer.
- Ancillary Benefits: DPMA use may lead to amenorrhea, which is advantageous in women with heavy menstrual bleeding and dysmenorrhea or anemia. Furthermore, DMPA is associated with decreased risks of endometrial, ovarian cancer, and pelvic inflammatory disease.
- Acceptability: DPMA works by inhibiting ovulation and by thickening the cervical mucous, impeding sperm motility. Women using Depo-Provera® typically gain 5.4 pounds during the first year of use, 8.1 pounds in year 2, and 13.8 pounds in year 3 *(1)*, but most women discontinue Depo-Provera for the menstrual irregularities it causes rather than because of the weight gain. Most women experience amenorrhea, but some women will experience vaginal spotting. DPMA, like all hormonal methods, offers no protection against sexually transmitted infections.
- Cost: DMPA costs approx $57 per injection plus the cost of an office visit.

INTRAUTERINE DEVICE

The intrauterine device (IUD) is enjoying a resurgence in popularity, in part because of the introduction of the levonorgestrel intrauterine system (LNG-IUS) Mirena®, which is available in the United States, joining the other IUD option, the Copper T 380A (ParaGard®).

- Effectiveness: The IUD is highly effective in preventing pregnancy; the Copper T 380A has a 0.8% failure rate with typical use and a 0.6% failure rate with perfect use, and the LNG-IUS has a 0.1% failure rate for both typical and perfect use.
- Safety: Risks include uterine perforation and infection with insertion, but have a very low incidence.
- Convenience: A trained clinician can insert this highly convenient method of contraception during a short office visit. After insertion, the Copper T 380A is approved for use for up to 10 years and the LNG-IUS is approved for use up to 5 years. A provider of the LNG-IUS must have special training in its insertion technique, which is available through the manufacturer.
- Ancillary Benefits: Mirena® is useful in women with heavy menstrual bleeding because it often causes amenorrhea, and it also reduces symptoms of

dysmenorrhea *(13)*. The Copper T 380A is also useful as emergency contraception if inserted up to 5 days after unprotected intercourse.

- Reversibility: Fertility is returned immediately on discontinuation of the IUD.
- Acceptability: The copper IUD works by creating an intrauterine and tubal environment that impairs sperm function and inhibits fertilization. The levonorgestrel intrauterine system prevents fertilization by thickening cervical mucous and suppressing the endometrium. Once inserted safely, modern IUDs rarely cause side effects. The copper device can cause irregular or heavy menstrual bleeding. In contrast, the LNG-IUS actually reduces the amount of menstrual bleeding and dysmenorrhea over time, often resulting in amenorrhea, but is associated with a higher incidence of ovarian cysts. Approximately 2 to 10% of women experience spontaneous expulsion, which is most likely to occur in the first year of use. IUDs do not protect against sexually transmitted infections and are not recommended for women with multiple sexual partners.
- Cost: The cost of each device, in addition to the fee for inserting the device, may seem prohibitive ($250–300 for the copper IUD and $300–400 for the LNG-IUS, plus the cost of the office visit and insertion). The IUD, however, has been shown to be cost-effective during the 5- to 10-year period of its use.

BARRIER METHODS

The barrier methods consist of the cervical cap, diaphragm, contraceptive sponge, female condom, and male condom. All are nonhormonal methods.

- Effectiveness: The effectiveness of each barrier method is highly dependent on its correct and consistent use.
  - The male condom, when used consistently and correctly, has a failure rate of 2%, but, for more typical use, has a failure rate of 15%. The female condom has a failure rate of 21% with typical use and 5% with perfect use.
  - The diaphragm has a failure rate of 16% with typical use and 6% with perfect use.
  - The cervical cap's failure rate varies from 16 to 32% for typical use and 9 to 26% for perfect use; the cervical cap is less effective in women who have had a vaginal delivery.
  - The contraceptive sponge's failure rate is similar to that of the cervical cap: 16 to 32% with typical use and 9 to 20% with perfect use.

  Overall, the contraceptive effectiveness of the barrier methods is much less than the hormonal methods or the IUD.

- Safety: Barrier methods are extremely safe.
- Convenience: Both male and female condoms and the contraceptive sponge are available without a prescription. The diaphragm and the cervical cap require fitting by a clinician. The condom requires placement just before intercourse; the diaphragm, cervical cap, and contraceptive sponge all may be placed in the vagina before the initiation of sexual activity. The diaphragm must be left in place for 6 hours after intercourse; it is recommended that additional

spermicide is inserted vaginally using an applicator before additional episodes of intercourse, although the evidence for spermicide use with the diaphragm in general is lacking *(14)*. The cervical cap may be left in place for 48 hours, with no additional spermicide required for additional episodes of intercourse. The contraceptive sponge provides protection against pregnancy for up to 24 hours, and must remain in place for 6 hours after intercourse.

- Reversibility: While using the barrier methods, fertility is maintained and pregnancy could result from the next occurrence of unprotected sexual intercourse.
- Ancillary Benefits: The male and female condoms offer protection against sexually transmitted infections, such as HIV, syphilis, gonorrhea, and chlamydia, however, *condoms do not protect against human papilloma virus*.
- Acceptability: Barrier methods prevent the sperm and egg from meeting by creating a physical barrier through which sperm cannot penetrate. The diaphragm, cervical cap, contraceptive sponge, and certain types of male condoms have the added mechanism of spermicide.
- Cost: Male condoms cost less than $1 per use and female condoms cost approx $3 per use. Health insurance does not cover the expense of condoms. The diaphragm costs $30 to $40 and the cervical cap costs $100 to $200 plus the cost of an office visit and spermicide. Spermicide costs approx $1 per use. At the current time, the contraceptive sponge is being reintroduced to the US market and no cost information is available.

FERTILITY AWARENESS-BASED METHODS

The oldest forms of birth control involve the determination of and avoidance of sexual intercourse during the periovulatory phase of menstrual cycle, or the use of barrier methods during that time. Methods differ in determining timing of ovulation (by calendar, basal body temperature, cervical mucous testing, or a combination of these methods), and the extent of the period of abstinence that they recommend. Other names for these methods are "natural family planning," "rhythm," or "periodic abstinence."

- Effectiveness: The failure rate for abstinence during fertile periods is estimated to be approx 25% with typical use and 1 to 9% with perfect use; the effectiveness of different methods cannot be rigorously compared because there have been too few adequately designed studies *(15)*.
- Safety: These methods have no risks other than unintended pregnancy.
- Convenience: These methods require a couple to be highly motivated because they require fertility monitoring and then adherence to multiple days of abstinence per ovulatory cycle.
- Reversibility: Fertility is never disrupted with fertility awareness-based methods.
- Ancillary Benefits: None.
- Acceptability: There is no interruption to ovulation, cervical mucous, or the endometrium because these are nonhormonal methods.
- Cost: None.

SURGICAL METHODS

Female sterilization is an option with considerable benefits for women, men, and couples who do not want to have children, and in women for whom pregnancy would be a grave medical risk. Surgical techniques for women include tubal ligation or occlusion, performed via laparoscopy, and hysteroscopic insertion of tiny coils (Essure) into the Fallopian tubes. Until obstruction caused by fibrosis is proven by hysterosalpingogram at 3 months, a back-up method is required. In men, the sterilization technique is vasectomy.

- Effectiveness: Effectiveness for female sterilization is similar to the IUD and implanted or injected hormones, with a failure rate of 0.5%, making female sterilization one of the most effective contraceptive options for women. Long-term effectiveness is not established yet for the Essure method. Male sterilization via vasectomy is also considered one of the most effective means of contraception, with a reported failure rate of 0.1 to 0.4% in the literature; these figures should be interpreted carefully, however, because the outcome studied is rarely unintended pregnancy, with many studies looking at sperm counts after the procedure *(1)*. In terms of cost, female sterilization is much more costly than male sterilization, but both methods are highly cost-effective compared with other methods of birth control.
- Safety: Male sterilization does not carry the associated risks of anesthesia that female sterilization does, and overall is considered a safer procedure. The Essure method is likewise performed in the outpatient setting without anesthesia; but the procedure is still in its early stages of use so that there are no data regarding long-term safety. With female sterilization performed in the operating suite, there are the usual surgical risks associated with anesthesia and surgical complications, such as infection and bleeding.
- Convenience: Once any of the procedures are performed, there is no need to consider contraception again. Men are generally counseled that they need 20 ejaculations (or 12 weeks after vasectomy) before they are considered sterile. Obstruction of the fallopian tubes needs to be confirmed by hysterosalpingogram at 3 months. If obstruction is not confirmed, the procedure needs to be repeated. Placement of coils is associated with pain due to cervical cramping and fallopian tube spasm.
- Reversibility: Although procedures exist to attempt to restore fertility after a sterilization procedure, both male and female sterilization procedures should be considered permanent.
- Ancillary Benefits: Studies have suggested that female sterilization via tubal ligation may protect against ovarian cancer *(1)*.
- Acceptability: Both male and female sterilization techniques work by preventing egg and sperm from meeting.
- Cost: Female sterilization costs $2500 to $4000; male sterilization costs $250 to $1000. Both procedures are considered highly cost-effective.

EMERGENCY CONTRACEPTION

Widespread use of emergency contraception, according to estimates, could prevent up to 50% of unintended pregnancies that now occur yearly in the United States. The FDA has approved three methods for emergency contraception: the combination oral contraceptive (Yuzpe regimen) used within 72 hours of unprotected intercourse, the progestin-only oral contraceptive (Plan B®) used within 72 hours of unprotected intercourse, and the copper T-380A inserted up to 5 days after unprotected intercourse. Multiple brands of combination oral contraceptives may be used for emergency contraception. For all methods, there are two doses, taken 12 hours apart. The number of pills taken with each dose varies depending on the oral contraceptive used: the required amount per dose of ethinyl estradiol is 100 μg; the required amount per dose of the progestin component is either 0.5 mg of levonorgestrel or 1 mg of norgestrel. Plan B® consists of two 0.75-mg tablets of levonorgestrel taken 12 hours apart.

- Effectiveness: Plan B® has been shown to be more effective at preventing pregnancy and is associated with fewer side effects as compared with the Yuzpe regimen. In a randomized controlled trial comparing the progestin-only regimen with the Yuzpe regimen, the failure rate with the progestin-only regimen was 1.1% and the failure rate for the Yuzpe regimen was 3.2% *(16)*. Both regimens are more effective the earlier they are taken after unprotected intercourse. Studies have shown that taking both doses of the Plan B regimen together in a single-dose is as effective as the two doses 12 hours apart *(17)*.
- Safety: Both emergency contraception regimens seem to be safe.
- Convenience: Whether emergency contraception should be available over-the-counter without a prescription is controversial. Currently, California, Alaska, Maine, New Mexico, and Hawaii have followed the example set by Washington State and allow pharmacists to dispense emergency contraception without a prescription. Studies have shown in other countries that the over-the-counter availability of emergency contraception did not increase high-risk sexual behaviors. In August of 2006, the FDA approved nonprescription status for Plan B, making it available over-the-counter to both women and men aged 18 and older in the United States.
- Acceptability: Although the exact mechanism of action of emergency contraception is disputed, it seems that the hormones inhibit ovulation and prevent implantation. Emergency contraception does not interfere with an established pregnancy. Nausea and vomiting are significantly higher in the combined hormone dose compared with the levonorgestrel-only dose. Anti-emetics, such as metoclopramide, taken 1 hour before the emergency contraceptive dose may prevent or minimize vomiting. If vomiting occurs within 1 hour of taking either dose, the dose be can repeated.
- Cost: Plan B® costs approx $30, which is similar to the cost of a pack of oral contraceptive pills required for the Yuzpe regimen.

Table 1
Summary of Contraceptive Methods

Method	*Specific Type*	*Effectiveness*	*Safety*	*Convenience*	*Reversibility*	*Ancillary Benefit*	*Acceptability*	*Cost*
Oral contraceptive	Combination estrogen–progestin	0.3% perfect use; 8% typical use	Smoking increases risk of thrombosis, stroke, and myocardial infarction	Must be taken every day at approximately the same time	Immediate on discontinuation	Can help with dysmenorrhea and acne; protects against ovarian and endometrial cancer	Prevents ovulation; may also thicken cervical mucous and change endometrium to prevent implantation; not for breastfeeding women; side effects	\$20–50 per 28 d cycle; \$115 for extended cycle pill (Seasonale®)
	Progestin-only	0.3% perfect use; 8% typical use	Safer than combination pills in patients at risk for cardiovascular disease	Must be taken at nearly the same exact time daily for maximum effectiveness	Immediate on discontinuation	Safe for use in breastfeeding women	Thickens cervical mucous to inhibit sperm motility	\$30–50 per 28 d cycle
IUD	LNG-IUS	0.1% for both perfect and typical use	Low incidence of uterine perforation or infection at time of insertion	Provides up to 5 yr of highly effective contraception with no concern regarding compliance	Immediate on discontinuation	Useful in women with heavy menstrual bleeding and dysmenorrhea	Causes changes in cervical mucous to inhibit sperm motility	\$300–400 every 5 yr plus cost of insertion

	ParaGard T380-A	0.6% perfect use; 0.8% typical use	Low incidence of uterine perforation or infection at time of insertion	Provides up to 5 yr of highly effective contraception with no concern regarding compliance	Immediate on discontinuation		Creates an intrauterine and tubal environment that impairs sperm function and inhibits fertilization	$250–300 every 10 yr plus cost of insertion
Contraceptive patch		0.3% perfect use; 8% with typical use	Same as the combination oral contraceptive	Requires once-weekly dosing	Immediate on discontiuation	Same as combination oral contraceptive	Same as combination oral contraceptive; patch may cause local skin irritation	$40 per 28 d cycle
Trans-vaginal		0.3% perfect use; 8% with typical use	Same as the combination oral contraceptive	Ring remains in place for 3 wks at a time	Immediate on discontinuation	Same as combination oral contraceptive	Same as combination oral contraceptive; ring may cause vaginal irritation or discharge	$38 per 28 d cycle
Injectable	DMPA	0.3% perfect use; 3% typical use	No increased risk of thromboembolism; associated with loss of bone-mineral density	Requires office visit every 3 mo for injection	Delayed for 6–12 mo after discontinuation	Use may lead to amenorrhea which may be beneficial in women with heavy menstrual bleeding and dysmenorrhea	Inhibits ovulation and inhibits sperm motility by thickening cervical mucous; cause weight gain	$57 per injection plus office visit

(Continued)

Table 1 (*Continued*)

Method	*Specific Type*	*Effectiveness*	*Safety*	*Convenience*	*Reversibility*	*Ancillary Benefit*	*Acceptability*	*Cost*
Emergency contra-ception	Plan B®	1.1% failure rate	No safety concerns have been identified	Few states allow phar-macists to dispense without a prescription, otherwise requires an office visit; must be taken within 72 h of unprotected intercourse	Does not affect future fertility	None	Thought to work by preventing ovulation but may also alter endometrium, thereby hindering implantation; nausea and vomiting are common side effects	$30
	Yuzpe regimen	3.2% failure rate	No safety concerns have been identified	Same as Plan B	Same as Plan B	None	Same as Plan B	$20–50 (same as 28-d pack of oral contrcep-tive pills)
Barriers	Diaphragm	6% perfect use; 16% typical use	No safety concerns	Must be inserted prior to intercourse	Fertility is not interrupted	None	Prevents fertiliza-tion by acting as a barrier between sperm and egg	$30–40 plus cost of office visit and spermi-cide

	Cap	9–26% perfect use; 16–32% typical use	No safety concerns	Must be inserted before intercourse	Fertility is not interrupted	None	Same as diaphragm	$100–200 plus cost of office visit and spermicide
	Sponge	9–20% perfect use; 16–32% with typical use	No safety concerns	Must be inserted before intercourse	Fertility is not interrupted	None	Same as diaphragm	No cost information available
	Male and female condom	2% perfect use and 15% typical use for male condom; 5% perfect and 21% typical use for female condom	No safety concerns	Must be placed just before intercourse	Fertility is not interrupted	Protects against sexually transmitted infections	Same as diaphragm	Male condom: $0.25–1 per use; Female condom: $3 per use
Surgical	Vasectomy	0.1–0.4%	Safe outpatient procedure, no anesthesia risks	Method is permanent and requires no further consideration of contraception	Not reversible	None	Creates permanent inability of sperm to come into contact with egg	$250–1000

(Continued)

Table 1 (*Continued*)

Method	*Specific Type*	*Effectiveness*	*Safety*	*Convenience*	*Reversibility*	*Ancillary Benefit*	*Acceptability*	*Cost*
	Female tubal ligation	0.5%	Surgical risks associated with anesthesia, infection, bleeding	Method is permanent and requires no further consideration of contraception	Not reversible	May protect against ovarian cancer	Creates permanent inability of sperm to come into contact with egg	$2500–4000
	Transcervical female sterilization (tubal occlusion)	Long-term effectiveness not established yet	Long-term safety not established	Method is permanent and requires no further consideration of contraception	Not reversible	No long-term data available	Creates permanent inability of sperm to come into contact with egg	$2000–3000
Fertility awareness-based methods		1–9% perfect use; 25% typical use	No safety concerns	Does not allow for spon taneity; best for highly motivated couples	Fertility is not interrupted	None	Failure rate is high	None

[a]IUD, intrauterine device; LNG-IUS, levonorgestrel intrauterine system; DMPA, Medroxyprogesterone acetate.

WHAT THE FUTURE MAY HOLD

The main innovations on the horizon are implantable contraceptive methods similar to Norplant®, which is a six-rod progestin implant that is no longer being manufactured after an advisory in 2000 warned about the contraceptive efficacy of certain suspected lots of Norplant systems (which were subsequently found to be effective). Implant systems of contraception are highly efficacious and convenient, but newer systems are not readily available in the United States.

- Jadelle® is a two-rod subdermal levonorgestrel system implanted in the inner aspect of the nondominant upper arm. It has been approved by the FDA for 5 years of use but has not been marketed in the United States. Up to 65% women using Jadelle® experience abnormal bleeding, including prolonged heavy bleeding, irregular spotting, or amenorrhea. The discontinuation rate is 20% and is related to abnormal bleeding.
- Implanon® is a single-rod progestin implant available in Europe and approved in the United States by the FDA in 2006. It releases etonogestrel and provides contraception for up to 3 years. Studies have shown it to be highly efficacious and rapidly reversible; it is discontinued most frequently for irregular bleeding *(18)*.

REFERENCES

1. Hatcher RA, Trussell J, Stewart FH, et al. Contraceptive Technology. 18th revised ed. Ardent Media, Inc., New York; 2004.
2. Consumer Reports: Your comparative guide to contraceptives. 2005 (Accessed 11 June, 2005, at http://www.consumerreports.org/main/content/display_report.jsp?FOLDER%3C%3Efolder_id=551091&ASSORTMENT%3C%3East_id=333141#).
3. Gallo M, Nanda K, Grimes DA, Schulz K. 20 mcg versus >20 mcg Estrogen combined oral contraceptives for contraception. Cochrane Database Syst Rev 2005(2):CD003989.
4. Holt VL, Scholes D, Wicklund KG, Cushing-Haugen KL. Body mass index, weight, and oral contraceptive failure risk. Obstet Gynecol 2005;105(6):1492–1493.
5. Petitti DB. Clinical practice. Combination estrogen-progestin oral contraceptives. N Engl J Med 2003;349(15):1443–1450.
6. Marchbanks PA, McDonald JA, Wilson HG, et al. Oral contraceptives and the risk of breast cancer. N Engl J Med 2002;346(26):2025–2032.
7. Truitt ST, Fraser AB, Grimes DA, Gallo MF, Schulz KF. Combined hormonal versus non-hormonal versus progestin-only contraception in lactation. Cochrane Database Syst Rev 2003(2):CD003988.
8. Cromer BA, Stager M, Bonny A, et al. Depot medroxyprogesterone acetate, oral contraceptives and bone mineral density in a cohort of adolescent girls. J Adolesc Health 2004; 35(6):434–441.
9. Choice of contraceptives. Treatment Guidelines from The Medical Letter 2004;2(24):55–62.
10. FDA Updates Labeling for Ortho Evra Contraceptive Patch, FDA News November 10, 2005 (Accessed 5 February, 2006 at http://www.fda.gov/bbs/topics/news/2005/NEW01262.html).
11. Gallo MF, Grimes DA, Schulz KF. Skin patch and vaginal ring versus combined oral contraceptives for contraception. Cochrane Database Syst Rev 2003(1):CD003552.

12. Scholes D, LaCroix AZ, Ichikawa LE, Barlow WE, Ott SM. Change in bone mineral density among adolescent women using and discontinuing depot medroxyprogesterone acetate contraception. Arch Pediatr Adolesc Med 2005;159(2):139–144.
13. Jensen JT. Noncontraceptive applications of the levonorgestrel intrauterine system. Curr Womens Health Rep 2002;2(6):417–422.
14. Cook L, Nanda K, Grimes D. Diaphragm versus diaphragm with spermicides for contraception. Cochrane Database Syst Rev 2003(1):CD002031.
15. Grimes DA, Gallo MF, Grigorieva V, Nanda K, Schulz KF. Fertility awareness-based methods for contraception. Cochrane Database Syst Rev 2004(4):CD004860.
16. Randomised controlled trial of levonorgestrel versus the Yuzpe regimen of combined oral contraceptives for emergency contraception. Task Force on Postovulatory Methods of Fertility Regulation. Lancet 1998;352(9126):428–433.
17. Cheng L, Gulmezoglu AM, Oel CJ, Piaggio G, Ezcurra E, Look PF. Interventions for emergency contraception. Cochrane Database Syst Rev 2004(3):CD001324.
18. Funk S, Miller MM, Mishell DR Jr, et al. Safety and efficacy of Implanon, a single-rod implantable contraceptive containing etonogestrel. Contraception 2005;71(5):319–326.

2 Premenstrual Syndrome and Premenstrual Dysphoric Disorder

Harris B. Cohen, MD

Contents

INTRODUCTION

Premenstrual syndrome (PMS) was first mentioned in a paper by Dr. Robert Frank in 1931, and further described and defined in the *British Medical Journal* in 1953 *(1)*. PMS is a common condition characterized by physical and behavioral symptoms that occur during the luteal phase of the menstrual cycle. The luteal phase is defined as the time in the menstrual cycle that occurs between ovulation and menstruation. Symptoms include abdominal bloating, headaches, breast tenderness and fatigue, which do not significantly impair the day-to-day activities of the woman's lifestyle. These symptoms have been reported to affect as many as 75% of women of reproductive age.

In 1987, the *Diagnostic and Statistical Manual of Mental Disorders* (DSM)-III-R made mention of late luteal phase dysphoric disorder, but not until 1994, in the DSM-IV, was premenstrual dysphoric disorder (PMDD) first described.

From: *Current Clinical Practice: Women's Health in Clinical Practice*
Edited by: Clouse and Sherif © Humana Press Inc., Totowa, NJ

In this edition, PMDD is classified as a "depressive disorder not otherwise specified." Criteria for diagnosis include the following:

During most menstrual periods in the previous year, presence of at least five of the following symptoms for most of the last week of the luteal phase, with improvement in symptoms a few days after onset of the follicular phase, and absence of symptoms during the week after menstruation; at least one of the first four symptoms must be included:

- Markedly depressed mood, feelings of hopelessness, or self-deprecating thoughts
- Marked anxiety
- Marked affective lability
- Persistent and marked anger or irritability or increased interpersonal conflicts
- Decreased interest in usual activities
- Concentration difficulty
- Lethargy or lack of energy
- Marked change in appetite
- Insomnia or hypersomnia
- Feeling overwhelmed
- Other physical symptoms (breast tenderness or swelling, headache, myalgias or arthralgias, bloating, or weight gain
- Marked interference with work, school, social activities, or interpersonal relationships
- Disturbance of another mood disorder, and not a mere exacerbation

Confirmation of the three criteria above by using ratings scales during at least two consecutive menstrual cycles *(2)*.

It is debatable whether PMS and PMDD are two diagnoses along one spectrum of pathology or two clinically distinct entities. PMS generally refers to the more mild emotional and physical symptoms that occur during the luteal phase of the menstrual cycle. PMDD causes symptoms severe enough to disrupt the woman's normal daily functioning. This distinction is important in establishing a correct diagnosis, as approximately one woman out of eight who presents to her physician for PMS symptoms actually meets PMDD criteria. The premenstrual worsening of an underlying, preexisting mood disorder does not qualify as PMDD.

EPIDEMIOLOGY

PMDD is thought to affect 3 to 8% of women of reproductive age, markedly less than the 75% of women thought to be affected by PMS. These numbers are supported by several community studies, showing a 1-year prevalence of 5.8% and a lifetime incidence of 7.4% *(3)*.

Interestingly, prevalence of disease does not seem to be dependent on cultural or socioeconomic differences. Onset of symptoms is generally in late adolescence, but maximum severity does not manifest until the woman reaches her late twenties to mid thirties. Currently, there does not seem to be a genetic predisposition to disease, although there is a higher concordance of disease in monozygotic twins versus dizygotic twins and in sisters versus nonrelated cohorts.

ETIOLOGY

The exact cause of PMDD is currently unknown. There seems to be a complex interplay of psychological, biological, and environmental factors that all take part in the manifestation of symptomatology. Initially, there was thought to be an imbalance in estrogen-to-progesterone ratios; however, current consensus favors normal hormonal function.

Current theory suggests that the normal variation in ovarian hormones and their interaction with central neurotransmitters is the inciting factor in PMDD *(4)*. The normal cyclic variation in estrogen and progesterone during a regular menstrual cycle has been shown to cause changes in the γ-amino butyric acid (GABA), serotonin, and opioid responses of the central nervous system.

The role of GABA in PMDD has not been thoroughly examined; however, a study looking at the progesterone metabolite allopregnenolone showed that this GABAergic neurotransmitter is found in lower concentrations in those women with PMDD than in healthy controls *(5)*. A deficiency of this metabolite can lead to increased anxiety levels, especially in times of stress. A GABA agonist, alprazolam, has been shown to be effective in improvement of these anxiety symptoms.

Of all of the neurotransmitter studies thus far, serotonin seems to be the most important in the etiology of PMDD. Central levels of this neurotransmitter are low during the luteal phase of the menstrual cycle in women with PMDD. Additionally, symptoms are exacerbated through depletion of tryptophan—serotonin's precursor. In addition to changes in serotonin levels, it is thought that postsynaptic serotonergic response may be altered during the late luteal phase of the menstrual cycle *(6)*.

Vitamin deficiencies have also been proposed as a cause of PMDD. However, studies have not shown any differences in levels of vitamins E, A, or B_6 in symptom sufferers versus controls. In addition, magnesium has not shown to be deficient in women with PMDD.

DIAGNOSIS

The diagnosis of PMDD can be challenging because of the constellation of somewhat nonspecific complaints that define this disorder. A thorough history and physical examination are essential to help exclude other causes of symptomatology, because there are no pathognomonic signs on physical exam or confirmatory laboratory findings associated with PMDD. In addition, the clinician must differentiate between PMDD and the possibility that the presenting symptoms are a premenstrual exacerbation of another underlying comorbidity. It is important to note that, in premenstrual exacerbation of medical or psychiatric illness, the symptoms are present throughout the entire menstrual cycle but are magnified premenstrually. Whereas, in PMDD, symptoms are only present in the luteal phase and completely resolve after menstruation. This differentiation is essential to correctly diagnosing true PMDD.

Other conditions that may mimic PMDD include:

- Psychiatric conditions: Major depression, dysthymia, bipolar II, cyclothymic disorder, panic disorder, generalized anxiety disorder, bulimia, posttraumatic stress disorder, and history of mental or physical abuse.
- Medical conditions: Hypothyroidism or hyperthyroidism, diabetes mellitus, autoimmune diseases, anemia, chronic fatigue syndrome, and endometriosis *(7)*. Fibromyalgia, irritable bowel syndrome, and migraine disorder (especially menstrual migraine) also share many features with PMDD. A pelvic exam in patients with lower abdominal or pelvic symptoms may help exclude pelvic inflammatory disease and other causes of secondary dysmenorrhea. Checking thyroid function tests, a complete blood cell count, and a follicle-stimulating hormone (FSH) level can help exclude thyroid disease, anemia, and perimenopause/menopause as being causal or contributory to the patient's symptoms.

DSM-IV criteria suggest confirmation of symptoms through the use of prospective daily rating scales for two menstrual cycles. There are several daily ratings scales that are commonly used, and patients may use one or several of these before seeking treatment. There is no consensus regarding which scale is best, and a simple internet search will allow the patient to view and download several examples. The patient can then complete these scales at home, before discussion with their physician.

The most commonly used scales are the Calendar of Premenstrual Experiences, the Daily Record of the Severity of Problems, the Premenstrual Syndrome Diary, and the Prospective Record of the Severity of Menstruation. By recording emotional and physical symptoms for two consecutive menstrual cycles, the clinician can more easily confirm diagnosis when there is a paucity of symptoms in the follicular phase, and an increase during the luteal phase. If the patient does not demonstrate a symptom-free period during the follicular phase of the cycle, an evaluation for an underlying mood or anxiety disorder should be initiated.

NONPHARMACOLOGICAL TREATMENT

Lifestyle modification should be first-line treatment for those patients with symptoms of PMDD that are less severe or in those women who are prediagnosis. Although evidence-based studies are scant, there are simple lifestyle measures that can be recommended that should not have untoward side effects or cause worsening of symptoms.

Dietary recommendations should include the reduction of salt, fat, caffeine, and refined sugar. This simple change may reduce the bloating and fluid retention that occur premenstrually. Frequent meals with small complex carbohydrate-packed snacks have been postulated to elevate tryptophan levels (a serotonin precursor). Reduction of alcohol may reduce irritability and decrease serotonergic inhibition.

The American College of Obstetricians and Gynecologists recommends magnesium, vitamin E, and calcium as nutritional supplements to help with premenstrual symptoms *(8)*. A meta-analysis of nine trials evaluated the efficacy of vitamin B_6; this study showed that dosages up to 100 mg/d are likely to help with luteal phase emotional and physical symptoms *(9)*. Calcium supplementation has also been examined, and dosages of 1000 to 1200 mg/d of elemental calcium have been shown to be effective in symptom reduction. The use of over-the-counter TUMS® as a calcium-delivery system may also reduce some of the bloating associated with PMDD. Smaller studies have shown some efficacy with magnesium in doses of 200-360 mg/d and vitamin E in dosages of 400 to 800 IU/d. Recent studies that show an increased risk of heart failure in older patients taking vitamin E should give the clinician pause before recommending this supplement in certain PMDD patients.

Several herbal therapies have been examined in the literature. There is conflicting data on evening primrose oil as an herbal remedy for PMDD. Initial studies showed symptom improvement, likely through increased levels of prostaglandin E_1 *(10)*. The extract of agnus castus fruit (chasteberry), through reduction of prolactin levels, may ameliorate breast tenderness in some women. Other herbs, including gingko biloba, St. John's wort, and kava kava have also been examined, but the data to support their efficacy is scant. It is important to note that the Food and Drug Administration (FDA) has not approved any herbal remedy for PMDD, and use of herbal remedies is strictly experimental.

Increased aerobic activity has been shown to benefit PMS sufferers, although this has not been studied extensively in PMDD. Exercise functions to increase endorphin release, promote self-esteem, and increase a sense of well-being, all of which may be at decreased levels in the PMDD patient. Patients should be encouraged to start slowly, with a final goal of 30 to 45 minutes of cardiovascular exercise three to four times per week.

Relaxation therapy, yoga, and meditation have shown to decrease the symptoms logged by women on their daily scales. Cognitive-behavioral therapy for patients with negative thoughts and self-blame may be effective. Bright-light therapy administered daily during the luteal phase has shown to be effective in one study, possibly through its indirect elevation of serotonin levels through the melatonin pathway *(11)*.

PHARMACOLOGICAL TREATMENT

Selective Serotonin Reuptake Inhibitors

Selective serotonin reuptake inhibitors (SSRIs) are first-line treatment for PMDD. These medications ease both the emotional and physical symptoms that are present in PMDD sufferers. Although most SSRIs have been shown to be effective in ameliorating PMDD symptoms, only fluoxetine (Sarafem® and Prozac®), extended-release paroxetine (Paxil CR®), and sertraline (Zoloft®) are FDA-approved for this indication.

The initial SSRI receiving FDA approval was fluoxetine, branded as Sarafem® by Eli Lilly. Effective dosing is between 20 and 60 mg/d, with a therapeutic dose of 20 mg.

More recently, the extended-release form of paroxetine (Paxil CR®) and sertraline (Zoloft®) have received approval. Efficacious dosing ranges are 12.5 to 25 mg/d for extended-release paroxetine *(12)* and 50 to 150 mg for sertraline *(13)*. Other SSRIs, including citalopram (Celexa®) and escitalopram (Lexapro®), have also been shown to be effective for PMDD symptom reduction, however, they are not FDA-approved at this time, and their use is strictly off-label. One small trial of fluvoxamine (Luvox®) found no benefit in PMDD *(14)*.

Interestingly, when compared with SSRI dosing for depressive disorder, the effective dosing for PMDD is usually lower. Although positive results are usually observed within the first month of treatment, sometimes in as few as 2 to 3 days, three menstrual cycles should be observed before considering a change in medication. Once clinical remission is achieved, continuing the effective medication is important, because studies have shown a worsening of symptoms after discontinuation of an SSRI *(15)*.

There are several dosing options for the SSRIs, because benefit is seen both with continuous (daily) dosing and luteal-phase (ovulation through menstruation) dosing *(16)*. Luteal phase dosing is an attractive choice for those patients looking to minimize cost, because medication is taken only for 2 weeks each month. In addition, SSRIs are associated with sexual side effects (decreased libido and anorgasmia), gastrointestinal side effects (nausea), and weight gain. Although these side effects are more common at higher dosages, luteal phase dosing may help to minimize these undesired side effects in women who derive emotional and other physical benefits from an SSRI. An attractive luteal phase dosing option is 90 mg fluoxetine administered once weekly for 2 weeks, which showed efficacy in a recent study *(17)*.

Non-SSRI Antidepressants

Other non-SSRI antidepressants have been evaluated for PMDD. Two receiving the most attention are clomipramine (Anafranil®) and venlafaxine (Effexor®). Clomipramine has been shown to be effective in dosages of 25 to 75 mg/d, but its use is limited by its anticholinergic side effects *(18)*. These may include dry mouth, urinary retention, constipation, blurred vision, and confusion. Venlafaxine in dosages of 75 to 112.5 mg/d has been shown to be efficacious and well-tolerated *(19)*.

Anxiolytics

Alprazolam, lorazepam, and clonazepam have all been evaluated in PMDD. These benzodiazepine anxiolytics function as GABA agonists in the central nervous system. Interestingly, GABA levels may be lower in women with PMDD *(20)*. Alprazolam has been the most studied agent in this category, with most studies showing more efficacy than placebo *(21)*. These medications are most effective in treating the anxiety aspect of PMDD, but caution is advised because of their addictive potential and should be viewed as second-line treatment. If prescribed, luteal phase treatment with taper at menses is recommended.

Hormonal Agents

Hormonal treatment of PMDD is postulated to work through suppression of ovulation, which leads to reduction of premenstrual symptomatology. The gonadotropin-releasing hormone (GnRH) agonists downregulate GnRH receptors and cause pharmacological suppression of ovulation.

Agents in this category include leuprolide, goserelin, and histrelin. These GnRH agonists have shown efficacy in PMDD, but are limited by their menopause-like side effects, which include hot flashes, vaginal dryness, irritability, and decreased bone density. Through their suppression of luteinizing hormone (LH) and FSH, estrogen and progesterone are also diminished. Studies which "add back" estrogen and/or progesterone to limit these side effects have shown a return of the PMDD symptoms that they were initially used to treat *(22)*. These medications are only available in an injectable or implantable form, and their costs can be substantial. Use of the GnRH agents should be reserved for those women who fail SSRI or anxiolytic therapy and have refractory PMDD symptoms.

Oral contraceptives also work through suppression of LH and FSH, resulting in anovulatory cycles. Limited evidence of their use in PMDD is conflicting, but there may be a weak class effect. One study examined a combination pill containing drospirenone and ethinyl estradiol (Yasmin®), which showed improvement in PMDD symptoms *(23)*. Oral contraceptives are generally more effective in the reduction of physical complaints, and may worsen the emotional symptoms of PMDD. More research is needed to further evaluate the efficacy of oral contraceptives in PMDD.

Danazol is a weak synthetic androgen that inhibits LH and FSH. Doses of up to 100 mg twice per day for up to 6 months may show some efficacy in symptom reduction *(24)*. However, weight gain, acne, and nausea may limit its use.

Other Therapies

Bromocriptine, a dopamine agonist, may be effective in reducing symptoms of breast tenderness when used preovulation through menstruation. Suggested dosages range from 2.5 mg one to three times per day. Spironolactone, a diuretic with antiandrogenic properties, has been used during the luteal phase to reduce bloating, breast tenderness, and acne. Dosing recommendations vary from 50 to 100 mg/d. If used frequently, serum potassium should be followed.

Nonsteroidal anti-inflammatory drugs are used for a multitude of premenstrual symptoms, including headache, abdominal cramping, breast tenderness, and joint pain, because these are all mediated by prostaglandins. Benefits include low cost and easy access; however, nonsteroidal anti-inflammatory drugs only show efficacy with the physical, and not the emotional, symptoms of PMDD.

Surgical therapy has been used for extreme cases of PMS, because hysterectomy with bilateral salpingo-oopherectomy has been shown to be curative. With the multitude of treatment options that now exist, surgical intervention no longer has a place in the treatment of PMDD.

CONCLUSION

Although popular culture has embraced and popularized PMS, the more severe and debilitating form of this disease has now entered the medical lexicon. PMDD is a prevalent disease with debilitating physical and emotional symptomatology. As we learn more about this disease, we can empower women to take control of their symptoms through pharmacological and nonpharmacological interventions. Patient education and proper diagnosis are essential, and treatment options must be thoroughly discussed on a patient-by-patient basis. The recent use of SSRIs as first-line pharmacotherapy has shown extremely promising results, and the increased clinical attention to PMDD is certain to yield future treatment breakthroughs.

REFERENCES

1. Dalton K, Greene R. The premenstrual syndrome. Brit Med J 1953;1:1007.
2. Adapted from Diagnostic and Statistical Manual of Mental Disorders, 4th Ed. Washington DC: American Psychiatric; 1994.
3. Wittchen H, Becker E, Lieb R, Krause P. Prevalence, incidence, and stability of premenstrual dysphoric disorder in the community. Psychol Med 2002;32(1):119–132.
4. Steiner M, Born L. Diagnosis and treatment of premenstrual dysphoric disorder: an update. Int Clin Psychopharmacol 2000;15:S5–S17.
5. Girdler S, Straneva P, Light KC, Pedersen CA, Morrow AL. Allopregnanolone levels and reactivity to mental stress in premenstrual dysphoric disorder. Biol Psychiatry 2001;49(9): 788–797.
6. Haslbreich U, Tworek H. Altered serotonergic activity in women with dysphoric premenstrual syndromes. Int J Psychiatry Med 1993;23(1):1–27.
7. Endicott, J. Differential diagnosis and comorbidity. In: Premenstrual Dysphorias: Myths and Realities (Gold J, Severino S, eds.). American Psychiatric, Washington DC, 1994; pp. 3–17.
8. American College of Obstetricians and Gynecologists. Premenstrual syndrome: clinical management guidelines for obstetrician-gynecologists. ACOG Practice Bulletin 2000;15: 1–9.
9. Wyatt K, Dimmock P, Jones PW, Shaughn O'Brien PM. Efficacy of vitamin B6 in the treatment of the premenstrual syndrome: systematic review. BMJ 1999;318:1375–1381.
10. Hardy M. Herbs of special interest to women. J Am Pharm Assoc 2000;40:234–242.
11. Lam R, Carter D, Misri S, Kuan AJ, Yatham LN, Zis AP. A controlled study of light therapy in women with late luteal phase dysphoric disorder. Psychiatry Res 1999;86:185–192.
12. Cohen L, Soares C, Yonkers KA, Bellew KM, Bridges IM, Steiner M. Paroxetine controlled release for premenstrual dysphoric disorder: a double-blind, placebo controlled trial. Psychosomatic Med 2004;66:707–713.
13. Cohen L. Sertraline for premenstrual dysphoric disorder. JAMA 1998;279:357–358.
14. Veeninga AT, Westenberg HG, Weusten JT. Fluvoxamine in the treatment of menstrually related mood disorders. Psychopharmacol 1990;102:414–416.
15. Pearlstein T, Joliat M, Brown EB, Miner CM. Recurrence of symptoms of premenstrual dysphoric disorder after the cessation of luteal-phase fluoxetine treatment. Am J Obstet Gynecol 2003;188:887–895.
16. Lin J, Thompson D. Treating premenstrual dysphoric disorder using serotonin agents. J Womens Health Gen Based Med 2001;10:745–750.
17. Miner C, Brown E, McCray S, Gonzales J, Wohlreich M. Weekly luteal-phase dosing with enteric-coated fluoxetine 90 mg in premenstrual dysphoric disorder: a randomized, double-blind, placebo-controlled clinical trial. Clin Ther 2002;24:417–433.
18. Sundblad C, Modigh K, Andersch B, Eriksson E. Clomipramine effectively reduces premenstrual irritability and dysphoria. Acta Psychiatr Scand 1992;85:39–47.
19. Cohen LS, Soares CN, Lyster A, Cassano P, Brandes M, Leblanc GA. Efficacy and tolerability of premenstrual use of venlafaxine (flexible dose) in the treatment of premenstrual dysphoric disorder. J Clin Psychopharm 2004;24(5):540–543.
20. Halbreich U, Petty F, Yonkers K, Kramer GL, Rush AJ, Bibi KW. Low plasma gamma-aminobutyric acid levels during the late luteal phase of women with premenstrual dysphoric disorder. Am J Psychiatry 1996;153:718–720.
21. Evans S, Haney M, Levin FR, Foltin RW, Fischman MW. Mood and performance changes in women with premenstrual dysphoric disorder: acute effects of alprazolam. Neuropsychopharmacology 1998;19:499–516.

22. Leather A, Studd J, Watson NR, Holland EF. The treatment of severe premenstrual syndrome with goserelin with and without add-back estrogen therapy. Gynecol Endocrinol 1999;13: 48–55.
23. Freeman E, Kroll R, Rapkin A, et al. Evaluation of a unique oral contraceptive in the treatment of premenstrual dysphoric disorder. J Womens Health Gen Based Med 2001;10: 561–569.
24. Hahn P, Van Vugt D, Reid R. A randomized, placebo-controlled, crossover trail of danazol for the treatment of premenstrual syndrome. Psychoneuroendocrinology 1995;20:193–209.

3 Menopause

Janice E. Nevin, MD, MPH
and Deborah Ehrenthal, MD, FACP

Contents

INTRODUCTION

It is estimated that more than 40 million women will experience menopause during the next 20 years. For most women, approximately one-third of their life will occur in the postmenopausal period *(1)*. Menopause represents a distinct event or stage in the life of a woman that is normal and may have a positive and liberating effect. For a health care provider and for the woman herself. menopause represents an opportunity to assess concerns and implement important disease prevention and health maintenance interventions.

DEFINITION

Menopause is a natural, biological event that is defined clinically by the absence of menses for 12 months or greater. Most women will experience menopause in their late 40s or early 50s, although the age range for normal menopause is 40 to 60 years of age, with an average age of 51 years *(2)*. During

From: *Current Clinical Practice: Women's Health in Clinical Practice*
Edited by: Clouse and Sherif © Humana Press Inc., Totowa, NJ

the period of time leading up to menopause, referred to as perimenopause, and during menopause itself, a woman will experience multiple endocrine, somatic, and psychological changes. More than half of women (51%) will describe menopause as a period of happiness and fulfillment, although increased anxiety about aging and body change may occur. Of importance to the woman and her health care provider is the recognition that this phase of life is accompanied with an increased risk of chronic disease. CVD, including the presence of metabolic syndrome; certain cancers; and osteoporosis are particular health concerns that should be specifically addressed during menopause *(3)*. Women will depend on their primary care provider for recommendations regarding prevention and screening. In addition, many women will seek treatment for menopausal-related symptoms, such as hot flashes, night sweats, vaginal dryness, insomnia, mood swings, and depression.

The physiological hallmark of menopause is the decline in estrogen. The gradual withdrawal of estrogen can have significant short- and long-term consequences and directly contributes to the symptoms of menopause. The cause and effect of estrogen on chronic diseases association with menopause is not well-understood. Recent studies have shown that estrogen replacement is not always the best approach to preventing or treating medical conditions associated with aging.

SYMPTOMS

A wide variety of symptoms are reported as being associated with the menopausal transition. These include vasomotor symptoms, vaginal dryness, sleep disturbance, mood symptoms, cognitive disturbances, uterine bleeding, sexual dysfunction, urinary complaints, and various somatic complaints, such as nervous tension, palpitations, and headaches, lack of energy, fluid retention, backache, difficulty in concentrating, dizziness, and an overall reduced quality of life *(4)*. However, although the prevalence of many of these problems and complaints increases for women during the time of menopause, they are not necessarily the result of the hormonal changes of menopause *(5)*. Evidence to date has shown that the complaints specifically related to the hormonal changes of menopause are changes in the menstrual cycle, vasomotor symptoms, and symptoms of vaginal dryness *(6)*.

Changes in the Menstrual Cycle

The most common clinical change a woman will notice as the menopausal transition begins will be changes in the menstrual cycle. During the early stage, there is no change in menstrual cycle regularity. Instead, women may notice a shorter cycle, a lighter or heavier flow, or a longer or shorter duration of menstrual flow *(7)*. These changes may be noted as early as age 30 years or as late as age 54 years, but they will occur most commonly between the ages of 40 and 44 years and, in the majority of women, by age 45 years.

As the menopausal transition proceeds, irregularity of the menstrual cycle becomes the characteristic feature. Anovulatory cycles become more common and, eventually, episodes of amenorrhea may develop. Long periods of amenorrhea may occur during the perimenopausal transition, only to be followed by a resumption of regular menses. Some cycles are associated with high levels of estrogen and low progesterone, which can lead to a heavy menses *(8)*.

Predicting the date of menopause, something many patients desire, is difficult and not aided by the measurement of hormone levels *(9,10)*. The changes patients have noted in their menstrual cycle can serve as a guide. Women who have missed more than 3 but fewer than 12 menses are very likely to complete the menopausal transition within the next 4 years *(11)*. Women who have a "running range" (the difference between the shortest and longest cycle) of more than 42 days are very likely to complete the menopausal transition within the next 12 months *(12)*.

Vasomotor Symptoms

Hot flushes and night sweats are one of the most identifiable symptoms of menopause and occur at some point in a majority of women during the menopausal transition. There is variability in reporting of symptoms among various cultures, with hot flushes reported less frequently among Japanese and Chinese women *(13)*. Symptoms are more common with increasing body mass index (BMI), and have a higher prevalence among smokers, women with a more sedentary lifestyle, and women under "financial strain" *(14)*. In addition, women who report premenstrual syndrome seem to be at greater risk of menopausal hot flushes, depressed mood, poor sleep, and decreased libido *(15)*.

The hot flush is experienced as a strong sense of warmth in the chest, which spreads upward toward the face and head before it fades, and is followed by sweating. It is created by a sudden vasodilation of skin capillaries and lasts up to several minutes. They occur unpredictably day or night, can be extremely bothersome, and may interrupt sleep. The cause of vasomotor symptoms is not known, but it is thought that hormonal changes during the menopausal transition increase the lability of the hypothalamic thermoregulatory center *(16)*.

Hot flushes can be experienced at any stage during the menopausal transition, but become more common as the date of the final menstrual period approaches. A recent review of four population-based cohort studies and 33 cross-sectional studies examined the association and prevalence of hot flushes with stage of menopause. Prevalence rates ranged from 14 to 51% for premenopausal women, approx 50% for perimenopausal women, and between 30 and 80% for postmenopausal women, and depended on the age and the population studied *(4)*.

It is important for the clinician to remember that not all symptoms reported as hot flushes are related to the menopausal transition. Systemic diseases, such as thyroid disease, carcinoid syndrome, and pheochromocytoma, as well as some neoplastic conditions and infections can causes hot flushes. This is especially important to consider when evaluating women who are under 45 years or women who are not yet experiencing changes in their menstrual cycle *(17,18)*.

GU Changes

Low levels of estrogen during the menopausal period lead to thinning of the vaginal epithelium, which can cause vaginal dryness and atrophic vaginitis. The prevalence of GU symptoms increases through the menopausal transition, with up to one-third of perimenopausal and postmenopausal women experiencing vaginal dryness *(4)*. Women with atrophic vaginitis may experience vaginal dryness, itching, burning, and dyspareunia. They may also have symptoms of vaginal bleeding or post-coital spotting. Other urinary symptoms associated with menopause include urgency, frequency, both urge and stress urinary incontinence, and increased incidence of recurrent urinary tract infection *(19)*.

Breast Tenderness

Breast tenderness is a bothersome complaint that improves during the menopausal transition, especially during the late perimenopausal and postmenopausal periods *(6)*.

Sleep Disturbance, Mood Change, Cognitive Disturbances

Changes in sleep, mood symptoms, and cognitive disturbances have all been associated with menopause. A recent review of the literature found that the prevalence of sleep disturbance is higher among perimenopausal and postmenopausal women, possibly because of vasomotor symptoms. This same review did not find support in the literature for the association of mood change and cognitive disturbances with menopause *(4)*.

EVALUATION OF THE MENOPAUSAL WOMAN

Evaluation of the perimenopausal and menopausal woman provides the clinician with the opportunity to assess health risk, address long-term prevention, evaluate perimenopausal and menopausal symptoms, and to provide anticipatory counseling for women approaching the change.

History

Health risks and opportunities for prevention can be assessed by obtaining a complete personal and family history, with attention to risk factors for CVD, osteoporosis, diabetes, and the common cancers (breast, colon, and lung). Cardiovascular risk factors include a personal history of hypertension, diabetes, hyperlipidemia, or tobacco use. Women with a family history of CVD in first-degree male relatives at the age of 55 years or younger or female relatives age 65 years or younger are at increased risk. Women should also be assessed for a history of fragility fractures as well as osteoporosis risk. In addition, women should be screened for depression, domestic violence, problem drinking, and a sedentary lifestyle.

Menopausal symptoms should be elicited, with specific questions directed toward vasomotor symptoms, menstrual changes, urogenital symptoms (dyspareunia, incontinence, vaginal discharge, or bleeding), and symptoms of depression. The extent to which these symptoms affect the quality of life should be discussed explicitly with the patient.

A complete menstrual history will help the clinician identify a perimenopausal bleeding pattern, define menopause, and elicit symptoms of abnormal uterine bleeding or postmenopausal bleeding. A woman older than 40 years with new changes in her menstrual cycle is most likely beginning the menopausal transition, especially if she has accompanying vasomotor symptoms. However, because there is such a large variation in the signs and symptoms of the menopausal transition, it is essential to exclude underlying pathology. The regularity and the length of the menstrual cycle, changes in menstrual flow, symptoms of intermenstrual bleeding or post-coital bleeding, and the presence or absence of symptoms of hot flushes or vaginal dryness will help direct evaluation.

For women who are experiencing a lighter menses or less-frequent menses (oligomenorrhea), the possibility of pregnancy and thyroid disease must be considered *(20)*. Symptoms pointing to other causes of amenorrhea or oligomenorrhea, such as previously unrecognized polycystic ovary syndrome, prolactinoma, and eating disorders, should be sought. Finally, the use of some commonly used medications can lead to oligomenorrhea or amenorrhea *(21)*.

For women with increased bleeding, a thorough menstrual bleeding history will help identify women with bleeding between menstrual cycles (intermenstrual bleeding), irregular bleeding (metrorrhagia), heavy bleeding (menorrhagia), or bleeding after intercourse (post-coital bleeding), who may have underlying anatomic pathology and who will require further evaluation. The absence of symptoms of breast tenderness and bloating before menses and cramping with menses (moliminal symptoms) in a woman with irregular menses suggests bleeding caused by chronic anovulation. In addition, a complete bleeding history should be sought because heavier menses may be caused by an underlying coagulopathy, such as unrecognized von Willebrand's Disease.

For women who are postmenopausal, the presence of postmenopausal bleeding should be specifically elicited because it may be the only symptom of endometrial cancer. Many women think it can be normal to have spotting and do not report this symptom until the bleeding is heavy, potentially resulting in a delay in evaluation and treatment.

Physical Exam

The height, weight, and blood pressure will enable screening for obesity and hypertension. The BMI should be determined. A complete exam should include an examination of the thyroid gland and an evaluation of signs of thyroid dysfunction because this may cause menstrual irregularity and sweating. A clinical breast exam should be performed as a component of breast cancer screening, as well as a cardiovascular exam. A pelvic exam, including a speculum exam and a bimanual exam, should be performed to evaluate any vaginal bleeding that has been reported and to assess the degree of vaginal atrophy as well as the presence of prolapse.

Testing

If there is any possibility of pregnancy, a urine or serum human chorionic gonadotropin levels should be measured if a woman presents with amenorrhea, oligomenorrhea, or irregular bleeding. Thyroid-stimulating hormone levels are generally measured as well if there are changes in the menstrual cycle, unless one has been obtained recently.

For most menopausal women, it is not necessary to obtain a blood test to confirm menopause. During the perimenopausal transition, the follicular-stimulating hormone (FSH) is quite variable and is not a reliable indicator of when menopause will occur *(22)*. It is, however, very useful in clearly identifying menopause for women who are experiencing hot flushes and have had a hysterectomy with intact ovaries. It is also used to identify premature ovarian failure in young women with amenorrhea.

For women who are taking combined hormonal contraceptives, the typical symptoms of menopause are masked by the hormones. A clinician can look for evidence of menopause by checking an FSH annually beginning at age 50 to 52 years. Because combined hormonal contraceptives will suppress the FSH, it must be measured on the sixth or seventh day of the placebo or pill-free week. An FSH greater than 20 IU/L suggests menopause, but, unfortunately, is not entirely accurate because of the fluctuations typically seen during perimenopause *(23)*. The risk to stopping hormones is the risk of pregnancy. An alternative approach is to continue combined hormonal contraceptives until the woman is in her mid-fifties, when the risk of ovulation and conception is very low. At that time, hormones can be stopped, and the woman can watch for recurrence of menses while using a back-up method for birth control.

Women with abnormal bleeding patterns will require further evaluation to exclude an underlying cause of bleeding before it can be attributed to the perimenopause. This includes women with bleeding that is prolonged or heavier than usual, women with bleeding between menses, and women with post-coital bleeding *(17)*. It is important to note that the risk of endometrial hyperplasia and endometrial cancer rises after age 40 years; women with hypertension, obesity, and diabetes are at an even higher risk *(14)*. Women who have had irregular periods for much of their life have likely had years of chronic anovulation. This places them at an increased risk for the development of endometrial hyperplasia and cancer. Regardless of a woman's age, an evaluation of heavy or intermenstrual bleeding should be pursued. All postmenopausal bleeding requires a diagnostic evaluation to exclude the presence of endometrial hyperplasia or endometrial cancer. This can be performed with transvaginal ultrasound, endometrial biopsy, or hysteroscopy.

Lipids typically increase during perimenopause and early menopause, and should be reassessed at this time *(24)*. Screening recommendations for type 2 diabetes vary. The American Diabetes Association recommends screening all women older than 45 years with a fasting blood glucose every 3 years, especially those who have an elevated BMI *(25)*. The United States Preventive Services Task Force (USPSTF) recommends screening those with hypertension and hyperlipidemia *(26)*. Women with a family history of osteoporosis, with a medical condition that increases their risk for osteoporosis, or a personal history that confers risk, should undergo screening for osteoporosis with a dual-energy X-ray absorptiometry scan. Once a woman has reached age 65 years, the USPSTF recommends routine screening for osteoporosis *(27)*.

Cancer screening continues through the menopausal period. For most women, screening mammography is recommended yearly from the age of 40 years *(28,29)*. Screening for cervical cancer with a Papanicolaou (Pap) smear continues, but may be performed every 2 to 3 years for women at low risk for cervical cancer *(30)*. Women with a history of abnormal Pap smears, human papilloma virus infection, other sexually transmitted diseases, or high-risk sexual behavior should continue with annual screening. Pap tests can be discontinued for women who have had a hysterectomy for benign disease. The age at which screening for cervical cancer should stop is controversial. The USPSTF recommends against screening for women 65 years and older who have had adequate recent screening with normal Pap smears and are not otherwise at high risk for cervical cancer. The American College of Obstetrics and Gynecology does not set an upper age limit, but the American Cancer Society recommends stopping at age 70 years for women who are at low risk and have been well-screened *(30)*. Screening for colon cancer begins for most women at age 50 years *(31)*. If there is a history of colon cancer in a first-degree relative, screening may begin earlier.

TREATMENT OF MENOPAUSAL SYMPTOMS

Vasomotor instability and urogenital changes of menopause are related to the withdrawal of estrogen, therefore, the most effective treatment of these symptoms is HRT. In the wake of the findings of the Women's Health Initiative (WHI), which raised concerns regarding increased risks of CVD and breast cancer, many physicians and patients have struggled with decision making with regard to HRT. Evidence continues to emerge to help clinicians better understand the risk–benefit profile and guide patients toward informed clinical decision making.

Hormone Replacement Therapy

For those women experiencing moderate-to-severe symptoms that interfere with the quality of their life, especially with the quality of their sleep, HRT remains an appropriate option. Estrogen has been shown to reduce the symptoms of menopause by 70 to 95% and is the most important indication to prescribe HRT. No other treatment is as effective.

Various options for prescribing HRT exist, including cyclical or continuous regimens, and oral or transdermal preparations *(16)*. Table 1 lists some of the formulations of estrogen and progesterone, including combination therapy, and the mechanisms of delivery that are available. In general, oral estrogens have a greater effect on the liver because of the first-pass effect and, as a result, increase high-density lipoproteins and triglycerides. The estrogen patch may be preferred in women who may need to avoid the impact on liver metabolism, for example, those with a tendency to venous thromboembolism, or gallbladder or hepatic disease. These women will not experience the potential beneficial effect on high-density lipoprotein cholesterol. Estrogen is also available in the form of an intravaginal ring (Femring®), which delivers 50 to 100 mg of estradiol daily and is effective for both vasomotor and GU symptoms. A new intranasal 17-β estradiol spray has been developed and is available in other countries.

Women with an intact uterus should be prescribed a progestogen (micronized progesterone or medroxyprogesterone acetate [MPA]) in addition to estrogen

Table 1
Types of Estrogens and Progestogens[a]

Estrogens	
Conjugated equine estrogens (CEE)	Oral, intravaginal cream
17-β estradiol	Oral, transdermal patch and gel, intravaginal ring, tablet and cream
Progestogens	
Medroxyprogesterone acetate (MPA)	Oral
Micronized progesterone	Oral, cream
Norethindrone acetate	Oral
Norgestimate	Oral
Levonorgestrel	Oral
Combinations	
CEE and MPA	Oral
Estradiol and norgestimate	Oral
Estradiol and norethindrone	Oral, transdermal patch
Estradiol and levonorgestrel	Transdermal patch

[a]Dosage and delivery method may vary depending on the need for systemic treatment of vasomotor symptoms or local treatment of genitourinary symptoms. Women with an intact uterus must be prescribed progesterone in addition to estrogen to prevent endometrial cancer.

to reduce the risk of endometrial cancer. In general, the lowest dose of both estrogen and progestogen that relieves symptoms should be prescribed, and for the shortest duration of time. Typically, this means 0.05 mg/d of weekly estradiol transdermal patch, 0.625 mg of oral conjugated equine estrogens (CEE), or 1 mg of oral 17-β estradiol. For long-term therapy, a reduction in dose to 0.025 mg/d weekly patch, 0.3 mg of CEE, or 0.5 mg of 17-β estradiol should be considered if symptoms permit. Progestogens can be administered in a cyclic or continuous regimen or as part of combination therapy. MPA can be started at 2.5 mg/d administered daily or for 10 to 14 days per month. Micronized progesterone may be administered as 100 mg daily (before bed) or 200 mg for 10 to 14 days per month. Unlike MPA, micronized progesterone does not attenuate estrogen's beneficial effects on lipids and has the lowest rate of unexpected bleeding. Some clinicians prefer to initiate therapy with cyclical dosing and move to continuous therapy once a bleeding pattern has been established and symptoms have been stable *(40)*.

Pregnancy, unexplained vaginal bleeding, acute or chronic liver disease, recent vascular thrombosis, and a history of breast or endometrial cancer are contraindications to HRT. A family history of breast cancer and a distant history of thromboembolism are relative contraindications and must be considered in the risk–benefit analysis in deciding to prescribe HRT. Although hypertension, hypercholesterolemia, diabetes, and cigarette smoking are not contraindications, they represent significant cardiovascular risk factors and must be seriously considered in decision making.

HRT use and symptomatology should be assessed on an annual basis or more frequently if questions arise. Because the vasomotor symptoms of menopause typically resolve in less than 5 years from the onset of menopause, HRT should be tapered and discontinued within 5 years.

After HRT is initiated, maximal symptom benefit may take 2 to 4 weeks to achieve. Once a decision is made to discontinue HRT, the dose should be tapered over several weeks to minimize the recurrence of symptoms. Current data does not support initiating HRT in women longer than 10 years after menopause because of the increased risk of coronary artery disease in the age group.

HRT and Coronary Heart Disease

Several promising observational studies published since the mid-80s suggested that HRT reduced the risk of CVD significantly, leading health care providers to think that HRT was a powerful tool to combat the number one killer of women—heart disease *(32)*. These observational studies reflected typical patterns of use in the community. Most patients initiated HRT at the time of menopause or shortly thereafter for treatment of symptoms. In addition, these studies relied heavily on periodic surveys to collect information regarding hormone use and health outcomes. Because HRT is known to have a beneficial impact on cardiovascular risk factors, such as lipid profile and the health of the endothelial lining, it seemed biologically plausible that HRT would also impact the clinical outcomes of CVD *(33)*.

In the 1990s, several randomized, placebo-controlled, double-blinded clinical trials began to report a failure of combination oral HRT in secondary prevention of CVD. The Heart and Estrogen/Progestin Replacement Study and Estrogen Replacement and Atherosclerosis (ERA) trials both examined the effect of oral CEE-MPA on cardiovascular outcomes for women with existing heart disease. At the conclusion both trials, there was no benefit to the HRT-treated group. In the Heart and Estrogen/Progestin Replacement Study, there was an increased risk of CVD in the first year of use in women taking HRT *(34,35)*. However, there was no increased risk for the following 3 years of the study.

The WHI, which also tested orally administered CEE-MPA, enrolled healthy women (no known CVD) who were, on average, 10 years after menopause. Once again, an increased risk of CVD was demonstrated in the user group with the trend for higher risk early, then declining with time *(36)*. No increased risk was observed for women younger than 60 years of age. The CEE-only arm of the study demonstrated no adverse effect of CEE on CVD or breast cancer, and a trend to lower rates of cardiovascular events *(37)*. Although the WHI has been criticized for not including enough women in the 50 to 54 years or 50 to 59 years age groups to adequately assess the CVD risk for these younger women, HRT should not be recommended to prevent CVD in women either as primary or secondary prevention *(38)*. Research continues to better elucidate the impact of age, years on HRT, type of hormone, and route of administration.

HRT and Breast Cancer

The most concerning risk for many women considering HRT is the risk of breast cancer. Many studies, including observational studies and clinical trials, have produced mixed results, with fewer than half of the studies showing an increased risk of breast cancer among women taking estrogen. Those studies showing an increase in risk demonstrate an increased risk of 35%, generally occurring after 5 years of use *(39)*. The CEE-MPA arm of the WHI was stopped early because the incidence of breast cancer exceeded the established safety threshold for the study. The excess risk of breast cancer was less than 1 additional case per 1000 woman years of use. To put this in perspective, obesity has a considerably greater impact on breast cancer risk. A weight gain of 10% in adult life is associated with a risk of breast cancer of 2 per 1000 woman years or 2.5 times the risk found in the WHI CEE-MPA arm *(40)*. The CEE-only arm of the WHI did not find an increased risk of breast cancer. Indeed, there was a trend toward risk reduction in women assigned to the treatment arm *(37)*.

These findings support those studies that have implicated progesterone as the hormone culprit responsible for the increased risk. In addition, women who develop breast cancer while taking HRT seem to have localized disease with less histologically aggressive tumors *(41)*. Indeed the Breast Cancer Detection Demonstration Project reported a 40 to 60% reduction in breast cancer mortality lasting 12 years after diagnosis among women diagnosed with breast cancer while taking estrogen. This may be because HRT is a marker for medical care and indicates an interest in health in general.

HRT: Other Considerations

Additional risks of HRT demonstrated by the WHI included an increased risk of stroke and an increased risk of venous thromboembolism. Ischemic stroke was increased in both arms of the study, especially in older women *(42)*. In addition, the risk of venous thromboembolism, including pulmonary embolism, was doubled, supporting findings from previous studies. An increase in gallbladder disease was also noted in the CEE-MPA arm.

Benefits to HRT initiated in the years immediately after menopause included a reduction in osteoporotic fractures, a reduction in colon cancer, and a reduction in risk for cognitive decline. Improvement in the quality of life and a decreased risk of dementia were not demonstrated by the WHI, although other studies have shown such an effect *(43–48)*.

HRT: Making Decisions

Because of the complexities of the benefits and risks of prescribing HRT, it is imperative that decision making be shared between provider and patient. The patient's individual factors, including severity of symptoms, presence of cardiovascular risks, degree of osteoporosis risk, and perceived risk of breast cancer, should be assessed. A patient's health beliefs, nutrition, and acceptance of alternative treatments, such as antidepressants or complementary therapies, should also be addressed. It is most important that patients be provided with accurate information and have adequate time to discuss individual fears or misperceptions to allow for effective decision making.

Other Treatments

Lifestyle

Lifestyle approaches, such as dressing in layers, drinking plenty of water, strategically placing portable fans, and commandeering control of the thermostat may be less effective than HRT, but should be discussed because they are easy to do and have no side effects.

Non-HRT Pharmacological Therapies

The recent scrutiny of HRT for vasomotor symptoms has accentuated the need to find alternative treatments for reducing the severity of vasomotor symptoms. Selective serotonin reuptake inhibitors (SSRIs), including fluoxetine (20 mg) and controlled-release paroxetine (12.5 mg and 25 mg) have been studied as alternatives. Several trials have demonstrated a 50 to 60% decrease in symptoms among women using these agents *(49)*. In addition, 75 mg of extended-release venlaxafine, a combination serotonin and norepinephrine reuptake inhibitor, was shown to reduce hot flash activity by 61% in a randomized double-blinded, placebo-controlled trial. A lower dose of 37.5 mg was effective in some women, but doses of 150 mg increased toxicity without improving efficacy and are not recommended *(16)*.

Other Agents

Gabapentin, an anticonvulsant, has also been studied and demonstrated a 54% reduction in a hot flush composite score reflecting frequency and severity of symptoms *(16)*. Clonidine and megestrol have also been shown to improve symptoms, but to a lesser degree. Started at 0.05 mg twice a day and increased to 0.2 mg twice a day, clonidine may reduce frequency of symptoms by 30 to 40% *(50)*.

Table 2
Complementary and Alternative Therapies With No Proven Effectiveness for Treating Symptoms of Menopause

Vitamin E
Red clover
EPO
Dong quai (used alone)
Acupuncture
Wild Yam
Ginko biloba
Homeopathic preparations
Massage
Foot reflexology
Chiropractic manipulation
Licorice

CAM in Menopause

The use of CAM for symptoms of menopause is common. In a telephone survey of 886 women, 22.1% used CAM therapies specifically to manage vasomotor symptoms *(51)*. Other studies have shown that up to 48% of women use CAM for menopause *(52)*. Many commonly used therapies have not been proven effective. Some of the commonly used remedies with no demonstrated effectiveness are listed in Table 2. Because there is a considerable placebo effect in both studies of conventional and CAM therapies, it is not surprising that many women perceive that these therapies are effective.

Black cohosh, which was used traditionally by Native Americans for gynecological and other conditions, is one of the most popular herbs. It is also one of the most well-studied CAM therapies and has been found to be beneficial in treating hot flashes in three of four trials. Studies have also examined safety issues and have not demonstrated an adverse effect on breast cancer or vaginal cytology. However, these studies have been short-term (generally <6 months), therefore, long-term safety from several years of use has not been established *(53–57)*. Patients interested in using black cohosh should use a preparation that provides 40 mg/d and should expect to see results in 8 to 12 weeks. Patients with a history of breast cancer should be advised regarding the absence of studies demonstrating long-term safety.

Soy or isoflavone supplementation has also been studied for effect on symptoms of menopause. Only three of eight studies with treatment phases of more than 6 weeks have shown significant improvement in hot flashes *(58–60)*. Comparisons are difficult because of the considerable variations in product dosage and scoring methods for evaluating symptoms. Soy has been shown to reduce total and low-density lipoprotein cholesterol in women at doses of 60 g/d, although the impact is greatest after menopause and not as significant as in compared with men *(61–63)*. Long-term safety of soy in women with breast cancer has not been established. Whole soy foods that contain 40 to 80 mg/d of isoflavones could be considered by healthy women who wish to use soy for the control of menopausal symptoms.

In addition, three prospective, randomized controlled trials demonstrated a 50% reduction in hot flash frequency using paced respirations. Paced respiration is a breathing technique used in yoga in which the participant breathes deeply and fully using the diaphragm, retains the breath for a few seconds, then exhales slowly and completely while standing or sitting erect. Because this technique is risk free, it can be recommended to all women *(64)*.

Treatment of GU Symptoms

Vaginal dryness is a common complaint during menopause. The loss of estrogen causes decreased vascularity and thinning of the estrogen dependent tissues of the lower vagina, labia, urethra, and trigone. Dyspareunia, vaginismus and decreased sexual satisfaction, discharge, burning, and itching may result. In addition, patients may experience an increase in urinary incontinence and infections.

HRT is the most effective treatment for these symptoms. Systemic therapy will treat both vasomotor and GU symptoms. For patients who desire treatment of GU symptoms only, intravaginal estrogen is effective in low doses. Types of intravaginal estrogens include 17-β estradiol cream, estradiol tablets, or CEE cream. All can be used daily in the vagina for 3 weeks and then dosed twice a week to maintain the benefit. A new intravaginal ring, Estring®, delivers 6 to 9 μg of estrogen daily for a period of 3 months *(65)*. Although the systemic absorption of the low-dose intravaginal products is minimal, regular use does increase the risk of endometrial cancer, therefore, progesterone should be prescribed to women with an intact uterus. Lubricants, especially water-soluble products, such as Astroglide, are also helpful for GU symptoms.

SUMMARY

Menopause represents a transition in the life of a woman marked by the cessation of menses. It also represents an important change in health risks, especially for chronic diseases, such as diabetes, heart disease, certain cancers, and osteoporosis. Women may seek medical attention for the vasomotor and GU symptoms that are characteristic and common in menopause. Although HRT remains the most effective treatment for menopausal symptoms, concerns regarding risks for breast cancer and CVD may cause the woman and her physician to seek alternatives. Most importantly, the provider can use the time with the patient to assess overall health risk, recommend screening tests, and provide counseling to optimize health and quality of life.

REFERENCES

1. Paoletti R, Wenger NK. Review of the international position paper on women's health and menopause: a comprehensive approach. Circulation 2003;107(9):1336–1339.
2. Stenchever M, Droegemuellor W, Herbst A, et al. Comprehensive Gynecology. Mosby, St. Louis, 2001.
3. Carr MC. The emergence of the metabolic syndrome with menopause. J Clin Endocrinol Metab 2003;88(6):2404–2411.
4. Nelson HD, Haney E, Humphrey L, et al. Management of Menopause-Related Symptoms. Summary, Evidence Report/Technology Assessment No. 120 (prepared by the Oregon Evidence-based practice center, under contract No. 290-02-0024) AHRQ Publication no. 05-E016-1. Agency for Healthcare Research and Quality, Rockville, MD, March 2005.
5. Soares CN, Joffe H, Steiner M. Menopause and mood. Clin Obstet Gynecol 2004;47(3): 576–591.
6. Dennerstein L, Dudley EC, Hopper JL, Guthrie JR, Burger HG. A prospective population-based study of menopausal symptoms. Obstet Gynecol 2000;96(3):351–358.
7. Mitchell ES, Woods NF, Mariella A. Three stages of the menopausal transition from the Seattle Midlife Women's Health Study: toward a more precise definition. Menopause: The Journal of the North American Menopause Society 2000;7(5):334–349.
8. Santoro N. The menopause transition: an update. Hum Reprod Update 2002;8(2):155–160.
9. Landgren BM, Collins A, Csemiczky G, Burger HG, Baksheev L, Robertson DM. Menopause transition: Annual changes in serum hormonal patterns over the menstrual cycle in women during a nine-year period prior to menopause. J Clin Endocrinol Metab 2004;89(6): 2763–2769.
10. Burger HG, Dudley EC, Hopper JL, et al. Prospectively measured levels of serum follicle-stimulating hormone, estradiol, and the dimeric inhibins during the menopausal transition in a population-based cohort of women. J Clin Endocrinol Metab 1999;84(11):4025–4030.
11. Dudley EC, Hopper JL, Taffe J, Guthrie JR, Burger HG, Dennerstein L. Using longitudinal data to define the perimenopause by menstrual cycle characteristics. Climacteric 1998;1(1): 18–25.
12. Taffe JR, Dennerstein L. Menstrual patterns leading to the final menstrual period. Menopause 2002;9(1):32–40.
13. Gold EB, Sternfeld B, Kelsey JL, et al. Relation of demographic and lifestyle factors to symptoms in a multi-racial/ethnic population of women 40-55 years of age. Am J Epidemiol 2000;152(5):463–473.
14. Santoro N, Chervenak JL. The menopause transition. Endocrinol Metabol Clin North Am 2004;33(4):627–636.
15. Freeman EW, Sammel MD, Rinaudo PJ, Sheng L. Premenstrual syndrome as a predicator of menopausal symptoms. Obstet Gynecol 2004;103(5 Pt 1):960–966.
16. American College of Obstetricians and Gynecologists. Vasomotor symptoms. Obstet Gynecol 2004;104(4 Suppl):106S–117S.
17. Kaunitz AM. Gynecologic problems of the perimenopause: evaluation and treatment. Obstet Gynecol Clin North Am 2002;29(3):455–473.
18. Mohyi D, Tabassi K, Simon J. Differential diagnosis of hot flashes. Maturitas 1997;27: 203–214.

19. American College of Obstetricians and Gynecologists. Genitourinary tract changes. Obstet Gynecol 2004;104(4 Suppl):56S–61S.
20. Ouhilal S, Harrison E, Santoro N. Perimenopausal Bleeding in Menstrual Disorders: A Practical Guide. ACP Press, Philadelphia. In press.
21. Leclair C, Ehrenthal D, Adams Hillard P. Amenorrhea and Oligomenorrhea, in Menstrual Disorders, A Practical Guide. ACP Press, Philadelphia, PA. In press.
22. Landgren BM, Collins A, Csemiczky G, Burger HG, Baksheev L, Robertson DM. Menopause transition: annual changes in serum hormonal patterns over the menstrual cycle in women during a nine-year period prior to menopause. J Clin Endocrinol Metabol 2004;89:2763.
23. Speroff L. Clinical Gynecologic Endocrinology and Infertility, 6th ed. Lipincott Williams and Wilkins, 1999, p. 662.
24. Edmunds E, Lip GY. Cardiovascular risk in women: the cardiologist's perspective. Quart J Med 2000;93(3):135–145.
25. American Diabetes Association. Screening for Type 2 Diabetes. Diabetes Care 2004; 27(Suppl 1):S11–S14.
26. United States Preventive Services Task Force, Screening for Diabetes, Adult Type 2. www.ahrq.gov/clinic/uspstfix.htm.
27. Nelson HD, Helfand M, Woolf SH, Allan JD. Screening for postmenopausal osteoporosis: a review of the evidence for the US Preventive Services Task Force. Ann Intern Med 2002; 137:529–541.
28. Smith RA, Saslow D, Sawyer KA, et al. and the American Cancer Society High-Risk Work Group; American Cancer Society Screening Older Women Work Group; American Cancer Society Mammography Work Group; American Cancer Society Physical Examination Work Group; American Cancer Society New Technologies Work Group; American Cancer Society Breast Cancer Advisory Group. American Cancer Society guidelines for breast cancer screening: update 2003. CA Cancer J Clin 2003;53(3): 141–169.
29. ACOG practice bulletin. Clinical management guidelines for obstetrician-gynecologists. Number 42, April 2003. Breast cancer screening. Obstet Gynecol 2003;101(4):821–831.
30. Waxman AG. Guidelines for cervical cancer screening: history and scientific rationale. Clin Obstet Gynecol 2005;48(1):77–97.
31. Walsh JME, Terdimamn JP. Colorectal cancer screening clinical applications. JAMA 2003; 289(10):1297–1302.
32. Speroff L, Massaferri EL. Hormone replacement therapy: clarifying the picture. Hosp Pract 2001;36(5):37–46.
33. Mendelsohn ME, Karas RH. The protective effects of estrogen on the cardiovascular system. NEJM 1999;340:1801–1811.
34. Hully S, Grady D, Bush T, et al. Randomized trial of estrogen plus progestin for secondary prevention of coronary heart disease in postmenopausal women: Heart and Estrogen/Progestin Replacement Study (HERS) Research Group. JAMA 1998;280:605–652.
35. Grady D, Herrington D, Bittner V, et al. Cardiovascular disease outcomes during 6.8 years of hormone therapy. JAMA 2002;288(1):49–57.
36. Writing group for the women's health initiative investigators. Risks and benefits of estrogen plus progestin in healthy postmenopausal women. JAMA 2002;288(3):321–333.
37. The Women's Health Initiative Steering Committee. Effects of conjugated equine estrogen in postmenopausal women with hysterectomy: the Women's Health Initiative Randomized Controlled Trial. JAMA 2004;291(14):1701–1712.
38. Grodstein F, Clarkson TB, Manson JE. Understanding the divergent data on postmenopausal hormone therapy. NEJM 2003;348(7):645–650.

39. Schairer C, Lubin J, Troisi R, et al. Menopausal estrogen and estrogen-progestin replacement therapy and breast cancer risk. JAMA 2000;283:485–491.
40. Langer RD. Postmenopausal hormone therapy: what's appropriate today. CME Bulletin. American Academy of Family Physicians 2005;4(1):1–12.
41. Gapstur SM, Morrow M, Sellers TA. Hormone Replacement therapy and risk of breast cancer with a favorable histology: results of the Iowa Women's Health Study. JAMA 1999;281: 2091–2097.
42. Grady D, Wngern NK, Herrington D, et al. Postmenopausal hormone therapy increases risk for venous thromboembolic disease: the heart and estrogen/progestin replacement study. Ann Intern Med 2000;132:689–696.
43. Viscoli CM, Brass LLM, Kernn WN, Sarrel PM, Suissa S, Horwitz RI. Estrogen therapy and risk of cognitive decline; results from the women's estrogen for stroke trial (WEST). Am J Obstet Gynecol 2005;192(2):387–393.
44. Grodstein F, Martinez ME, Platz EA, et al. Postmenopausal hormone use and risk for colorectal cancer and adenoma. Ann Intern Med 1998;128(9):705–712.
45. Hayes J, Ockene JK, Brunner RL, et al. Effects of estrogen plus progestin on health-related quality of life. NEJM 2003;348(19):L1839–L1854.
46. Rapp SR, Espeland MA, Shumaker SA, et al. Effect of estrogen plus progestin on global cognitive function in postmenopausal women: the women's health initiative memory study; a randomized controlled trial. JAMA 2003;289(20):2663–2672.
47. Shumaker SA, Legault C, Rapp SR, et al. Estrogen plus progestin and the incidence of dementia and mild cognitive impairment in postmenopausal women: the women's health initiative memory study; a randomized controlled trial. JAMA 2003;289(20):2651–2662.
48. Zandi PP, Carlson MC, Plassman BL, et al. Hormone replacement therapy and incidence of Alzheimer disease in older women: the Cache County study. JAMA 2002;288(17):2123–2129.
49. Stearns V, Beebe KL, Iyengar M, Dube E. Paroxetine controlled release in the treatment of menopausal hot flashes: a randomized controlled trial. JAMA 2003;289(21):2827–2834.
50. Nevin JE, Pharr ME. Preventive care for the menopausal woman. Prim Care Clin Office Pract 2002;29:583–597.
51. Newton KM, Buist DS, Keenan NL, Anderson LA, LaCroix AZ. Use of alternative therapies for menopause symptoms: results of a population-based survey. Obstet Gynecol 2002;100(1): 18–25.
52. Kronenberg F, Fugh-Berman A. Complementary and alternative medicine for menopausal symptoms: a review of randomized, controlled trials. Ann Intern Med 2002;137(10):805–813.
53. Liske E, Hanggi W, Henneicke-von Zepelin HH, Boblitz N, Wustenberg P, Rahifs VW. Physiological investigation of a unique extract of black cohosh (cimicifugae racemosae rhizoma): a 6 month clinical study demonstrates no systemic estrogenic effect. J Womens Health Gend Based Med 2002;11(2):163–174.
54. Lupu R, Mehmi I, Atlas E, et al. Black cohosh, a menopausal remedy, does not have estrogenic activity and does not promote breast cancer cell growth. Int J Oncol 2003;23(5): 1407–1412.
55. Pockaj BA, Loprinzi CL, Sloan JA, et al. Pilot evaluation of black cohosh for the treatment of hot flashes in women. Cancer Invest 2004;22(4):515–521.
56. Huntley A, Ernst E. A systematic review of the safety of black cohost. Menopause 2003; 10(1):58–64.
57. Jacobson JS, Troxel AB, Evans J, et al. Randomized trial of black cohosh for the treatment of hot flashes among women with a history of breast cancer. J Clin Oncol 2001;19(10): 2739–2745.
58. Krebs EE, Ensrud KE, MacDonald R, Wilt TJ. Phytoestrogens for treatment of menopausal symptoms: a systematic review. Obstet Gynecol 2004;104(4):824–836.

59. Albertazzi P, Pansini F, Bonaccorsi G, Zanotti L, Forini E, DeAloysio D. The effect of dietary soy supplmentation on hot flushes. Obstet Gynecol 1998;91(1):6–11.
60. Han KK, Soares JM Jr., Haidar MA, DeLima GR, Garacat EC. Benefits of soy isoflavone therapeutic regimen on menopausal symptoms. Obstet Gynecol 2002;99(3):389–394.
61. Anderson JW, Johnstone BM, Cook-Newell ME. Meta-analysis of the effects of soy protein intake on serum lipids. N Engl J Med 1995;333(5):276–282.
62. Roughead ZK, Hunt JR, Johnson LK, Badger TM, Lykken GI. Controlled substitution of soy protein for meat protein; effects on calcium retention, bone, and cardiovascular health indices in postmenopausal women. J Clin Endocrinol Metab 2005;90(1):181–189.
63. Kreijkamp-Kaspers S, Kok L, Grobbee DE, et al. Effect of soy protein containing isoflavones on cognitive function, bone mineral density and plasma lipids in postmenopausal women; a randomized controlled trial. JAMA 2004;292(1):65–74.
64. Irvin JH, Domar AD, Clark C, et al. The effects of relaxation response training on menopausal symptoms. J Psychosom Obstet Gynaecol 1996;17(4):202–207.
65. Casper F, Petri E. Local treatment of urogenital atrophy with an estradiol-releasing vaginal ring: a comparative and placebo-controlled multicenter study. Vaginal Ring Study Group. Int Urogynecol J Pelvic Floor Dysfunct 1999;10(3):171–176.

4 Osteoporosis

Colleen Veloski, MD

CONTENTS

INTRODUCTION

Fractures caused by osteoporosis are among the most serious health risks women face as they age. Osteoporosis affects eight million American women, causing approximately 1.5 million osteoporotic fractures per year, with a direct annual expenditure of nearly $18 billion *(1)*. Fewer than 50% of women who suffer a hip fracture will recover their previous level of function *(2)*. A 50-year-old woman's lifetime risk of dying from a hip fracture is equal to her risk of dying from breast cancer *(3)*. The enormity of the impact of osteoporotic fractures on the health and quality of life of women underscores the importance of preventing and treating osteoporosis.

Half of the calcium in the adult skeleton is deposited between the ages of 13 and 17 years. Although peak bone mass is achieved in the third decade of life, loss of estrogen at menopause triggers rapid bone loss. Clearly, the assessment and optimization of bone health are vital components of the routine health care

From: *Current Clinical Practice: Women's Health in Clinical Practice*
Edited by: Clouse and Sherif © Humana Press Inc., Totowa, NJ

of women of all ages. Important advances in the prevention, diagnosis, and treatment have transformed the management of this disease in clinical practice.

DEFINITION

Osteoporosis is defined as a skeletal disorder characterized by compromised bone strength predisposing to an increased risk of fracture *(4)*. Bone strength is comprised of bone density and bone quality. Bone quality is determined by the degree of calcification, microarchitecture, bone turnover, and structure. Currently, bone quality cannot be measured directly and is not apparent unless a patient suffers a fragility fracture (a fracture occurring with minimal trauma, such as a fall from a standing height or less). However, bone mineral density (BMD) can be measured safely and reliably by dual-energy X-ray absorptiometry (DXA). The World Health Organization (WHO) defines osteoporosis and osteopenia using BMD measurement by DXA. The WHO definitions compare a patient's BMD with the mean for a normal young adult population of the same sex and race. The resultant T-score represents the number of standard deviations above or below the mean BMD for normal young adults, as shown in Table 1 *(5)*.

The WHO classification is applicable only to measurements of BMD at the hip, spine, and forearm in postmenopausal women. The lowest T-score of the posteroanterior (PA) spine, femoral neck, trochanter, or total hip is used to classify patients using the WHO criteria *(6)*. The WHO classification does not apply to peripheral measurements of BMD *(7)*.

Although not part of the WHO classification, the presence of a fragility fracture establishes the clinical diagnosis of osteoporosis, regardless of T-score, provided other causes for the fracture (e.g., pathological fracture, trauma, and so on) have been excluded.

The International Society for Clinical Densitometry (ISCD) recommends that Z-scores be used in premenopausal women *(8)*. The Z-score compares a patient's BMD with age-matched controls and expresses the difference in terms of a standard deviation score.

PATHOGENESIS OF OSTEOPOROSIS

Bone mass in adults is determined by the peak bone mass achieved at maturity, the rate of bone formation, and the rate of resorption. Poor nutrition, genetic factors, physical inactivity, and endocrine abnormalities can cause low peak bone mass, thereby increasing the risk of age-related osteoporosis.

Changes in bone mass are caused by an imbalance between bone formation and bone resorption. Healthy bone is continuously remodeling as small areas

Table 1
WHO Criteria for Diagnosing Osteoporosis Using Bone Density Measurements[a]

Category	*T-Score*
Normal	Not more than 1.0 SD[b] below the young adult mean
Low bone mass (osteopenia)	Between 1.0 and 2.5 SD below the young adult mean
Osteoporosis	More than 2.5 SD below the young adult mean
Severe or established osteoporosis	More than 2.5 SD below the young adult mean with a fracture

[a]Ref. *(5)*.
[b]SD, Standard deviation.

of bone are resorbed by osteoclasts and new bone is deposited by osteoblasts. The remodeling cycle is regulated by parathyroid hormone (PTH), estrogen, vitamin D, growth factors, and cytokines. Bone resorption is accelerated by the loss of estradiol at menopause, vitamin D or calcium deficiency, hyperparathyroidism, and other endocrine abnormalities. Inadequate bone formation occurs as osteoblast function declines with age and excessive resorption depletes the template on which new bone is formed *(9)*.

Recently, researchers identified a system of proteins that are involved in the cell–cell interaction between osteoblasts and osteoclasts. The receptor activator of nuclear factor-κB ligand (RANKL) expressed on the surface of osteoblasts causes activation of osteoclasts when it binds to receptor activator of nuclear factor-κB (RANK) on the surface of osteoclasts. The binding of RANKL to RANK and the subsequent activation of osteoclasts and resorption can be prevented by osteoprotegerin (OPG), a receptor protein produced by the osteoblasts *(10)*. OPG inhibits osteoclast activation by acting as a decoy receptor for RANKL. The convergence hypothesis proposed by Hofbauer et al. *(11)* suggests that the RANK/OPG system may function as a common final pathway for the regulation of osteoclast functions. The use of OPG or a similar protein as a therapeutic agent for osteoporosis is currently under investigation.

RISK ASSESSMENT

Careful risk assessment often provides opportunities for prevention, early detection, and therapeutic intervention. Risk factors for osteoporosis and fracture, as well as conditions and medications predisposing to bone loss, should be considered.

Table 2
Risk Factors for Osteoporotic Fractures in Postmenopausal Women[a]

Major Risk Factors	*Additional Risk Factors*
Personal history of fracture as an adult	Estrogen deficiency at an early age (<45 yr)
History of a low trauma fracture in a first degree relative	Dementia
Low body weight (<127 lb)	Impaired vision
Current smoking	Poor health status (frailty)
Use of oral corticosteroid for >3 mo	Life-long low calcium intake
	Low physical activity/poor mobility
	Alcohol excess (>2 drinks per d)

[a]From ref. *(13)*.

Risk Factors for Osteoporosis and Fracture

Risk factors for low BMD are different than the risk factors for fracture. Fractures of the hip and spine are the most significant clinical end points associated with osteoporosis. Low BMD is the best predictor of fracture in asymptomatic untreated women *(12)*. However, clinical risk factors for low BMD do not reliably predict osteoporosis and are not a substitute for BMD testing. The risk factors for osteoporosis related fractures are listed in Table 2 *(13)*.

Several studies have quantified the risk associated with the various risk factors. The National Osteoporosis Risk Assessment (NORA) study is the largest study of postmenopausal women in the United States. This cohort of more than 200,000 postmenopausal women included more than 18,000 minority women. The NORA study confirmed the association of advanced age, low body weight, maternal history of osteoporosis or fracture, personal history of fracture, cigarette smoking, lack of exercise, use of glucocorticoids, and non-use of estrogen with low BMD. Age was found to be the most important risk factor predicting low BMD, even after controlling for other fractures and body mass index (BMI). Hispanic and Asian women were more likely to have osteoporosis, but the risk of fracture was no different for Hispanics and lower for Asians. African American heritage, higher BMI, estrogen use, diuretic use, and exercise were identified as factors protective against osteoporosis (14).

The NORA study also provided information regarding fracture risk. A personal history of fragility fracture was found to be the most important risk factor, nearly doubling the risk of future fracture. Patients with a history of fragility fracture are at highest risk for subsequent fracture in the first year or two after the initial event *(15)*. Because of its high predictive value for future

Table 3
Medical Conditions That May Increase Risk

Endocrine	Hyperparathyroidism, hypercalciuria, hyperthyroidism, diabetes mellitus, Cushing's syndrome, adrenal insufficiency, acromegaly
Genetic	Ehlers-Danlos, Marfan's syndrome, Gaucher's disease, hemachromatosis, osteogenesis imperfecta
Hypogonadal states	Hyperprolactinemia, athletic amenorrhea, panhypopituitarism, premature menopause, Turner's syndrome, androgen insensitivity
Rheumatologic diseases	Ankylosing spondylitis, rheumatoid arthritis, systemic lupus erythematosis
Gastrointestinal fiseases	Gastrectomy/bariatric surgery, celiac disease, malabsorption, cirrhosis
Hematological fisorders	Mutliple myeloma, leukemia, hemophilia, thalassemia, mastocytosis, sickle cell anemia
Nutritional	Vitamin D deficiency, eating disorders, vitamin B12 deficiency
Miscellaneous	Amyloidosis, AIDS/HIV, organ transplantation, renal disease, alcoholism

fractures, a previous fragility fracture should prompt BMD testing and perhaps a search for secondary causes of osteoporosis in any woman, regardless of age or menstrual status.

Secondary Causes of Osteoporosis

In addition to the established risk factors for osteoporosis and fracture, many medical conditions are known to cause secondary osteoporosis, that is, osteoporosis that is caused or worsened by other disorders or medications. Up to 30% of postmenopausal women with osteoporosis have been found to have secondary causes *(16)*. Because many of the medical conditions known to cause bone loss require treatment and are potentially reversible, recognition and diagnosis are critical. A partial list of conditions that may increase the risk of osteoporosis is shown in Table 3 *(13,17)*.

Medications

Medications associated with an increased risk of accelerated bone loss are shown in Table 4 *(13)*. Glucocorticoids are the most common cause of secondary osteoporosis. Some anticonvulsants, such as phenytoin phenobarbital, and carbamazepine, stimulate hepatic enzymes that degrade vitamin D. Patients receiving long-term therapy with these anticonvulsant medications should receive vitamin D supplementation to maintain 25-hydroxyvitamin D levels in the optimal range. Women who receive aromatase inhibitors as adjuvant therapy

Table 4
Medications Predisposing Patients to Bone Loss[a]

Glucocorticoids and adrenocorticotropin
Aromatase inhibitors
Gonadotropin-releasing hormone agonists
Anticonvulsants
Cytotoxic drugs
Immunosuppressants
Long-term heparin
Lithium
Long-acting progestin

[a]From Ref. *(13)*.

for breast cancer or suppressive doses of thyroxine are also at an increased risk for fracture. Organ transplant patients are an especially high-risk group because of the use of glucocorticords, heparin, and immunosuppressives, such as cyclosporine and tacrolimus *(17)*.

SELECTING PATIENTS FOR SCREENING

Nearly 40% of postmenopausal women older than 50 years of age have undiagnosed osteopenia and an additional 7% have osteoporosis *(14)*. Although universal screening of all postmenopausal women has not been shown to be cost-effective or improve outcomes, targeted screening of women at increased risk is warranted. Clinical practice guidelines have been issued by several groups including the US Preventive Services Task Force, the National Osteoporosis Foundation (NOF), the National Institute of Health, and the American Association of Clinical Endocrinologists (AACE). Almost all guidelines recommend screening postmenopausal women age 65 years or older, in accordance with evidence of increased fracture risk in these women. The guidelines regarding screening of postmenopausal women younger than 65 years of age vary considerably. The US Preventive Services Task Force recommends screening women age 60 to 65 years with increased risk for osteoporotic fractures *(19)*. The NOF and AACE recommend testing for any postmenopausal woman with one or more risk factors *(13,20)*.

The benefit of BMD testing in premenopausal women is less clear, given the lack of evidence regarding the fracture risk in this age group. The AACE and the ISCD recommend BMD testing for the following:

1. Any woman who suffers a fragility fracture.

2. Premenopausal women with a disease or condition known to cause secondary osteoporosis (*see* Table 3), or who are taking a medication associated with bone loss (*see* Table 4) *(20,21)*.

SCREENING TESTS

The techniques for measuring bone density can be divided into those used to measure at central skeletal sites (e.g., spine and hip) and those used to measure at peripheral skeletal sites (e.g., heel, forefinger, and forearm).

Measurement of BMD at Central Skeletal Sites

DXA

Central DXA is the most accurate method for predicting low BMD. Typically, measurements are taken at both the PA lumbar spine (L1–L4) and the hip. The femoral neck and total proximal femur are the most useful hip measurements in predicting fracture, whereas Ward's area is unreliable and should not be used for diagnosis *(21)*. Spinal measurements may be artificially increased in older women with arthritis, but may show osteoporotic values earlier than the hip in younger postmenopausal women because cancellous bone loss is rapid in early menopause. Measurement at the 1/3 radius of the nondominant forearm is the preferred site for patients with disorders that affect mostly cortical bone (e.g., hyperparathyroidism).

DXA results are expressed both graphically and as T- and Z-scores. Both scores compare the patient's bone density to a gender- and race-matched healthy population. However, Z-scores compare the patient's bone density to an age-matched population, whereas T-scores compare it to a young population at peak bone mass. T-scores are used to diagnose osteoporosis (*see* Table 1). A low T-score at any one of the measured sites is considered diagnostic of osteoporosis. When BMD is measured in young women, the Z-score is more appropriate than the T-score. A Z-score of –2 or less is generally accepted as a strong indication to search thoroughly for secondary causes of osteoporosis. Some authors advocate an investigation in all premenopausal and perimenopausal women with a Z-score less than –1 *(17)*. Because there is no evidence to support a specific cut-point to evaluate for secondary causes, the need for further investigation should be guided by the clinical indications.

Quantitative Computed Tomography

Quantitative computed tomography is another method used to measure bone density. In the lateral projection, trabecular bone is analyzed separately without interference from the cortical bone of the spinous processes, yielding a sensitive measure of early bone loss. Quantitative computed tomography is seldom used because it is more expensive, requires more radiation than DXA, and its correlation with fracture risk is not standardized.

Measurement of BMD at Peripheral Sites

Central DXA equipment is large, expensive, and not always available. Smaller, less costly, portable technologies that test peripheral BMD provide greater access to testing. Low BMD by peripheral densitometry and ultrasonography is predictive of fracture risk but less predictive than BMD at the hip *(14,22)*. T-scores obtained from peripheral devices may not be applicable to the WHO's definitions of osteoporosis and osteopenia. Patients found to have abnormal BMD at peripheral sites should be referred for central DXA testing. Peripheral measurements should not be used for the diagnosis or follow-up of osteoporosis *(21)*.

Single-Photon Absorptiometry

A single type of photon passes through a peripheral bone. Bone density is estimated by the degree of attenuation. Because the technology cannot discriminate between attenuation by soft tissue or bone, single-photon absorptiometry can only be used at peripheral sites such as the heel or the radius.

Dual-Photon Absorptiometry

Two different photons are passed through peripheral bone. The two photons are attenuated differently by bone and soft tissue allowing measurement of bone density that is more accurate, at central as well as peripheral sites.

Peripheral DXA

DXA can be used at either peripheral or central skeletal sites. Two photons are emitted from an X-ray tube rather than a radioactive source, resulting in better accuracy than dual-photon absorptiometry. The finger, forearm, or heel are the usual measurement sites.

Quantitative Ultrasound

Quantitative ultrasound indirectly estimates bone density by measuring the transmission of ultrasound through bone or the reflectance of ultrasound waves from the surface of bone at a peripheral site (usually the heel, finger, or tibia).

CLINICAL EVALUATION OF THE PATIENT

A thorough history and physical exam often offers opportunities for primary prevention, screening, and treatment.

Medical History

The medical history should include elucidation of the risk factors for osteoporosis and related fractures (*see* Table 2). Key information to elicit in each part of the medical history is:

1. Medical history.
   a. Personal history of fragility fractures.
   b. Presence of any conditions associated with secondary osteoporosis (*see* Table 3).
   c. Medications associated with accelerated bone loss (*see* Table 4).
   d. Age at menopause.
   e. History of falling.
   f. Lifetime number of fractures.
2. Family history.
   a. First degree relatives with osteoporosis or osteoporotic fractures.
   b. Strong family history of fractures, kidney stones, or autoimmune disease (e.g., celiac sprue).
3. Social history.
   a. Lifelong calcium/vitamin D intake.
   b. Exercise habits.
   c. Frequent dieting or significant weight loss.
   d. Smoking.
   e. Nutrition (intake of dairy products, use of multi-vitamins and supplements).
   f. Alcohol use.
   g. Sun exposure/sunscreen use.

Review of Systems

The review of systems is directed toward detecting symptoms associated with secondary causes of osteoporosis listed in Table 3. Loss of height or a history of the abrupt onset of back pain that subsides over weeks may indicate a previous vertebral fracture. The presence of weight loss and palpitations suggests hyperthyroidism. Gastrointestinal (GI) symptoms, such as diarrhea, abdominal pain, or nausea, may be present in patients with inflammatory bowel disease or malabsorptive syndromes.

Physical Exam

A careful physical exam may reveal signs of symptomatic osteoporosis or provide clues for the presence of systemic disease associated with secondary osteoporosis. For example, moon facies, truncal obesity, and striae suggest Cushing's syndrome. Weight loss could indicate an eating disorder, malignancy, or a malabsorptive syndrome.

Table 5
Basic Laboratory Evaluation of Secondary Osteoporosis

Complete blood count
Renal function
Chemistry panel including calcium
Liver function tests
Intact parathyroid hormone
Thyroid function tests
24-h urinary calcium and creatinine excretion
25-hydroxyvitamin D

Height and weight are key measurements to obtain and follow over time. Weight less than 127 pounds is an independent risk factor for low BMD. The height measurement should be compared with the patient's height as a young adult. A loss of height of 1 inch or more or the presence of significant kyphosis is suspicious for multiple vertebral fractures. Similarly, a rib–pelvis overlap or chest deformity suggests height loss caused by vertebral compression fractures.

Laboratory Evaluation

Laboratory evaluation to exclude secondary causes of osteoporosis is appropriate for all women diagnosed with low BMD. A basic laboratory evaluation suggested for all patients being evaluated for osteoporosis is presented in Table 5.

A study by Tannenbaum et al. *(23)* found previously undiagnosed disorders of bone and mineral metabolism in 32% of postmenopausal women with osteoporosis who lacked known risk factors for low bone mass. This study also found that a testing strategy consisting of measurement of serum calcium, PTH, 25-hydroxyvitamin D, and a 24-hour urine calcium for all women, plus a thyroid-stimulation hormone for women on thyroid replacement therapy, would have been sufficient to diagnose 98% of the affected women, at an estimated cost of $116 per patient screened.

An elevated alkaline phosphatase level suggests either liver or bone pathology. A bone-specific alkaline phosphatase or a γ-glutamyl transpeptidase can distinguish between a hepatic or skeletal source (e.g., Paget's disease, hyperparathyroidism, or any state of increased bone turnover). Increased urinary excretion of calcium (>300 mg/d) indicates a state of accelerated bone resorption, for instance, hyperthyroidism, malignancy, absorptive hypercalciuria, or renal leak hypercalciuria *(24)*.

Specialized laboratory testing is warranted if the results of the basic laboratory testing or the clinical picture suggest a secondary cause of osteoporosis.

Table 6
Directed Laboratory Assessment for Secondary Osteoporosis

Suspected Condition	*Test*
Cushing's syndrome	24-h free cortisol or overnight dexamethasone suppression test
Multiple myeloma	Serum and urine protein electrophoresis Immunoelectrophoresis Bone marrow aspirate
Celiac sprue	Tissue transglutaminase antibody, IgA Small bowel biopsy
Hemachromatosis	Serum iron and ferritin
Systemic mastocytosis	Transiliac bone biopsy Patients with unusual features

Examples of specialized laboratory tests for suspected secondary causes of osteoporosis are listed in Table 6.

Markers of Bone Turnover

Bone is a metabolically active organ that undergoes a finely regulated process of continuous remodeling. Remodeling activity can be assessed by measuring the biochemical markers of bone turnover outlined in Table 7 *(25)*. In general, high levels of bone markers in the serum or the urine are associated with a greater risk of rapid bone loss. Important exceptions include the growth period early in life, and treatment with PTH that results in an overall increase in bone turnover favoring bone formation.

Currently, there are no definitive guidelines on the use of bone markers. Although markers of bone turnover are not useful for making the diagnosis of osteoporosis, they can be useful in assessing the efficacy of antiresorptive therapy. BMD changes may not become apparent for 2 years, whereas the effect of antiresorptive drugs on bone markers occur within 3 to 6 months.

Because there is wide variability in the values of bone markers according to the time of day, season, age, sex, and so on, large differences between samples are required for a change to achieve significance. For example, a decrease of greater than 40 to 50% in urinary N-terminal telopeptide excretion, after 6 months of antiresorptive therapy, is considered significant *(25,26)*.

To assess the efficacy of antiresorptive treatment, bone resorption markers should be measured at the initiation of therapy and 6 months thereafter. Ideally, the baseline measurement should be the mean of two samples collected consecutively in the same week. Check with your clinical lab or the manufacturer's

Table 7
Commonly Used Markers of Bone Turnover[a]

Resorption Markers	*Formation Markers*
Pyridinoline	Osteocalcin
Deoxypyridinoline	Bone-specific alkaline phosphatase
N-terminal telopeptide	
C-terminal telopeptide	Procollagen type I N-terminal propeptide

[a]From ref. *(25)*.

specification to determine the proper handling of specimens (e.g., time of collection, fasting, requirements, and so on) and the least significant change.

PREVENTION AND TREATMENT OF OSTEOPOROSIS

The goals of preventing and treating osteoporosis are to reduce the likelihood of fractures, decrease bone loss, and preserve or increase bone strength.

Nonpharmacological Therapy

Calcium and Vitamin D

Adequate calcium and vitamin D intake is essential for the prevention and treatment of osteoporosis. Adult premenopausal women should receive 1000 to 1200 mg calcium daily from diet or supplements *(27)*. A total calcium intake of 1200 to 1500 mg daily is recommended for postmenopausal women *(28)*. Vitamin D is necessary for the efficient absorption of calcium. Without vitamin D, the intestinal absorption of calcium is not sufficient to cover obligate calcium losses. Although the Institute of Medicine recommends 400 to 600 IU/d for middle aged and older adults, and the NOF advises 400 to 800 IU/d for women with osteoporosis, the amount of vitamin D intake required to achieve bone health is an area of uncertainty.

Vitamin D is a fat-soluble vitamin that maintains calcium homeostasis and regulates bone health. Cutaneous synthesis of vitamin D by solar UVB irradiation of 7-dehydrocholesterol provides 90% or more of the human body's vitamin D requirement *(29)*.

Adequate endogenous vitamin D can generally be obtained by exposure to midday sun, without sunscreen, for 10 to 15 minutes twice weekly *(30)*. However, sunlight is insufficient for cutaneous vitamin D synthesis during the winter months at latitudes above 37° (roughly north of North Carolina) *(31)*. Anything that interferes with the penetration of UVB radiation into the skin, such as sunscreen use, darkly pigmented skin, or the age-related decline of 7-dehydrocholesterol in the skin, will decrease cutaneous vitamin D production significantly. Very few foods contain vitamin D naturally, however, in the United States, milk, infant formula, and some cereals are fortified with vitamin D. Patients with limited sunlight exposure, or factors that impair cutaneous production of vitamin D, may be wholly dependent on supplementation and dietary sources of the vitamin.

Measurement of serum 25-hydroxyvitamin D is the best test to assess bodily stores of vitamin D. Although 1,25 dihydroxyvitamin D is the biologically active form, it has a short half-life and does not accurately reflect bodily stores. Opinions vary concerning the 25-hydroxyvitamin D level and the total daily vitamin D intake required to optimize skeletal health. Many labs still use 10 to 15 ng/mL (25–37.5 nmol/L) as the lower limit of normal for serum 25-hydroxyvitamin D. Several studies have shown that PTH levels are suppressed at an optimum stable level as serum 25-hydroxyvitamin D levels approach 30 ng/mL (75 nmol/L) *(32–35)*. Other studies have shown that, in the absence of sun exposure, an intake of 1000 IU of cholecalciferol (vitamin D3) is necessary to achieve these levels *(36–38)*. In summary, measurement of 25-hydroxyvitamin D to assess and adjust vitamin D supplementation is useful in patients at risk for deficiency including those with osteoporosis, limited sun exposure, dark skin, malabsorptive syndromes, and the elderly. Patients found to be severely deficient (<20 ng/mL) should be treated with 50,000 IU of oral vitamin D weekly for 8 weeks *(30)*.

Some, but not all, studies have found that vitamin D supplementation with or without calcium reduces fracture risk. A meta-analysis that included only double-blinded, randomized, controlled trials concluded that 700 to 800 IU/d vitamin D, with or without calcium, reduced fracture risk, but 400 IU/d did not *(39)*. In two recent randomized trials, 1000 mg calcium and 800 IU/d of vitamin D did not reduce nonvertebral fracture risk in older women *(40,41)*. Given the high estimated prevalence of vitamin D deficiency, and a recent finding that 52% of postmenopausal women receiving therapy for osteoporosis had suboptimal vitamin D levels, supplementation with at least 800 IU/d is still a mainstay of therapy *(42)*. Consider higher doses in patients with little or no sun exposure, an inadequate serum 25-hydroxyvitamin D level, or other risk factors.

Behavior Modification

Because cigarette smoking is positively associated with the development of osteoporosis, patients who smoke should be counseled regarding smoking cessation. Similarly, excessive consumption of caffeine and alcohol should be

Table 8
Medications Associated with Increased Fall Risk

Benzodiazepines
Serotonin reuptake inhibitors
Tricyclic antidepressants
Neuroleptics
Anticonvulsants
Some antiarrhythmics

discouraged. Regular weight-bearing and muscle-strengthening activity has been shown to maintain and increase BMD, improve muscle strength, and reduce the risk of falling *(43–45)*. Examples of effective activities include brisk walking or jogging, weight lifting and resistance training, and rhythmic movement, such as dancing or Tai Chi. Thirty to 60 minutes of physical activity three times weekly is recommended to improve BMD.

Fall Prevention

Falls are a major health problem for all older adults, resulting in fractures, head injuries, fear of falling, and, in some cases, loss of independence. Women with osteoporosis are at particularly high risk of sustaining a fracture from a fall. The most effective fall-prevention strategy is a multifactorial risk assessment linked to targeted intervention, such as balance and gait training, review of medications, and modifications of home hazards *(46)*. The medications strongly associated with increased fall risk are shown in Table 8 *(47,48)*.

Undergarments with hip protective padding have been shown to reduce the risk of hip fracture. Hip protectors should be considered for patients at high risk of falling, or who have sustained a hip fracture in the past. Although the use of hip protectors has been shown to reduce the risk of hip fracture, compliance is generally poor *(49)*.

Pharmacological Treatment Recommendations

The pharmacological treatment recommendations of the NOF and the AACE are outlined in Table 9. Both groups agree that patients with a T-score less than −1.5 with risk factors should receive pharmacological treatment. The recommendations differ for the patients without risk factors. The NOF recommends treating patients with no risk factors at a T-score of –2.0 or less, whereas AACE recommends treating those with a T-score of –2.5 or lower *(13,20)*.

Regardless of the T-score, two risk factors deserve special consideration. A history of fragility fracture is a strong predictor of future fracture and should be treated accordingly whether or not the T-score is below –2.5. Patients who

Table 9
Pharmacologic Treatment Recommendations

Organization	*Whom to Treat*
NOF	T-score below –2.0
	T-score below – 1.5 with one or more risk factors
	Any spine or hip fracture
AACE	T-score below –2.5
	T-score below –1.5 with risk factors
	T-score below –1.0 with fragility fracture

NOF, National Osteoporosis Foundation; AACE, American Association of Clinical Endocrinologists

have fragility fractures often have T-scores above –2.5 *(50,51)*. Age is another important independent risk factor. For any given T-score, the risk of fracture is much higher in older patients.

Pharmacological Therapy

The two classes of drugs used to prevent and treat osteoporosis are antiresorptive agents that block osteoclastic bone resorption, and anabolic agents that stimulate osteoblastic bone formation. The Food and Drug-approved pharmacological options for the prevention and treatment of osteoporosis include alendronate, risidronate, and raloxifene. Teriparatide and calcitonin are approved for treatment only. Estrogens are approved for prevention only *(52)*.

BISPHOSPHONATES

Bisphosphonates are stable pyrophosphate analogs that bind permanently to the surface of mineralized bone and inhibit osteoclastic bone resorption. Because of their clinical efficacy and safety profile, bisphosphonates are considered first-line therapy for the treatment of postmenopausal osteoporosis. Both alendronate and risidronate increase lumbar spine BMD by 5 to 7%, and hip BMD by 3 to 6% when used for 3 years *(53,54)*. Both agents also reduce the incidence of vertebral and hip fractures by 30 to 50% *(55)*. Both are oral preparations that can be taken daily or weekly. Alendronate is administered at 5 mg daily, or 35 mg weekly for prevention, and 10 mg daily or 70 mg weekly for treatment. Risidronate is administered at 5 mg daily or 35 mg weekly for both indications.

A 10-year study of alendronate and a 7-year study of risidronate found that increases in BMD and decreases in markers of bone turnover were maintained for the duration of the study *(56,57)*. Patients receiving bisphosphonates should also receive 1200 to 1500 mg calcium and at least 800 IU of vitamin D daily from diet and supplements. The adverse effects of alendronate and risidronate are similar; heartburn, esophageal irritation, and esophagitis are common. To avoid the GI side effects, the medication must be taken with 8 oz of water before eating or taking other medications. Patients must remain upright and take nothing by mouth except water for 30 minutes after taking the drug. Infrequent adverse events associated with bisphosphonates include myalgias, arthralgias, and ocular inflammation. Osteonecrosis of the jaw is a serious adverse event that has been reported in patients receiving intravenous pamidronate and zolendrate for treatment of hypocalcaemia associated with malignancy and metastatic osteolytic lesions. However, osteonecrosis of the jaw has also very rarely been reported in some women taking oral alendronate or risedronate for osteoporosis *(58)*.

Ibandronate is the newest bisphosphonate to be approved for the prevention and treatment of osteoporosis and has been shown to significantly reduce vertebral fractures in women with osteoporosis *(59)*. The dosage is 2.5 mg daily or 150 mg monthly for both prevention and treatment. Similar to other bisphosphonates, it is poorly absorbed and can cause GI disturbances, such as esophagitis. It also must be taken with 8 oz of water after an overnight fast. Patients must remain upright and take nothing by mouth except water for 60 minutes.

Postmenopausal Hormone Therapy

Estrogen slows bone resorption, increases BMD, and reduces osteoporotic fractures. The Women's Health Initiative trial found that women who received estrogen with or without a progestin had 33% fewer hip and vertebral fractures *(60,61)*.

Although approved for the prevention of osteoporosis, estrogen is no longer recommended for osteoporosis prevention because the WHI trial found no cardiovascular benefit and an increased risk of breast cancer, thromboembolic events, and stroke *(60)*. The risks and benefits of treatment must be weighed when considering hormone replacement therapy (HRT) for the prevention of osteoporosis. Studies have shown that accelerated bone loss occurs when estrogen therapy is withdrawn, *(62)* clinicians should consider initiating bisphosphonate therapy when discontinuing estrogen treatment in women taking HRT for the prevention of osteoporosis.

Selective Estrogen-Receptor Modulators. Similar to estrogen, selective estrogen receptor modulators (SERMs) bind to estrogen receptors, inhibit bone resorption, and increase BMD in the spine and hip. The antiresorptive effect of SERMs on bone is not as potent as the effect of estrogen. Raloxifene is the only SERM approved for the prevention and treatment of osteoporosis. Raloxifene significantly reduces the incidence of new vertebral fractures, but nonvertebral fractures are not reduced *(63)*. The risk of breast cancer was significantly reduced in postmenopausal women with osteoporosis treated with raloxifene for 4 years *(64)*. The side effects associated with raloxifene include increased hot flashes and increased risk of venous thromboembolism.

Calcitonin. Calcitonin is a naturally occurring peptide hormone derived from the parathyroid glands that affects serum calcium levels by inhibiting bone resorption. Compared with other antiresorptive agents, the action of calcitonin is mild. Because it is a peptide, calcitonin must be taken by injection or intranasally. The PROOF study found that a daily dose of 200 IU of nasal salmon calcitonin significantly reduced vertebral fractures, but nonvertebral fractures were not affected *(65)*. Calcitonin also decreases the pain associated with recent vertebral fractures *(66)*. Generally, calcitonin should only be used in women at least 5 years postmenopausal who are unable or unwilling to use other osteoporosis medications *(13)*.

Anabolic Agents

Parathyroid Hormone. Synthetic PTH is the only anabolic agent approved for the treatment of osteoporosis. In contrast to antiresorptive agents that inhibit bone resorption, synthetic PTH stimulates bone formation through an increase in bone remodeling.

PTH 1–34 (teriparatide) is the biologically active N-terminal of the first 34 amino acids of PTH. Although chronic exposure to elevated PTH, as in hyperparathyroidism causes increased bone catabolism, intermittent exposure increases bone density.

Teriparatide is indicated for postmenopausal women with osteoporosis who are at high risk of fracture, that is, those with previous osteoporotic fractures, multiple risk factors, or failure or intolerance of other osteoporosis therapies. A large randomized clinical trial by Neer et al. *(67)* found that 20 μg of teriparatide daily significantly increased BMD and reduced vertebral fractures by more than 50% in postmenopausal women with previous vertebral fractures. This trial was terminated prematurely after 20 months because of the development of osteosarcoma in a toxicology study in rats. Although no cases of osteosarcoma have been reported in humans, the Food and Drug Administration (FDA) assigned a black box warning to the drug and limited treatment duration to 2 years.

Teriparatide is only available as an injection in a dose of 20 μg daily. It is contraindicated in patients with an increased risk of skeletal malignancy. Because of a small transient increase in calcium, teriparatide is contraindicated in patients with hypocalcaemia or hyperparathyroidism.

In summary, teriparatide is a potent anabolic agent that significantly increases BMD and reduces vertebral and nonvertebral fractures. In contrast to the bisphosphonates, there are no data demonstrating significant reduction in hip fractures. In view of the high cost, need for daily subcutaneous injections, and the availability of other drugs with proven efficacy, teriparatide use is likely to remain limited to postmenopausal women with severe osteoporosis refractory to other treatment modalities or those unable to tolerate other treatments.

Combination Therapy

Several studies have found that combination or sequential therapies increase BMD more than monotherapy, however, there are no data showing reduced fractures. A 3-year randomized placebo controlled study comparing HRT alone to alendronate, or alendronate plus HRT, found that BMD was significantly greater at all femoral and vertebral sites in women treated with combination therapy *(68)*. A 1-year randomized double-blinded study assessed the effects of raloxifene alone versus alendronate alone or combined raloxifene and alendronate. In this study, combination therapy was superior to raloxifene alone and to alendronate alone at the femoral neck *(69)*.

In summary, the efficacy and safety of combination therapy with antiresorptive agents have not been proven. The use of two antiresorptive agents is difficult to justify given the lack of data on fractures, increased expense, and increased potential for side effects.

Combination or Sequential Therapies with PTH

Because bisphosphonates inhibit bone resorption, and PTH stimulates bone formation, combination therapy offers the possibility of synergy. However, a well-designed randomized controlled study, consisting of 238 postmenopausal women, comparing PTH or alendronate alone or in combination found no significant difference in the increase in BMD at the spine between the PTH group and the combination therapy group *(70)*. In fact, changes in volumetric density and markers of bone turnover suggest that the concurrent use of a bisphosphonate and PTH may attenuate the anabolic effects of PTH.

In a continuation of the same trial, women who had received PTH monotherapy for 1 year were then assigned to receive either 1 year of placebo or alendronate. Women treated with placebo after PTH therapy lost much of the previous gain in BMD, whereas women treated with alendronate maintained or increased BMD gains *(71)*.

In summary, the combination of PTH and a bisphosphonate is not superior to either agent alone, and may attenuate the anabolic effects of PTH. After discontinuation of PTH monotherapy, increases in BMD are rapidly lost. Treatment with a bisphosphonate immediately after discontinuation of PTH preserves or increases BMD.

Monitoring Response to Therapy

The NOF recommends measuring BMD by central DXA 1 to 2 years after the initiation of therapy. Certain high-risk patients, such as those treated with glucocorticoids, or who have sustained a fracture, may require more frequent follow-up. The value of measuring BMD is limited by the rate of response to therapy and the inherent precision error of DXA. Changes of less than 2 to 4% in the vertebrae and 3 to 6% at the hip can be caused by measurement error, depending on the equipment used *(13)*. In addition, BMD changes in response to antiresorptive therapy are often small and occur slowly. Consequently, changes that exceed the precision error of the DXA may not occur until after 2 to 3 years of therapy. Markers of bone turnover may be used to monitor treatment response earlier, as described in the markers of bone turnover section of this chapter.

Treatment with antiresorptive agents has been found to reduce fracture risk more than would be predicted by the increase in BMD. To interpret DXA results meaningfully, clinicians must know the least significant change as determined by the inherent precision error of the equipment. It is not possible to compare DXA results performed on different machines unless cross calibration between the old and the new machine is performed. Similarly, results of a DXA performed at one institution cannot be compared with one performed at another institution because of differences in the least significant change between machines.

Clinicians must interpret DXA results carefully, realizing that the lack of an apparent significant response to therapy is not indicative of treatment failure. Bone losses greater than the least significant change are indicative of treatment failure, but may not be detected for 2 years or more.

REFERENCES

1. Gabriel SE, Tosteson AN, Leibson CL, et al. Direct medical costs attributable to osteoporotic fractures. Osteoporos Int 2002;13:323–330.
2. Office of Technology Assessment. Hip Fracture Outcomes in people age 50 and over. Washington, DC: US Government Printing Office; 1994. Background paper OTA-BP-H-120.
3. Cummings SR, Black DM, Rubin SM. Lifetime risks of hip, Colles', or vertebral fracture and coronary heart disease among white postmenopausal women. Arch Int Med 1989;149: 2445–2448.
4. NIH Consensus Development Panel on Osteoporosis. JAMA 2001;285:785–795.
5. World Health Organization. Assessment of fracture risk and its application to screening for postmenopausal osteoporosis. WHO Technical Report Series. No. 843; Geneva, Switzerland: World Health Organization; 1994.
6. Handy RC, Petak SM, Lenchik L. International Society for Clinical Densitometry Position Development Panel and Scientific Advisory Committee. Which central dual X-ray absorptiometry skeletal sites and regions of interest should be used to determine the diagnosis of osteoporosis? J Clin Densitom 2002;5(Suppl):S11–S18.

7. Miller PD, Njeh CF, Jankowski LG. International Society for Clinial Densitometry Position Development Panel and Scientific Advisory Committee. What are the standards by which bone mass measurement at peripheral skeletal sites should be used in the diagnosis of osteoporosis? J Clin Densitom 2002;5(Suppl):S39–S45.
8. Writing Group for the ISCD Position Development Conference. Diagnosis of osteoporosis in men, premenopausal women, and children. J Clin Densitom 2004;7(1):17–26.
9. Raisz LG, Rodan GA. Pathogenesis of osteoporosis. Endocrinol Metab Clin North Am 2003;32:15–24.
10. Simonet WS, Lacey DL, Dunstan CR, et al. Osteoprotegerin: a novel secreted protein involved in the regulation of bone density. Cell 1997;89:309–319.
11. Hofbauer LC, Khosla S, Dunstan CR, et al. The roles of osteoprotegerin and osteoprotegerin ligand in the paracrine regulation of bone resorption. J Bone Miner Res 2000;15(1): 2–12.
12. Kanis JA, Meton LJ, Christiansen C, et al. The diagnosis of osteoporosis. J Bone Miner Res 1994;9:1137–1141.
13. National Osteoporosis Foundation. Physician's Guide to Prevention and Treatment of Osteoporosis. Washington DC: National Osteoporosis Foundation, 2003.
14. Siris ES, Miller PD, Barrett-Connor E, et al. Identification and fracture outcomes of undiagnosed low bone mineral density in postmenopausal women: results from the National Osteoporosis Risk Assessment. JAMA 2001;286:2815–2822.
15. Lindsay R, Silverman SL, Cooper C, et al. Risk of new vertebral fracture in the year following a fracture. JAMA 2001;285:320–323.
16. Orlil ZC, Raisz LG. Causes of secondary osteoporosis. J Clin Densitometry 1999;2:79–92.
17. Stein E, Shane E. Secondary osteoporosis. Endocrinol Metab Clin North Am 2003;32: 115–134.
18. Preventive Services Task Force, Screening for osteoporosis in postmenopausal women: recommendations and rationale. Ann Int Med 2002;137:526–528.
19. Hodgson SF, Watts NB, Bilezikian JP, et al. American Association of Clinical Endocrinologists medical guidelines for clinical practice for the prevention and treatment of postmenopausal osteoporosis: 2001 edition, with selected updates for 2003. Endocr Pract. 2003;9:544–564. Erratum in: Endocr Pract 2004;10:90.
20. Leib ES, Lewiecki EM, Binkley H, et al. Official positions of the International Society for Clinical Densitometry. J Clin Densitom 2004;7:1–6.
21. Picard D, Brown JP, Rosenthal L, et al. Ability of peripheral DXA measurement to diagnose osteoporosis as assessed by central DXA measurement. J Clin Densitom 2004;7:111–118.
22. Tannebaum C, Clark J, Schwartzman K, et al. Yield of laboratory testing to identify secondary contributors to osteoporosis in otherwise healthy women. J Clin Endocrinol Metab 2002;87:4431–4437.
23. Becker C. Clinical evaluation for osteoporosis. Clin Geriatr Med 2003;19:299–320.
24. Hammett-Stabler CA. The use of biochemical markers in osteoporosis. Clin Lab Med 2004;24:175–197.
25. Rosen HN, Moses AC, Garker J, et al. Utility of biochemical markers of bone turnover in the follow-up of patients treated with bisphosphonates. Calcif Tissue Int 1998; 63:363–368.
26. Office of Dietary Supplements. NIH. Dietary supplement fact sheet. http://ods.od.nih.gov/ fact sheets/calcium asp. Last accessed 3/16/07.
27. Office of the Surgeon General. Bone health and osteoporosis: report of the surgeon general. Department of Health and Human Services, Rockville MN, 2004, pp. 436.
28. Holick MF. Vitamin D: importance in the prevention of cancers, type 1 diabetes, heart disease, and osteoporosis. Am J Clin Nutr 2004;79:362–371. Erratum in: Am J Clin Nutr 2004;79:890.

29. Holick MF. Vitamin D: the underappreciated D-lightful hormone that is important for skeletal and cellular health. Curr Opin Endocrinol Diabetes 2002;9:87–98.
30. Webb AR, Kline L, Holick MF. Influence of season and latitude on the cutaneous synthesis of vitamin D3: exposure to winter sunlight in Boston and Edmonton will not promote vitamin D3 synthesis in human skin. J Clin Endocrinol Metab 1988;67:373–378.
31. Chapuy MC, Preziosi P, Maamer M, et al. Prevalence of vitamin D insufficiency in an adult normal population. Osteoporos Int 1997;7:439–443.
32. Thomas MK, Llyod-Jones DH, Thadhani RI, et al. Hypovitaminosis D in medical inpatients. N Engl J Med 1998;338:777–783.
33. Tangpricha V, Pearce EN, Chen TC, et al. Vitamin D insufficiency among free-living healthy young adults. Am J Med 2002;112:659–662.
34. Dawson-Hughes B, Heaney RP, Holick MF. Estimates of optimal vitamin D status. Osteoporos Int 2005;16:713–716.
35. Barger-Lux MJ, Heaner RP, Dowell S, et al. Vitamin D and its major metabolites: serum levels after graded oral dosing in healthy men. Osteoporos Int 1998;8:222–230.
36. Tangpricha V, Koutkia P, Rieke SM, et al. Fortification of orange juice with vitamin D: a novel approach for enhancing vitamin D nutritional health. Am J Clin Nutr 2003;77: 1478–1483.
37. Tangpricha V, Pearce EN, Chen TC, et al. Vitamin D insufficiency among free-living healthy young adults. Am J Med 2002;11:659–662.
38. Bischoff-Fearrari H, Willett WC, Wong JB, et al. Fracture prevention with vitamin D supplementation: a meta-analysis of randomized controlled trials. JAMA 2005;293: 2257–2264.
39. Grant AM, Avenell A, Campbell MK, et al. Oral vitamin D3 and calcium for secondary prevention of low-trauma fractures in elderly people (Randomised Evaluation of Calcium or Vitamin D, RECORD): a randomised placebo-controlled trial. Lancet 2005;365: 1621–1628.
40. Porthouse J, Cockayne S, King C, et al. Randomised controlled trial of calcium and supplementation with cholecalciferol (vitamin D3) for prevention of fractures in primary care. BMJ 2005;330:1003.
41. Holick MF, Siris ES, Binkley N, et al. Prevalence of vitamin D inadequacy among postmenopausal North American women receiving osteoporosis therapy. J Clin Endocrinol Metab 2005;90:3215–3224.
42. Beard A, Bravo G, Gauthier P. Meta-analysis of the effectiveness of physical activity for the prevention of bone loss in postmenopausal women. Osteoporos Int 1997;7:331–337.
43. Kelley GA. Exercise and regional bone mineral density in postmenopausal women: a meta-analytic review of randomized trials. Am J Phys Med Rehabil 1998;77:76–87.
44. Chang JT, Morton SC, Rubenstein LZ, et al. Interventions for the prevention of falls in older adults: systematic review and meta-analysis of randomised clinical trials. BMJ 2004;328:680.
45. Tinetti ME, Baker DI, McAvay G, et al. A multifactorial intervention to reduce the risk of falling among elderly people living in the community. N Engl J Med 1994;331: 821–827.
46. Leipzig RM, Cumming RG, Tinette ME. Drugs and falls in older people: a systematic review and meta-analysis: I. Psychotropic drugs. J Am Geriatr Soc 1999;47:30–39.
47. Leipzig RM, Cumming RG, Tinette ME. Drugs and falls in older people: a systematic review and meta-analysis: II. Cardiac and analgesic drugs. Am Geriatr Soc 1999: 47:40–50.
48. Parker MJ, Gillespie LD, Gilespie WJ. Hip protectors for preventing hip fractures in the elderly. Nurs Times 2001;97:41.

49. Wainwright SA, Marshall LM, Ensrund KE, et al. Study of Osteoporotic Fractures Research Group. Hip fracture in women without osteoporosis. J Clin Endocrinol Metab 2005;90: 2787–2793.
50. Schuit SC, van der Klift M, Weel AE, et al. Fracture incidence and association with bone mineral density in elderly men and women: the Rotterdam Study. Bone 2004;34:195–202.
51. Rosen CJ. Clinical practice. Postmenopausal osteoporosis. N Engl J Med 2005;353: 595–603.
52. Cranney A, Wells G, Willan A, et al. Meta-analyses of therapies for postmenopausal osteoporosis. II. Meta-analysis of alendronate for the treatment of postmenopausal women. Endocr Rev 2002;23:508–516.
53. Cranney A, Tugwell P, Adachi J, et al. Meta-analyses of therapies for postmenopausal osteoporosis. III. Meta-analysis of risedronate for the treatment of postmenopausal osteoporosis. Endocr Rev 2002;23:517–523.
54. Guyatt GH, Cranney A, Griffith L, et al. Summary of meta-analyses of therapies for postmenopausal osteoporosis and the relationship between bone density and fractures. Endocrinol Metab Clin North Am 2002;31:659–679.
55. Bone HG, Hosking D, Devogelaer JP, et al. Ten years' experience with alendronate for osteoporosis in postmenopausal women. N Engl J Med 2004;350:1189–1199.
56. Mellstrom DD, Sorenson OH, Goemaere S, et al. Seven years of treatment with risedronate in women with postmenopausal osteoporosis. Calcif Tissue Int 2004;75:462–468.
57. Ruggiero SL, Mehrota B, Rosenberg TJ, et al. Osteonecrosis of the jaws associated with the use of bisphosphonates: a review of 63 cases. J Oral Maxillofac Surg 2004;62:527–534.
58. Chestnut CH III, Skag A, Christansen C, et al. Effects of oral ibandronate administered daily or intermittently on fracture risk in postmenopausal osteoporosis. J Bone Miner Res 2004;19:1241–1249.
59. The Writing Group for the PEPI. Effects of hormone therapy on bone mineral density: results from the postmenopausal estrogen/progestin interventions (PEPI) trial. JAMA 1996;276:1389–1396.
60. The Women's Health Initiative Steering Committee. Effects of conjugated equine estrogen in postmenopaual women with hysterectomy, JAMA 2004;291:1701–1712.
61. Greenspan SL, Emkey RD, Bone HG, et al. Significant differential effects of alendronate, estrogen, or combination therapy on the rate of bone loss after discontinuation of treatment of postmenopausal osteoporosis. A randomized, double-blind, placebo-controlled trial. Ann Intern Med 2002;137:875–883.
62. Ettinger B, Black DM, Mitlak BH, et al. Reduction of vertebral fracture risk in postmenopausal women with osteoporosis treated with raloxifene: results from a 3-year randomized clinical trial. Multiple Outcomes of Raloxifene Evaluation (MORE) Investigators. JAMA1999;282:637–645. Erratum in: JAMA 1999;282:212.
63. Cauley J, Norton L, Lippman M, et al. Continued breast cancer risk reduction in postmenopausal women treated with raloxifene: 4-year results from the MORE trial. Multiple outcomes of raloxifene evaluation. Breast Cancer Res Treat 2001;65:125–134. Erratum in: Breast Cancer Res Treat 2001;67:191.
64. Chesnut CH III, Silverman S, Andriano K, et al. A randomized trial of nasal spray salmon calcitonin in postmenopausal women with established osteoporosis: the prevent recurrence of osteoporotic fractures study. PROOF Study Group.Am J Med 2000;109:267–276.
65. Silverman SL, Azria M. The analgesic role of calcitonin following osteoporotic fracture. Osteoporos Int 2002;13:858–867.
66. Neer RM, Arnaud CD, Zanchetta JR, et al. Effect of parathyroid hormone (1-34) on fractures and bone mineral density in postmenopausal women with osteoporosis. N Engl J Med 2001;344:1434–1441.

67. Greenspan SL, Resnick NM, Parker RA. Combination therapy with hormone replacement and alendronate for prevention of bone loss in elderly women: a randomized controlled trial. JAMA 2003;289:2525–2533.
68. Johnell O, Scheele WH, Lu Y. Additive effects of raloxifene and alendronate on bone density and biochemical markers of bone remodeling in postmenopausal women with osteoporosis. J Clin Endocrinol Metab 2002;87:985–992.
69. Black DM, Greenspan SL, Ensrud KE. The effects of parathyroid hormone and alendronate alone or in combination in postmenopausal osteoporosis. N Engl J Med 2003;349:1207–1215.
70. Black DM, Bilezikian JP, Ensrud KE. One year of alendronate after one year of parathyroid hormone (1-84) for osteoporosis. N Engl J Med 2005;353:555–565.

5 Women and Coronary Heart Disease

Susan Mather, MD

Contents

From: *Current Clinical Practice: Women's Health in Clinical Practice*
Edited by: Clouse and Sherif © Humana Press Inc., Totowa, NJ

INTRODUCTION

Cardiovascular disease (CVD), encompassing both coronary heart disease (CHD) and cerebrovascular disease, is a major health burden worldwide in men and women. Although historically considered a "man's disease," this myth is quickly fading and for good reason.

According to a world conference on women and CVD held in 2000, CVD is the leading cause of death in women in developed countries and is anticipated to be the leading cause of death in women in developing countries by the year 2020. Most of these estimated 10 million deaths in women worldwide occur in poor and developing countries; this may be because of the continued commonality of rheumatic heart disease. Similarly, morbidity caused by heart disease affects large numbers of women worldwide *(1)*.

Not only is CVD the most common cause of death in women, but it also is associated with significant economic costs. In the United States, the 2005 estimated total cost of CVD is more than 390 billion dollars; CHD alone represents more than 140 billion dollars. In 2002, the top two diagnoses for hospitalized patients were coronary atherosclerosis and acute myocardial infarction (AMI), at a cost of more than 66 billion dollars *(2)*.

CVD is associated with significant morbidity as well. Cerebrovascular disease and coronary artery disease (CAD) share similar risk factors. This chapter will focus on the risk factors for CAD and review prevention, diagnosis, and management of heart disease in women.

EPIDEMIOLOGY

During the past few decades, medical knowledge surrounding the pathophysiology, risks and treatment of CVD has grown tremendously. Cardiovascular death rates in men are finally beginning to decline; unfortunately, a similar decline is not occurring in women. In fact, for the past 20 years, more women than men have died per year of CVD disease in the United States. This is in part because the general population is aging and elderly women outnumber elderly men *(3)*.

Historically, reproductive issues dominated medical attention in women's healthcare; heart disease was considered more of an issue in men. Eventually, risk factors for men were recognized to be risk factors in women as well. One important sex difference is that women experience CVD later in life than men. The average age for first myocardial infarction (MI) is 65.8 years for men and 70.4 years for women *(2)*.

The medical community has increasingly recognized the significance of heart disease in women. Sex differences have also been observed in terms of heart disease in presentation, diagnosis, management, and prognosis. However, many of the recommendations for the management of heart disease in women are extrapolated from research performed mostly in white men.

In the past, clinical investigators and the Food and Drug Administration (FDA) excluded women of childbearing potential in many early studies of cardiovascular drugs, particularly phase 1 and phase 2 trials. Since 1986, however, the National Institutes of Health (NIH) made efforts to encourage inclusion of women in studies *(4)*. In fact, inclusion of women and outcome data analyzed by sex is now a requirement in studies sponsored by the NIH *(3)*.

RACE AND ETHNICITY

Racial differences in the risk, prevalence and mortality of CVD have been observed. For example, a survey of three ethnic groups of women (white, black and Mexican American) conducted between 1988 and 1994 showed that women in ethnic minority groups had a higher prevalence of CVD risk factors, such as hypertension (HTN), increased body mass index (BMI), lack of physical activity, and diabetes in comparison with white women. In addition, women of lower socioeconomic status had a higher prevalence of smoking, physical inactivity, higher BMI, and hyperlipidemia *(5)*.

In response to findings of racial/ethnic differences in risk factors, the Department of Health and Human Services (DHHS) launched an initiative in1998 to eliminate the existing disparities by 2010 *(6)*. To explore the scope of the mortality issue, data from death certificates of women who died of heart disease from 1991 to 1995 was collected. Five racial and ethnic groups were evaluated: American Indian/Alaska Native, Asian/Pacific Islander, black, Hispanic, and white. Of this sample, 64% of heart disease deaths were caused by ischemic heart disease. Although race and ethnicity information recorded on death certificates is not always reliable *(7)*, nonetheless, important general findings emerged from the study.

Overall findings indicated that American Indian/Alaska Native and black women had the highest proportion of "premature" heart disease deaths (deaths occurring at younger than 65 years of age). Black women had the highest rates of heart disease mortality, whereas Asian/Pacific Islanders had the lowest mortality; the difference was greater than twofold. Overall, the rate of heart disease deaths declined in the 1990s, but not as fast as the declines seen in the 1970s and 1980s.

Although this data describes ethnic differences in mortality, it does not identify the potential role of factors such as social class, culture, behavioral risk factors, psychological risk factors, and effects of racism *(8)*. To further explore what puts women at risk for CVD, we can look at established risk factors and how they specifically affect women.

RISK FACTORS AND PREVENTION

Multiple known risk factors exist for CHD and CVD. Some are modifiable with lifestyle changes or medication and some are not. Data from the Framingham Heart Study provides a method of calculating future risk of CHD events using the top CHD risk factors. Although the Framingham study cohort was mainly middle class and white, the prediction functions have been reliably applied to black men and women. There is, however, some indication that ethnic-specific recalibration may be needed to accurately apply these functions to other ethnic groups *(9)*.

The Third Report of the National Cholesterol Education Program (NCEP) Expert Panel on Detection, Evaluation, and Treatment of High Blood Cholesterol in Adults (Adult Treatment Panel [ATP] III) provides the following list of CHD risk factors *(10)*:

- Elevated low-density lipoprotein (LDL) cholesterol
- Low high-density lipoprotein (HDL) (<40 mg/dL)
- Age
  - Men ≥45 years
  - Women ≥55 years
- Family history of premature CHD
- Current cigarette smoking
- HTN (≥140/90 mmHg or on an antihypertensive medication)
- Male sex
- Diabetes mellitus
- Obesity
- Physical inactivity
- Atherogenic diet

Examples of emerging risk factors include:

- Elevated serum triglycerides (≥200 mg/dL)
- Elevated lipoprotein (a)
- Homocysteine
- Inflammatory markers, such as C-reactive protein (CRP)

Let us look more closely at the individual risk factors.

TYPE 2 DIABETES

Type 2 diabetes accounts for approx 90 to 95% of cases of diabetes and is a preventable risk factor. It is characterized initially by insulin resistance and progressive β-cell dysfunction. The American Diabetes Association (ADA) diagnostic criteria for type 2 diabetes are *(11)*:

1. Symptoms of diabetes (e.g., polyuria, polydipsia, unexplained weight loss) plus casual plasma glucose at least 200 mg/dL.
2. Fasting plasma glucose at least 126 mg/dL.
3. Oral glucose tolerance test with a 2-hour post-load glucose of at least 200 mg/dL.

Type 2 diabetes is currently an epidemic. Since 1990, the prevalence has increased by more than 60%. Statistics from 2002 reveal that approx 7% of US adults have type 2 diabetes, with the highest prevalence in Native Americans, Native Alaskans, black, and Mexican-American women *(2)*. Worldwide, there are approx 171 million people with diabetes, and the projected figure anticipated for 2030 is 366 million people with diabetes. Furthermore, in 2004, the DHHS reported that approx 40% of US adults have "prediabetes" (fasting blood glucose between 100 and 126 mg/dL), putting them at increased risk of diabetes *(2)*.

Diabetes is clearly an independent risk factor for CVD *(12)*. Being diabetic confers a high risk (>20%) of having a coronary event in 10 years time based on the Framingham Risk Score for women. This is a similar risk to women who have established CHD, cerebrovascular disease, and peripheral arterial disease *(13)*. Eighty percent of patients with diabetes die of thrombotic events and it is estimated that up to 75% of diabetic deaths are caused by cardiovascular complications *(14)*. Heart disease death rates are two to four times higher in diabetic patients than in nondiabetic individuals.

Some research has shown that the relative risk of CHD, heart failure, and intermittent claudication may be greater in female diabetic patients compared with male diabetic patients. Multiple studies have suggested that diabetes is a stronger risk factor for cardiovascular mortality in women *(15)*. However, a meta-analysis of 16 studies on CHD mortality in diabetic men and women found that, overall, the odds ratio for CHD mortality caused by diabetes was not significantly different between women and men. The authors of this meta-analysis reported that the apparent sex difference previously noted was most likely caused by inadequate control of other CHD risk factors in the studied populations. They revealed nonstatistically significant adjusted summary odds ratios for CHD mortality in women (odds ratio, 2.9) versus men (odds ratio, 2.3) *(16)*. Although this matter is not definitively resolved, it should be stressed that perhaps as important as a possible sex difference regarding who has a higher morbidity or mortality, the difference in cardiac risk between individuals with or without diabetes is substantial.

In diabetics, tight glucose control is associated with decreased cardiovascular morbidity and decreased mortality *(15)*. The ADA goal for hemoglobin A_{1c} is less than 7%, whereas the goal of the American Association of Clinical Endocrinologists is less than 6.5% *(13)*. To achieve this, lifestyle changes in addition to pharmacotherapy are usually needed in most diabetic patients. Although tight glucose control is essential, other factors play a role in the development of CAD *(12)*. Endothelial cell dysfunction in type 2 diabetics caused by hyperinsulinemia, platelet adhesion and aggregation, and a decrease in fibrinolytic activity that favors clotting promote atherosclerosis *(15,17)*.

Unfortunately, many patients with diabetes have other CVD risk factors. Although trends indicate that hyperlipidemia, HTN, and smoking rates seem to be decreasing, 50% of patients with diabetes have hyperlipidemia, more than 30% have HTN, and one of six smokes cigarettes. The direct and indirect cost of diabetes in the United States in 2002 was 132 billion dollars *(2)*.

The US Preventive Services Task Force recommends screening for type 2 diabetes in adults with HTN or hyperlipidemia, but found there was insufficient evidence to recommend for or against routine screening of asymptomatic adults *(18)*. The ADA recommends screening asymptomatic adults who are 45 years of age and older, particularly those who are overweight, and adults who are younger than 45 years with other risk factors. The ADA recommends a fasting plasma glucose as the initial screening test for nonpregnant adults because it is a less expensive, easier, and more convenient profile compared with the 2-hour 75-g glucose-load oral glucose tolerance test *(19)*.

METABOLIC SYNDROME

The metabolic syndrome, also known as the insulin resistance syndrome, is a constellation of risk factors that confer an increased risk of CVD morbidity and mortality. Some patients seem to be genetically prone to the syndrome, and most patients with metabolic syndrome are overweight. According to the NCEP ATP III, the syndrome is defined as three or more of the following *(20)*:

- Waist circumference greater than 40 inches in men and 35 inches in women
- Serum triglyceride level at least 150 mg/dL
- HDL level less than 40 mg/dL in men and less than 50 mg/dL in women
- Blood pressure at least 130/85 mmHg
- Fasting glucose level at least 110 mg/dL

The metabolic syndrome amplifies the risk that an elevated LDL confers and is associated with an increased risk of stroke and MI morbidity in both sexes even when age, race and smoking are taken into account *(10,20)*.

The Women's Ischemia Syndrome Evaluation (WISE) study found that in more than 700 women with suspected myocardial ischemia, each unit worsening of metabolic status (from normal metabolism to metabolic syndrome to diabetes) was associated with an approximately twofold adjusted risk of death and major adverse cardiovascular event (including death, nonfatal MI, stroke, and congestive heart failure). Furthermore, in those women who had angiographically significant CAD, presence of the metabolic syndrome resulted in a significantly increased 4-year risk of cardiovascular events versus women with normal metabolic status (hazard ratio 4.93 [95% confidence interval, 1.02–23.76; $p = 0.05$]). Women with the metabolic syndrome and without significant CAD on coronary angiography did not have an increased 4-year cardiovascular risk *(21)*.

The results of the WISE study support the theory that the metabolic syndrome is associated with an increased risk of CHD, although not as high as the risk associated with diabetes *(22)*.

A possible explanation for the association between the metabolic syndrome and increased risk of cardiovascular events is the presence of chronic systemic inflammation and, possibly, the presence of a procoagulant state. Elevated serum concentrations of inflammatory markers have been associated with the metabolic syndrome and with cardiovascular events. It is hypothesized that inflammation may destabilize atherosclerotic plaque in the coronary arteries, leading to increased thrombosis and cardiac events *(21,22)*.

Some of the components of the metabolic syndrome are modifiable; and, as the syndrome gains more recognition by physicians, the emphasis on appropriate risk modification should continue to gain strength.

HYPERTENSION

HTN, defined as systolic blood pressure of at least 140 mmHg, or diastolic blood pressure of at least 90 mmHg *(23)* is very common in the United States. Data collected from 1988 through 1991 found that 24% of the US adult population had HTN *(24)*. More recently, it is estimated that almost one-third of adults are affected. Before age 55 years, men with HTN outnumber women, however after age 55 years, the percentage of women with HTN exceeds that of men *(2)*.

Furthermore, patients who have normal blood pressure levels at age 55 years have a 90% lifetime risk of developing HTN. The higher the blood pressure. the higher the risk of heart (and other end organ) disease. In 2003, the Seventh Report of the Joint National Committee on Prevention, Detection, Evaluation, and Treatment of High Blood Pressure made the categories of blood pressure classification somewhat stricter. Notably, "normal" blood pressure for adults is defined as systolic blood pressure of *less than* 120 mmHg and diastolic blood pressure *less than* 80 mmHg. A new category called pre-HTN was added and is defined as systolic blood pressure of 120 to 139 mmHg and diastolic blood pressure of 80 to 89 mmHg. Patients with pre-HTN are at a higher risk for developing HTN *(23)*.

Black women bear a disproportionate burden of HTN. Studies have reported a higher incidence of both treated and untreated HTN in black women versus white women. Racial differences are most noticeable in younger age groups. In one study of women 25 to 34 years old, 23% of black women and 8% of white women were hypertensive. In women 35 to 54 years old, 39% of black women and 21% of white women were hypertensive. These age differences were almost eliminated in the 55 to 74 year age range *(25)*.

In both black and white women, baseline factors predictive of a higher incidence of HTN include older age, greater BMI, and fewer years of education. According to data from US National Health and Nutrition Examination Survey III, patient awareness of HTN and treatment increased significantly from 1988 through 1991 *(25)*.

Early diagnosis and treatment are important for women to reduce their risk of CVD. If lifestyle changes do not lower blood pressure, antihypertensive medication should be used. Benefits other than a decrease in blood pressure may be sought by the choice of antihypertensive, therefore, medication regimens should be individualized. The Antihypertensive and Lipid-Lowering Treatment of Prevent Heart Attack Trial was a large trial of hypertensive men and women older than age 55 years that compared treatment with a thiazide diuretic, a dihydropyridine calcium channel blocker or an angiotensin-converting enzyme inhibitor. After 5 years, there was no difference detected between groups in combined fatal CHD or nonfatal MI *(26)*. However, other trials have demonstrated differences in cardiovascular endpoints based on class of HTN medication.

Studies have demonstrated substantial reductions in major CVD events, CHD, and stroke in both sexes with reduction of blood pressure *(27)*.

CHOLESTEROL

Hyperlipidemia is underdiagnosed. A 2004 study revealed that only 60 to 70% of women had a lipid profile checked in the last 5 years *(28)*. Hyperlipidemia is also undertreated; most women on lipid-lowering medication are not at goal cholesterol.

Elevated LDL, total cholesterol, and triglycerides, and low HDL are established risk factors for CVD in both men and women *(29)*. ATP III identifies LDL as the primary target of therapy, although abnormal triglycerides and HDL may be more predictive in women.

Guidelines for management of hyperlipidemia are similar for both men and women. In women 45 to 75 years of age, the recommended goal LDL is less than

100 mg/dL in those with CHD or a CHD risk equivalent (e.g., peripheral arterial disease or diabetes) *(10)*. However, an update to the ATP III guidelines, based on emerging data from multiple clinical trials suggests a goal LDL less than 70 mg/dL when risk is very high *(30)*. For women with at least two risk factors, LDL should be less than 130 mg/dL and for women with no or one risk factor, LDL should be less than 160 mg/dL *(10)*. More recent trial data suggests that use of a statin in patients with CAD or diabetes, regardless of baseline LDL (i.e., even if LDL is <100 mg/dL) can reduce cardiac risk *(31)*. Based on these data, experts have suggested that a goal LDL less than 100 mg/dL may be reasonable in a patient with at least two risk factors and a 10-year risk for CHD of greater than 20% *(32)*.

In women, age is not considered a risk factor until age 55 years because the onset of CHD events is, in general, delayed by approx 10 to 15 years in women as opposed to men. LDL and triglyceride levels rise later in women, and HDL levels are usually approx 10 mg/dL higher. The higher HDL in women seems to confer protection from CHD *(10)*. There is also evidence that lipoprotein (a), a lipoprotein less amenable to treatment, is an independent risk factor for CHD events in premenopausal and postmenopausal women *(33)*. There is less than clear evidence for elevated triglyceride levels in women as an independent risk factor of CHD events *(10)*.

A meta-analysis of 13 studies performed to investigate the effects of lipid-lowering medication in the prevention of CHD events in women with and without CVD, found that women with known CVD who had their lipids lowered had significantly reduced CHD mortality, reduced nonfatal MI, fewer revascularization events, and reduced total CHD events. On the other hand, women without known CVD did not benefit from lipid-lowering medication in terms of mortality or cardiovascular events. This differs from findings in men. One possible reason that these primary prevention trials did not show a beneficial effect could be because relatively few events occurred in these trials. Because women have a lower risk in general for CVD compared with men, the number needed to treat to prevent one CHD event is higher in women. Therefore, more women than men need to be studied to see a primary preventive effect. The number needed to treat for secondary prevention in men and women, on the other hand, is similar. Short follow-up periods in some of the studies could have also limited power *(29)*.

Maintaining normal lipid levels should be promoted through lifestyle changes (i.e., diet and exercise) and, in high-risk women, with the help of pharmacotherapy.

OBESITY AND NUTRITION

Overweight is defined as a BMI of 25 or higher; obesity is defined as a BMI of 30 or higher. The prevalence of obesity has increased substantially since the early 1990s in every group, but particularly in black women. Almost 7 of every 10 adults in the United States are overweight and 3 of every 10 are considered obese.

Dietary Guidelines for Americans 2005 is a joint DHHS and US Department of Agriculture project that provides evidence-based guidelines for health and disease prevention through nutrition and physical activity. Current recommendations stand out from previous guidelines in that regular physical activity and weight control are strongly emphasized in addition to the usual discussion of food recommendations *(34)*.

The American Heart Association considers following a heart-healthy diet useful and effective in its evidence-based guidelines for CVD prevention in women. A heart-healthy diet is described as "…an overall healthy eating pattern that includes intake of a variety of fruits, vegetables, grains, low-fat or nonfat dairy products, fish, legumes, and sources of protein low in saturated fat (e.g., poultry, lean meats, plant sources)." It further restricts saturated fat intake to less than 10% of calories, cholesterol intake to less than 300 mg/d, and overall intake of *trans* fatty acids *(13)*.

Ingestion of fish has been associated with a decreased CVD risk, possibly because of the ingestion of omega-3 fatty acids. Women, particularly those of childbearing age, however, should be aware of the high levels of mercury found in some species of fish. They should consider eating fish with lower levels of mercury or consuming other sources of omega-3 fatty acids, such as walnuts, and flaxseed, walnut, canola, soybean, or distilled fish oils. It should be noted that the cardiovascular benefits of nonmarine omega-3 fatty acids are less well studied *(13)*.

Participants of the Nurses' Health Study, a very large cohort of registered nurses without diagnosed CVD, cancer, or diabetes at baseline enrollment, were evaluated for several lifestyle variables including diet during 14 years of follow-up. A healthy diet, alone and in conjunction with other healthy lifestyle habits, was found to be associated with a lower risk of CHD events. In this analysis, a healthy diet was one that was low in *trans* fat, had a low glycemic load, was high in cereal fiber, high in marine omega-3 fatty acids and folate, and had a high ratio of polyunsaturated to saturated fat *(35)*.

A more in-depth analysis of dietary patterns in the Nurses' Health Study cohort was performed to look at two major dietary patterns, a "prudent diet" and a "Western diet." The prudent diet was high in fruits, vegetables, whole grains, legumes, poultry, and fish. The Western diet contained more refined grains, processed meats, red meats, desserts, high-fat dairy products, and fried foods. The prudent diet pattern was inversely associated with the risk of CHD to a significant degree, even after adjustment for multiple variables such as age,

BMI, smoking, caloric intake, supplemental vitamin use, and hormone replacement therapy (HRT). The Western diet was associated with a significantly higher risk of fatal and nonfatal MI after multivariate adjustment. The findings were not appreciably different between smokers and nonsmokers, lean and overweight women, or those with and without a CHD family history. Study results were consistent with observations from the Health Professionals' Follow-up Study in men *(36)*.

Of the approx 2000 calories ingested daily per adult in the United States, roughly one-third are from fat. For women, the average daily intake of total fat is 67.3 g. On average, 23 g of that fat is saturated. Major sources of saturated fat in the American diet are red meat, butter, whole milk, and eggs. Overall, Americans are eating more meat (including red meat, poultry, and fish) than in 1970, but less red meat and more poultry and fish *(2)*. The average daily intake of dietary cholesterol in women in the United States is also too high, and the average daily intake of dietary fiber is too low.

More than 70% of women eat fewer than the recommended amount of fruits and vegetables daily. Those most likely to have a high intake of fruits and vegetables are white women 65 years of age and older who are college graduates, physically active, and nonsmokers. By and large, obese people have not been shown to observe the recommendations for fruit and vegetable intake *(2)*.

Observations of lower rates of CHD in Japan and the Mediterranean, where diets are similar to prudent and heart healthy diets, should encourage a change from our Western ways of eating *(37)*.

Less than adequate amounts of folate and vitamin B_6 in the diet may be unhealthy for the heart. Folate and vitamin B_6 are cofactors for metabolism of the amino acid homocysteine. Multiple studies have demonstrated a relationship between increased levels of serum homocysteine and increased risk of CVD in women *(38–41)*. Elevated levels of homocysteine are an established risk factor for CVD in men and have been found to be an independent risk factor for fatal and nonfatal MI in middle-aged women *(39)*. Potential mechanisms of action of homocysteine that may lead to increased risk of CHD include direct endothelial toxicity, decreased endothelial reactivity, stimulation of smooth muscle cell growth, and increased coagulation *(40)*.

SMOKING

Although cigarette smoking in adults has declined since the mid 1960s, approx 25% of American women smoke. Smoking independently raises the risk factor of sudden cardiac death in CHD. The vast majority of smokers start their addictive habit as teenagers; most are of a lower education and income level and most are white.

Smokers are two to four times more likely than nonsmokers to develop CHD. A dose relationship exists between smoking and MI risk; risk increases exponentially with the number of cigarettes smoked daily in women. It is important to note, however, that the risk of MI is increased even if only one to five cigarettes are smoked daily. Further, smokers are much more likely to develop other vascular diseases, such as stroke and peripheral vascular disease *(2)*. According to the Surgeon General, a woman who smokes dies approx 14.5 years earlier than a nonsmoking woman. Epidemiological data suggests that regardless of the length of smoking, an ex-smoker's risk of MI significantly declines with time *(42)*.

PHYSICAL INACTIVITY

Regular physical activity is associated with a reduced risk of high blood pressure, stroke, CAD, and type 2 diabetes. Sedentary behavior confers a risk of CHD equivalent to that of HTN, hyperlipidemia, and smoking. More than one-third of American adults are not physically active, and even more so in women. Higher education level and higher income are associated with increased leisure-time physical activity. Hispanic and black women seem to be least active, whereas white women are most active *(2)*. Exercise capacity has been found to be a stronger independent predictor of death in women compared with men *(43)*. In women, findings seem consistent regardless of ethnicity, age, or BMI. Even small amounts of exercise can be beneficial. It has been shown that walking at least 2.5 hours weekly reduces cardiovascular event risk significantly *(44)*. One study found that light-to-moderate activity had an association with lower CHD rates in women; this held true even in those at higher risk because of being overweight, having high cholesterol or using tobacco *(45)*. Another study showed that women who engaged in brisk walking for 1.5 hours weekly had a reduction in risk of coronary events that was as substantial as women who vigorously exercised for 45 minutes weekly. Sedentary women who become active show substantially lower rates of coronary events than women who remain sedentary *(46)*.

It is recommended that adults exercise for at least 30 minutes of moderate-intensity physical activity on most days of the week. Exercise that is more frequent may be needed for weight loss. In general, women older than 50 years old should consult with their physician before starting a physical activity program, particularly if the program is vigorous and the patient has known CVD or risk factors *(34)*.

ALCOHOL CONSUMPTION

Epidemiological data has shown a reduced CHD mortality in males that may be attributable to light-to-moderate alcohol intake. In the Nurses' Health Study, subjects without known CVD or cancer provided information regarding their alcohol intake and were followed for up to 12 years. Mortality results showed that light-to-moderate alcohol drinkers (1.5–29.9 g of alcohol daily) had an overall reduced mortality, mostly because of a lower risk of fatal CVD. A more than moderate intake of alcohol was associated with increased mortality *(47)*.

Patients with diabetes who participated in the Nurses' Health Study were examined further in terms of alcohol use and risk of CHD. An inverse association between alcohol consumption and CHD risk in these diabetic women was observed even after adjusting for multiple other CHD risk factors. The reduction in risk in fatal and nonfatal CHD events was observed in women who consumed 0.1 to 4.9 g/d and at least 5 g/d *(48)*.

In a study of women with known CAD, ingestion of wine (as opposed to spirits or beer) was found to be associated with increased heart rate variability; providing evidence that cardiac autonomic activity is affected by alcohol *(49)*. Effect on lipids likely also plays a role, specifically in increased levels of HDL. In a study of MI survivors compared with matched patients without CHD, an inverse relationship between alcohol consumption in the previous year and risk of MI was found. The reduced risk of MI seemed to be mediated by lipid values, particularly levels of whole HDL, and HDL-2 and HDL-3 subfractions. Other lipids, such as total cholesterol, LDL, and triglycerides, did not significantly alter the relationship between MI and alcohol consumption like HDL did *(50)*. An effect on coagulation may also play a role. A study in French men found that those who drank alcohol demonstrated a positive difference in platelet aggregation induced by thrombin adenosine disphosphate *(51)*.

Despite evidence of reduced CHD with alcohol intake, physicians must weigh the risks and benefits of making recommendations for alcohol consumption to their patients. Excessive alcohol use is associated with multiple physical, psychological, and social problems. Cancers (including breast cancer), stroke, gastrointestinal disorders, liver disease, HTN, accidents, and suicides all have associations with alcohol use. This makes some physicians understandably hesitant to recommend "medicinal" alcohol. Perhaps not all alcohol use should be discouraged, however, particularly in patients without addiction issues. Clearly, multiple factors must be considered in a woman's overall health plan, particularly with regard to alcohol use.

INFLAMMATORY MARKERS

There is growing belief that inflammation may contribute to the atherosclerotic process. Observational studies have looked at this possible relationship. This possible association opens the possibility of using plasma inflammatory markers to both identify people at increased risk for CVD and modify the inflammatory process to effect morbidity and mortality of CVD.

CRP is a marker of inflammation that may be independently associated with cardiovascular events in women *(52–54)*. CRP, however, is not necessarily specific to heart disease.

Another inflammatory marker, the cytokine, interleukin-6, increases levels of CRP as well as fibrinogen and platelets. Interleukin-6 has been associated with an increased risk of cardiovascular events and all-cause mortality in women *(52,53)*.

An elevated white blood cell (WBC) count is a known indicator of cellular response to an inflammatory process. The Women's Health Initiative (WHI) Observational Study followed baseline and 6-year WBC counts of more than 70,000 women aged 50 to 79 years without diagnosed CVD. After controlling for multiple CHD risk factors, a twofold elevated risk of CHD death was found in women with WBC counts in the upper quartile at baseline. Even when CRP was accounted for, the WBC count remained an independent predictor of CHD risk *(55)*. This possible relationship needs to be studied further before any conclusions can be made.

The idea of using inflammation markers to identify at-risk patients is exciting but one must remember that the vast majority of first MIs are attributable to the classic risk factors discussed *(56)*. Although it may be uncommon that inflammatory markers would be the only clues present to warn against the possible development of CVD, not all people who have cardiovascular events have traditional risk factors. Hopefully, further study of inflammation and CHD will help determine how to best use these biomarkers in patient care. Perhaps in the future, markers will be followed to assess changing risk of cardiac events during treatment or will be manipulated to actually promote CVD risk modification.

MENOPAUSE

Age and hormonal status are important risk factors for heart disease. Rates of CHD in postmenopausal women are two to three times higher than in women of the same age who have not undergone menopause *(2)*.

Starting in the 1980s, observational epidemiological studies suggested a favorable effect of postmenopausal estrogen replacement therapy in the reduction of all-cause mortality and cardiovascular mortality in women.

Focusing on heart disease, clinical trials to further study these observations included the Heart and Estrogen/Progestin Replacement Study (HERS) in the 1990s. HERS was a large secondary prevention study designed to evaluate the effect of estrogen and medroxyprogesterone acetate on the risk for CHD events in postmenopausal women with known CHD. After a follow-up of approx 4 years, results failed to show a difference between the HRT and placebo groups in the primary outcomes of nonfatal MI and CHD death. In the first year of the study, the reported incidence of these CHD events was higher in the HRT group. However, by the end of the study, the reported incidence was lower in the HRT group versus placebo *(57,58)*.

The NIH sponsored the WHI, a large study started in the 1990s that was designed to evaluate the effect of HRT on certain chronic disease endpoints in postmenopausal women aged 50 to 79 years (mean age, 63.3 ± 7.1 yr). One study arm received placebo or estrogen plus medroxyprogesterone acetate; another arm of hysterectomized women received placebo or estrogen alone.

After approx 5 years of follow-up, the estrogen and progestin arm was stopped early because the incidence of breast cancer exceeded preset stopping criteria and the global index, which took into account certain outcomes, did not support continuation. In regard to the end point of heart disease, final centrally adjudicated data showed an increased hazard ratio for CHD (nonfatal MI or CHD death) in the first year with a trend toward a lower risk with time *(59,60)*.

The WHI unopposed estrogen versus placebo trial was stopped early after almost 7 years of follow-up. In review of the data at that time, the hazard ratio showed that CHD (nonfatal MI or CHD death) was not increased in the subjects administered estrogen *(61)*.

Regarding hormone therapy and heart disease in postmenopausal women, current evidence-based recommendations are that HRT (estrogen alone or combined estrogen plus progestin) should not be initiated or continued for the prevention of CVD in postmenopausal women *(13)*.

DIAGNOSIS

Diagnosing cardiac ischemia and evaluating symptoms of cardiac disease may be more challenging in women than men. Women very often describe chest pain, one of the most common presenting symptoms of cardiac problems, atypically. The lack of a typical angina pectoris description may delay the correct diagnosis in a woman with unstable angina or an AMI *(27)*.

SYMPTOMS AT PRESENTATION

As stated, presenting symptoms of CHD may not be the same in women as in men. This has been demonstrated time and again in research and epidemiological studies. More often than men, women describe multiple symptoms, not just chest pain. They may complain of abdominal pain, dyspnea, nausea, and fatigue *(27)*. Men have been found to be significantly more likely to report diaphoresis, whereas women are significantly more likely to report back pain, jaw pain, neck pain, nausea, and shortness of breath in association with cardiac ischemia *(62)*.

In a retrospective study of mostly white women who had suffered an AMI, the majority of women experienced symptoms such as unusual fatigue, sleep disturbances, and shortness of breath intermittently for at least 1 month before their AMI *(63)*. At the time of their AMIs, the most common symptoms were shortness of breath, weakness, and unusual fatigue. Chest pain, the symptom most health care providers are trained to expect in association with the occurrence of an AMI, was reported in less than half of the women *(63)*.

A chart review of more than 300 patients older than age 35 years presenting to an emergency department (ED) with new-onset chest pain found that women were more likely to complain of chest pain that was pleuritic in nature. Another interesting finding was that women were significantly more likely to present to the ED later after onset of symptoms than men. This same review noted that although the men and women had similar risk factors, the men were more likely to receive a cardiology consultation, receive medication appropriate for cardiac chest pain, and be admitted to a unit capable of cardiac monitoring *(64)*. Another study has shown that women tend to wait longer after symptoms begin to go to the ED. This study also provided evidence that black women postpone going to the ED for evaluation even longer than white women *(65)*.

Presenting with "atypical" symptoms of cardiac chest pain, unless recognized by the women themselves or the health care professionals caring for them, may lead to a delay in appropriate or aggressive care or even result in misdiagnoses. The presence of underlying risk factors should always be sought to aid one in stratifying the risk of ischemic disease in a patient presenting with possible symptoms of cardiac ischemia.

These findings highlight the importance of patient education and health care provider education in interpretation of atypical signs and symptoms of acute coronary syndromes.

CARDIAC BIOMARKERS

In patients with acute coronary syndrome, cardiac biomarkers can be helpful in risk stratification and treatment decisions. The Treat Angina with Aggrastat and Determine Cost of Therapy with an Invasive or Conservative Strategy–Thrombolysis In Myocardial Infarction 18 study examined the sex differences in cardiac biomarkers in patients with acute coronary syndrome. Again, women's presentations differed from men. Broadly speaking, women were less likely to have elevated Creatine Kinase-MB or troponins (markers of myocyte destruction) and more likely to have elevated high-sensitivity CRP, a marker of inflammation, and brain natriuretic peptide, a peptide elevated in heart failure exacerbation. Other studies have found similar sex differences in the level of biomarkers present. Why this may occur is not clear; these findings do suggest that multiple cardiac biomarkers should be considered when women present with cardiac symptoms *(66)*.

NONINVASIVE CARDIAC TESTING

Stress tests are noninvasive methods of investigating the possible presence of CAD in patients at risk.

It is not clear that noninvasive exercise testing is as diagnostically accurate in women as in men. Many studies would suggest not and, therefore, the usefulness of noninvasive exercise tests in diagnosing women with CAD has been questioned. The methods and thresholds of ECG exercise stress testing were established, by and large, in men. In either sex, the test's sensitivity and specificity is not as accurate as other stress tests. However, meta-analyses have reflected better sensitivity and specificity in men than women. One possible reason for the lower diagnostic accuracy in women is the lower prevalence of CAD in women. However, in studies of men and women with similar CAD prevalence, tests on women still seem to be less accurate *(67)*. Other theories, such as estrogen effect, inappropriate catecholamine response, and the presence of breast tissue in women have been put forth *(68,69)*.

Maintaining the same stressor (exercise) but changing the imaging study to a nuclear medicine material, such as thallium, improves sensitivity compared with an ECG. However, breast attenuation of radioactivity may cause a study to be falsely interpreted as positive by the reviewer. Breast attenuation and the fact that women tend to have smaller left ventricular sizes, make exercise thallium stress tests more accurate in men than women *(27,67)*. Qualified and experienced physicians interpreting the images is very important to accuracy.

The use of technetium 99m Sestamibi, a higher energy agent than thallium, has been shown to lead to less breast attenuation in women and better accuracy in the detection of CAD *(2,67)*.

Exercise echocardiography is another stress-testing method with promising sensitive and specific results *(67)*. Sonographic imaging of the heart after exercising has the added benefit of allowing the imager to assess valvular function, chamber wall thickness, and ejection fraction. One caveat is that images will not be optimal in women with a large body habitus.

Electron beam computed tomography (EBCT), designed to detect calcified atherosclerotic coronary artery plaques, is a newer noninvasive test for CAD. Although it is not a time-honored screening tool and its usefulness has not been fully established, coronary calcium scores may help predict cardiac risk when used in conjunction with the Framingham Risk Score in intermediate risk asymptomatic patients *(70)*. This has not been thoroughly established, however, and calcium scores need to be calculated using references of the same sex and age. A low score may indicate a low probability of obstructive CAD but one must remember that uncalcified plaques cannot be assessed with this instrument.

The American College of Cardiology/American Heart Association's expert consensus panel on this topic found that EBCT has low specificity in diagnosing obstructive CAD and it has not been proven to be superior to alternative available noninvasive methods of diagnosing CAD. Furthermore, because of EBCT's prognostic uncertainties, the panel thinks it should not be made available to the public without a physician's request and that the role of EBCT in following progression or regression of CHD needs further study *(71)*.

INVASIVE CARDIAC TESTING

There are also sex differences regarding coronary angiography. In men and women who undergo cardiac catheterization for chest pain, not all have obstructive disease amenable to intervention. A coronary angiogram with no evidence of visible disease or non-obstructive atherosclerotic changes may lead to inappropriate reassurance for the patient and physician.

More than 10% of women presenting with acute coronary syndrome have normal or non-obstructive findings on catheterization; a greater incidence than found in men. It is estimated that 20% of women with "normal" findings do indeed have ischemic disease, possibly caused by atherosclerosis-related endothelial dysfunction, decreased reserve of coronary artery flow caused by microvascular dysfunction, or coronary spasm *(72,73)*.

These women are not without future risk of a cardiovascular event and, of course, worsening of coronary artery atherosclerosis. Patients with unstable angina and non-obstructive CAD have a 2% risk of death or MI at 30 days. Therapies to reduce future cardiac events have not been studied in these women. Current thinking is that treatment should be symptomatic (e.g., β-blocker for angina) and aimed at aggressive cardiac risk factor management *(72,73)*.

In general, approx 50% of women undergoing coronary angiography have no obstructive CAD found compared with 17% of men *(74)*. Because many women undergoing angiography have risk factors for CAD and persistent anginal pain, it is possible that the microvascular CAD referred to earlier is the culprit. Nuclear magnetic resonance spectroscopy cardiac stress testing is being studied in research trials to further explore the possibility of female-specific microvascular disease *(75)*.

In an Israeli study of 135 women 50 years of age or younger with chest pain referred for cardiac angiography, 58% were found to have angiographically significant CAD (≥50% narrowing of at least one coronary vessel). The group of women with significant CAD had a higher prevalence of known CAD (previous MI), high cholesterol, and postmenopausal status. In a subgroup of women who had previously undergone noninvasive testing, test results between the group having evidence of significant angiographic CAD and those who did not were not statistically different. In addition, the prevalence of typical and atypical chest pain in both groups of women did not differ significantly. In follow-up 4 to 5 years later, none of the women without CAD on angiogram had experienced an MI *(76)*.

MANAGEMENT

In the United States in 2002, there were almost 7 million cardiovascular operations or procedures performed, 4 million on men and 3 million on women. The number of cardiac catheterizations increased by 389% from 1979 to 2002 and more than 500,000 coronary artery bypass graft (CABG) surgeries were performed in 2002 *(2)*.

Some research has suggested that sex differences exist in the aggressiveness of CAD management, particularly in terms of invasive procedures *(77,78)*. Other research has not borne this out *(79)*.

Recent research suggests that when other variables are taken into account, women and men receive similar treatment after experiencing an acute MI. An Israeli study found that women received similar medications and had similar rates of thrombolysis, angiography, percutaneous transluminal coronary angioplasty and CABG surgery *(80)*. A study out of Canada found a similar lack of sex bias in access to CABG and percutaneous transluminal coronary angioplasty in women who had cardiac catheterizations *(81)*. Likewise, data review of 35 hospitals across the United States revealed that using accepted criteria for catheterization in the management of unstable angina, no sex differences existed in the rates of catheterizations.

Regarding coronary artery bypass surgery, fewer women who fit surgical criteria actually seem to have the surgery compared with men. Reasons such as socioeconomic issues and higher likelihood of procedure refusal have been postulated *(82)*.

MORTALITY AND PROGNOSIS

Epidemiological studies in women with AMI show higher short-term (during hospitalization) and long-term (2 year) mortality rates than men. A complete explanation for these findings does not exist. It is possible that these studies did not completely control for all risk factors. It is also possible that women are sicker than their male counterparts on presentation. There may be other, more difficultly measured, variables at play, such as psychosocial issues or socioeconomic issues *(83,84)*.

One study that suggests a difference in illness severity between the sexes at presentation is a Scottish epidemiological study of more than 200,000 male and female first MI survivors. In this study, female sex was associated with increased mortality in the short-term. The authors point to a possible selection bias. When AMI cases that did not survive to hospitalization were taken into account, women were actually less likely to die in the short-term than men. Men, they found, were less likely to survive to make it to hospitalization than women. Eliminating the men who did not survive to make it to the hospital resulted in a subset of men who were not as sick being compared with the entire cohort of women. Mortality at 1 year did not show a sex difference *(85)*. This long-term data is consistent with other longer-term mortality data.

The Third International Study of Infarct Survival in women and men hospitalized for AMI found that, at first look, women had significantly higher rates of cardiovascular complications and mortality than men at 35 days. However, when age was controlled, these higher rates decreased significantly. When other baseline differences between the men and women were controlled, the rates of morbidity and mortality became even more similar although a residual slightly increased morbidity and mortality for the women in the study remained. According to the authors, differences in inpatient management between men and women were too small to be relevant to differences in morbidity and mortality *(86)*.

Another study of long-term mortality showed that women at least 65 years of age who were followed after hospitalization for unstable angina had a lower risk of death than men at 5 years. This survival advantage did not hold true for women after AMI, particularly in those younger than 65 years of age *(87)*.

The existence of true long- and short-term mortality sex differences is not entirely certain, but it reinforces the importance of providing standard of care treatment to any patient with a cardiac presentation.

LOOKING TOWARD THE FUTURE

According to the US Census, there will be 40 million Americans at least 65 years old in 2010 *(2)*. Because the risk of CVD increases with age, it is of utmost importance from a public health standpoint to continue to improve efforts to prevent and treat CVD.

One way of improving control of the issue is by educating clinicians to recognize that men and women with heart disease may differ in presentation, response to treatment, and prognosis and to aggressively treat risk factors in women. Clinicians should be persistent in educating their female patients regarding heart disease prevalence and risk factors. Emerging risk factors, such as inflammatory markers and calcium scores, are of interest and may grow in usefulness as research continues, but focus should remain on identifying and modifying established and traditional risk factors, such as diabetes, hyperlipidemia, HTN, and smoking. Current data do not support the widely held view in the medical community that greater than 50% of patients with CHD lack conventional risk factors *(88–90)*.

Of equal importance to clinician awareness is getting women themselves to understand the importance of risk factor modification to prevent cardiac events and making them aware that CVD is a more likely culprit in the demise of their health than they probably perceive.

Public awareness of CVD is still not satisfactorily pervasive. In 1997, the American Heart Association initiated a national campaign to improve awareness of CVD risk among women. A follow-up survey in 2003 showed improvement in awareness of CHD as the leading killer in women (46% of women knew this as opposed to 30% in 1997). Likewise, the number of women who thought cancer was the leading killer of women decreased. On a more personal level, however, only 13% of women surveyed (from 7% in 1997) perceived heart disease as their greatest personal health threat. The perception that cancer, particularly breast cancer, is the most common life-threatening health problem for women still exists to a great extent. Older white women demonstrated the highest levels of CVD awareness even though DHHS data tells us that black women have the highest heart disease death rate in this country. Less than 40% of the women surveyed reported that their physicians had ever discussed heart disease with them. It seems that the media is a more likely source of information regarding heart disease than the doctor's office *(91)*. One opportunity for clinicians to begin discussing heart disease is during office visits for gynecological care, pre-pregnancy care and prenatal care. It is important for the medical system to promote opportunities to discuss these issues with women. Governmental policies and programs can certainly contribute to efforts aimed at reducing CVD morbidity and mortality. Provision of grants to support research on CVD prevention and treatment, ensuring healthcare access to all women, and development of programs to promote disease awareness and encourage healthier lifestyles are all ways to help accomplish the goal.

Many programs have been established with state and federal assistance. One example is the WISEWOMAN program. Established by the federal government, the program promotes CVD education, prevention, and treatment in women. The program targets middle-aged and poor minority women. Activities include screening, follow-up treatment, and establishment of community support for lifestyle changes. Results in terms of reducing cholesterol and blood pressure and decreasing smoking rates are promising *(92)*.

REFERENCES

1. Bonita R, Wilson E, Fodor G, et al. The First International Conference on Women, Heart Disease and Stroke: Science and Policy in Action. Victoria, British Columbia, Canada, May 7–10, 2000. (Accessed March 17, 2005, at http://www.medscape.com/viewprogram/897_pnt.)
2. American Heart Association. Heart Disease and Stroke Statistics–2005 Update. American Heart Association, Dallas, 2005.
3. Wenger NK, You've come a long way, baby–cardiovascular health and disease in women–problems and prospects. Circulation 2004;109:558–560.
4. Thomas JL, Braus PA. Coronary artery disease in women–a historical perspective. Arch Intern Med 1998;158:333–337.
5. Winkleby MA, Kraemer HC, Ahn DK, Varady AN. Ethnic and socioeconomic differences in CVD risk factors–findings for women from the third national health and nutrition examination survey, 1988-1994. JAMA 1998;280:356–362.
6. Casper ML, Barnett E, Halverson JA, et al. Women and Heart Disease: An Atlas of Racial and Ethnic Disparities in Mortality, 2nd ed. Office for Social Environment and Health Research, West Virginia University, Morgantown, WV, 2000.
7. Sorlie PD, Rogot E, Johnson NJ. Validity of demographic characteristics on the death certificate. Epidemiology 1992;3:181–184.
8. Williams DR, Collins C. U.S. socioeconomic and racial differences in health: patterns and explanations. Annu Rev Sociol 1995;21:349–386.
9. D'Agostino RB, Grundy S, Sullivan LM, Wilson P. Validation of the Framingham coronary heart disease predictions scores: results of a multiple ethnic groups investigation. JAMA 2001;286(2):180–187.
10. National Cholesterol Education Program. Third Report of the expert panel on detection, evaluation, and treatment of high blood cholesterol in adults (Adult Treatment Panel III). NIH Pub. No. 02-5215. National Heart, Lung, and Blood Institute, Bethesda, MD, 2002.
11. American Diabetes Association. Position paper: diagnosis and classification of diabetes mellitus. Diabetes Care 2005;28:S37–S42.
12. Blake GJ, Pradhan AD, Manson JE, et al. Hemoglobin A1C level and future cardiovascular events among women. Arch Intern Med 2004;164:757–761.
13. Mosca L, Appel LJ, Benjamin EJ, et al. Evidence-based guidelines for cardiovascular disease prevention in women. Circulation 2004;109:672–693.
14. Calles-Escandon J, Garcia-Rubi E, Mirza S, Mortensen A. Type 2 diabetes: one disease, multiple cardiovascular risk factors. Coron Artery Dis 1999;10:23–30.
15. Barrett-Connor E, Giardina EG, Gitt AK, Gudat U, Steinberg HO, Tschoepe D. Women and heart disease: the role of diabetes and hyperglycemia. Arch Intern Med 2004;164: 934–942.
16. Kanaya AM, Grady D, Barrett-Connor E. Explaining the sex difference in coronary heart disease mortality among patients with type 2 diabetes mellitus. Arch Intern Med 2002;162: 1737–1745.
17. Sowers JR. Diabetes mellitus and cardiovascular disease in women. Arch Intern Med 1998;158:617–621.

18. U.S. Preventive Services Task Force. Screening for diabetes mellitus, adult type 2. Release date: February 2003 (Accessed May 2, 2005, at http://www.ahrq.gov/clinic/uspstf/usps-diab.htm.).
19. American Diabetes Association. Standards of medical care in diabetes. Diabetes Care 2005;28(1):S4–S36.
20. Ninomiya JK, L'Italien G, Criqui MH, Whyte JL, Gamst A, Chen RS. Association of the metabolic syndrome with history of myocardial infarction and stroke in the third national health and nutrition examination survey. Circulation 2004;109:42–46.
21. Kip KE, Marroquin OC, Kelley DE, et al. Clinical importance of obesity versus the metabolic syndrome in cardiovascular risk in women: a report from the women's ischemia syndrome evaluation (WISE) study. Circulation 2004;109:706–713.
22. Marroquin OC, Kip KE, Kelley DE, et al. Metabolic syndrome modifies the cardiovascular risk associated with angiographic coronary artery disease in women: a report from the women's ischemia syndrome evaluation. Circulation 2004;109:714–721.
23. Chobanian AV, Bakris GL, Black HR, et al. for the National High Blood Pressure Education Program Coordinating Committee. The Seventh Report of the Joint National Committee on prevention, detection, evaluation, and treatment of high blood pressure. JAMA 2003;289: 2560–2572.
24. Burt VL, Whelton P, Roccella EJ, et al. Prevalence of hypertension in the US adult population: results from the third national health and nutrition examination survey, 1988-1991. Hypertension 1995;25:305–313.
25. Gillum RF. Epidemiology of hypertension in African American women. Am Heart J 1996;131:385–395.
26. Furberg CD, Wright JT, Davis BR, et al. Major outcomes in high-risk hypertensive patients randomized to angiotensin-converting enzyme inhibitor or calcium channel blocker vs diuretic: the antihypertensive and lipid-lowering treatment to prevent heart attack trial (ALLHAT). JAMA 2002;288:2981–2997.
27. Mosca L, Manson JE, Sutherland SE, Langer RD, Manolio T, Barrett-Connor E. Cardiovascular disease in women: a statement for healthcare professionals from the American Heart Association. Circulation 1997;96:2468–2482.
28. Grant AO, Jacobs AK, Clancy C. Cardiovascular disease in women–are there solutions? Circulation 2004;109:561.
29. Walsh JM, Pignone M. Drug treatment of hyperlipidemia in women. JAMA 2004;291: 2243–2252.
30. Grundy SM, Cleeman JI, Merz NB, et al. Implications of recent clinical trials for the National Cholesterol Education Program Adult Treatment Panel III guidelines. Circulation 2004;110(6):763.
31. Heart Protection Study Collaborative Group. MRC/BHF Heart protection study of cholesterol lowering with simvastatin in 20,536 high-risk individuals: a randomised placebo-controlled trial. Lancet 2002;360:7–22.
32. Amsterdam EA. At the intersection of cardiology and primary care. Patient Care 2005;46–57.
33. Orth-Gomer K, Mittleman MA, Schenck-Gustafsson K, Wamala SP, Eriksson M, Belkic K. Lipoprotein(a) as a determinant of coronary heart disease in young women. Circulation 1997;95:329–334.
34. 2005 Dietary Guidelines Advisory Committee Report. Dietary Guidelines for Americans 2005: U.S. Department of Health and Human Services, U.S. Department of Agriculture (last accessed May 2, 2005, at http://www.health.gov/dietaryguidelines).
35. Stampfer MJ, Hu FB, Manson JE, Rimm EB, Willett WC. Primary prevention of coronary heart disease in women through diet and lifestyle. N Engl J Med 2000;343:16–22.

36. Fung TT, Willett WC, Stampfer MJ, Manson JE, Hu FB. Dietary patterns and the risk of coronary heart disease in women. Arch Intern Med 2001;161:1857–1862.
37. Iso H, Stampfer MJ, Manson JE, et al. Prospective study of fat and protein intake and risk of intraparenchymal hemorrhage in women. Circulation 2001;103:856–863.
38. Ridker PM, Manson JE, Buring JE, Shih J, Matias M, Hennekens CH. Homocysteine and risk of cardiovascular disease among postmenopausal women. JAMA 1999;281:1817–1821.
39. Zilberstein DE, Bengtsson C, Björkelung C, et al. Serum homocysteine in relation to mortality and morbidity from coronary heart disease: a 24-year follow-up of the population study of women in Gothenburg. Circulation 2004;109:601–606.
40. Rimm EB, Willett WC, Hu FB, et al. Folate and Vitamin B6 from diet and supplements in relation to risk of coronary heart disease among women. JAMA 1998;279:359–364.
41. Knekt P, Alfthan G, Aromaa A, et al. Homocysteine and major coronary events: a prospective population study amongst women. J Int Med 2001;249:461–465.
42. Rosenberg L, Palmer JR, Shapiro S. Decline in the risk of myocardial infarction among women who stop smoking. N Engl J Med 1990;322:213–217.
43. Gulati M, Pandey DK, Arnsdorf MF, et al. Exercise capacity and the risk of death in women: the St. James women take heart project. Circulation 2003;108:1554–1559.
44. Manson JE, Greenland P, LaCroix AZ, et al. Walking compared with vigorous exercise for the prevention of cardiovascular events in women. N Engl J Med 2002;347:716–725.
45. Lee IM, Rexrode KM, Cook NR, Manson JE, Buring JE. Physical activity and coronary heart disease in women: is "no pain, no gain" passé? JAMA 2001;285:1447–1454.
46. Manson JE, Hu FB, Rich-Edwards JW, et al. A prospective study of walking as compared with vigorous exercise in the prevention of coronary heart disease in women. N Engl J Med 1999;341:650–658.
47. Fuchs CS, Stampfer MJ, Colditz GA, et al. Alcohol consumption and mortality among women. N Engl J Med 1995;332:1245–1250.
48. Solomon CG, Hu FB, Stampfer MJ, et al. Moderate alcohol consumption and risk of coronary heart disease among women with type 2 diabetes mellitus. Circulation 2000;102: 494–499.
49. Janszky I, Ericson M, Blom M, et al. Wine drinking is associated with increased heart rate variability in women with coronary heart disease. Heart 2005;91:314–318.
50. Gaziano JM, Buring JE, Breslow JL, et al. Moderate alcohol intake, increased levels of high-density lipoprotein and its subfractions, and decreased risk of myocardial infarction. N Engl J Med 1993;329:1829–1834.
51. Renaud SC, Beswick AD, Fehily AM, Sharp DS, Elwood PC. Alcohol and platelet aggregation: the Caerphilly prospective heart disease study. Am J Clin Nut 1992;55:1012–1017.
52. Ridker PM, Hennekens CH, Buring JE, Rifai N. C-reactive protein and other markers of inflammation in the prediction of cardiovascular disease in women. N Engl J Med 2000;342: 836–843.
53. Davison S, Davis SR. New markers for cardiovascular disease risk in women: impact of endogenous estrogen status and exogenous postmenopausal hormone therapy. J Clin Endo Metab 2003;88:2470–2478.
54. Rifai N, Buring JE, Lee IM, Manson JE, Ridker PM. Is C-reactive protein specific for vascular disease in women? Ann Intern Med 2002;136:529–533.
55. Margolis KL, Manson JE, Greenland P, et al. Leukocyte count as a predictor of cardiovascular events and mortality in postmenopausal women: the women's health initiative observational study. Arch Intern Med 2005;165:500–508.
56. Yusuf S, Hawken S, Ounpuu S, et al. Effect of potentially modifiable risk factors associated with myocardial infarction in 52 countries (the INTERHEART study): case-control study. Lancet 2004;364:937–952.

57. Barrett-Connor E. An epidemiologist looks at hormones and heart disease in women. J Clin Endo Metab 2003;88:4031–4042.
58. Hulley S, Grady D, Bush T, et al. Randomized trial of estrogen plus progestin for secondary prevention of coronary heart disease in postmenopausal women. JAMA 1998;280:605–613.
59. Manson JE, Hsia J, Johnson KC, et al. Estrogen plus progestin and the risk of coronary heart disease. N Engl J Med 2003;349:523–534.
60. Rossouw JE, Anderson GL, Prentice RL, et al. Risks and benefits of estrogen plus progestin in healthy postmenopausal women: principal results from the Women's Health Initiative randomized controlled trial. JAMA 2002;288:321–333.
61. Anderson GL, Limacher M, Assaf AR, et al. Effects of conjugated equine estrogen in post-menopausal women with hysterectomy: the Women's Health Initiative randomized controlled trial. JAMA 2004;291:1701–1712.
62. Goldberg RJ, O'Donnell C, Yarzebski J, Bigelow C, Savageau J, Gore JM. Sex differences in symptom presentation associated with acute myocardial infarction: a population-based perspective. Am Heart J 1998;136:189–195.
63. McSweeney JC, Cody M, O'Sullivan P, Elberson K, Moser DK, Garvin BJ. Women's early warning symptoms of acute myocardial infarction. Circulation 2003;108:2619–2623.
64. Lehmann JB, Wehner PS, Lehmann CU, Savory LM. Gender bias in the evaluation of chest pain in the emergency department. Amer J Card 1996;77:641–644.
65. Massey CV, Hupp CH, Kreisberg MS, Burpo SS, Hoff CJ, Alpert MA. Race affects time to presentation, but not diagnostic evaluation of women with suspected coronary artery disease. JACC (Abstract). February 1995;982–117:267A–268A.
66. Wiviott SD, Cannon CP, Morrow DA, et al. Differential expression of cardiac biomarkers by gender in patients with unstable angina/non-ST-elevation myocardial infarction. Circulation 2004;109:580–586.
67. Kwok Y, Kim C, Grady D. Segal M, Redberg R. Meta-analysis of exercise testing to detect coronary artery disease in women. Am J Cardiol 1999;83:660–666.
68. Marwick TH, Anderson T, Williams MJ, et al. Exercise echocardiography is an accurate and cost-efficient technique for detection of coronary artery disease in women. J Am Coll Card 1995;26:335–341.
69. Sketch MH, Mohiuddin SM, Lynch JD, Zencka AE, Runco V. Significant sex differences in the correlation of electrocardiographic exercise testing and coronary arteriograms. Am J Card 1975;36:169–173.
70. Greenland P, LaBree L, Azen SP, Doherty TM, Detrano RC. Coronary artery calcium score combined with Framingham score for risk prediction in asymptomatic individuals. JAMA 2004;291:210–215.
71. O'Rourke RA, Brundage BH, Froelicher VF, et al. American College of Cardiology/American Heart Association expert consensus document on electron-beam computed tomography for the diagnosis and prognosis of coronary artery disease. J Am Coll Cardiol 2000;36:326–340.
72. Bugiardini R, Merz CN. Angina with "normal" coronary arteries: a changing philosophy. JAMA 2005;293:477–484.
73. Reis SE, Holubkov R, Conrad-Smith AJ, et al. Coronary microvascular dysfunction is highly prevalent in women with chest pain in the absence of coronary artery disease: results from the NHLBI WISE study. Am Heart J 2001;141:735–741.
74. Shaw LJ, Gibbons RJ, McCallister B, et al. Gender differences in extent and severity of coronary disease in the ACC-National Cardiovascular Data Registry (abstract). J Am Coll Cardiol 2002;39:321A.
75. Johnson BD, Shaw LJ, Buchthal SD, et al. Prognosis in women with myocardial ischemia in the absence of obstructive coronary disease. Circulation 2004;109:2993–2999.

76. Gurevitz O, Jonas M, Boyko V, Rabinowitz B, Reicher-Reiss H. Clinical profile and long-term prognosis of women <50 years of age referred for coronary angiography for evaluation of chest pain. Am J Cardiol 2000;85:806–809.
77. Steingart RM, Packer M, Hamm P, et al. Sex differences in the management of coronary artery disease. N Engl J Med 1991;325:226–230.
78. Shaw LJ, Miller DD, Romeis JC, Kargl D, Younis LT, Chaitman BR. Gender differences in the noninvasive evaluation and management of patients with suspected coronary artery disease. Ann Int Med 1994;120:559–566.
79. Hachamovitch R, Berman DS, Kiat H, et al. Gender-related differences in clinical management after exercise nuclear testing. J Am Coll Cardiol 1995;26:1457–1464.
80. Gottlieb S, Harpaz D, Shotan A, et al. Sex differences in management and outcome after acute myocardial infarction in the 1990s: a prospective observational community-based study. Circulation 2000;102:2484–2490.
81. Ghali WA, Faris PD, Galbraith PD, et al. Sex differences in access to coronary revascularization after cardiac catheterization: importance of detailed clinical data. Ann Intern Med 2002;136:723–732.
82. Scirica BM, Moliterno DJ, Every NR, et al. Differences between men and women in the management of unstable angina pectoris (the GUARANTEE registry), Am J Cardiol 1999;84:1145–1150.
83. Vaccarino V, Parsons L, Every NR, et al. Sex-based differences in early mortality after myocardial infarction. N Engl J Med 1999;341:217–225.
84. Vaccarino V, Horwitz RI, Meehan TP, Petrillo MK, Radford MJ, Krumholz HM. Sex differences in mortality after myocardial infarction: evidence for a sex-age interaction. Arch Intern Med 1998;158:2054–2062.
85. MacIntyre K, Stewart S, Capewell S, et al. Gender and survival: a population-based study of 201,114 men and women following a first acute myocardial infarction. J Am Coll Cardiol 2001;38:729–735.
86. Malacrida R, Genoni M, Maggioni AP, et al. A comparison of the early outcome of acute myocardial infarction in women and men. N Engl J Med 1998;338:8–14.
87. Chang WC, Kaul P, Westerhout CM, et al. Impact of sex on long-term mortality from acute myocardial infarction vs unstable angina. Arch Int Med 2003;163:2476–2484.
88. Greenland P, Knoll MD, Stamler J, et al. Major risk factors as antecedents of fatal and nonfatal coronary heart disease events. JAMA 2003;290:891–897.
89. Khot UN, Khot MB. Prevalence of conventional risk factors in patients with coronary heart disease. JAMA 2003;290:898–904.
90. Canto JG, Iskandrian AE. Major risk factors for cardiovascular disease–debunking the "only 50%" myth. JAMA 2003;290:947–949.
91. Mosca L, Ferris A, Fabunmi R, Robertson RM. Tracking women's awareness of heart disease: an American Heart Association national study. Circulation 2004;109:573–579.
92. National Women's Law Center, University of Pennsylvania School of Medicine, Oregon Health & Science University. Making the grade on women's health: a national and state-by-state report card. 2001. (Available at http://www.nwlc.org/pdf/2001ReportCardChapter4.pdf).

6 Sexual Problems

Leonore Tiefer, PhD

Contents

INTRODUCTION: WHAT DOES A PRIMARY CARE PHYSICIAN NEED TO KNOW ABOUT SEXUAL PROBLEMS OF WOMEN?

Expectations and standards for women's sexual lives are a matter of wide cultural variation and continual historical change *(1–3)*. At the beginning of the 21st century, cultural and social shifts that affect women's sexuality are being brought about by globalization, women's liberation, commercialization, medicalization, and new media technologies. In the midst of all this, general and specialist physicians are called on to play an active role in dealing with sexual problems.

For example, a course for primary care physicians recently (May, 2005) posted on the website of the Canadian Society for Obstetrics and Gynecology

From: *Current Clinical Practice: Women's Health in Clinical Practice*
Edited by: Clouse and Sherif © Humana Press Inc., Totowa, NJ

(4) urged physicians to bring up sexual questions and routinely take a sexual history, insisting that this would benefit both patient and physician. This advice is now heard routinely in medical meetings: "Don't wait for the patient to raise the subject! Always include a sexual history!"

But the field of sexual medicine itself is new, language and classification schemes for sexual problems continue to change, sexual problems and satisfactions are often idiosyncratic and subjective, medical education on sexuality is still usually limited to pathophysiology, sexuality interviewing skills are not well developed, and there is a very real danger that overenthusiasm by the unspecialized physician can add to a patient's problems.

For example, several questions in the pretest for the course on the website of the Canadian Society for Obstetrics and Gynecology course mentioned above imply, incorrectly, that there is reliable prevalence data regarding sexual problems and dysfunctions. The first question asks, "Which of the following is true? (a) Rates of sexual dysfunction are higher among men than women. (b) Rates of sexual dysfunction are higher among women than men. (c) Men and women have about equal rates of sexual dysfunction." The correct answer is given as (a), although no reference is offered. Any one reference, in fact, would be easy to challenge because of the lack of consensus regarding definition and measurement issues *(5)*.

Vague prevalence statistics are just one example of a complex picture. When physicians talk with their patients regarding sexual problems and solutions, they are "no longer talking exclusively about scientific facts, but unavoidably enter the world of value judgments" *(6)*. What sexual activities and desires are normal? What sexual frequencies are normal? How important is orgasm? How are age-related sexual changes experienced and adapted to? No scientific or medical research can determine what should be considered normal or important in terms of sexual experience.

Thus, a chapter on sexuality for primary care physicians begins not with "Epidemiology" or "Differential Diagnosis" or other classic ways of discussing a medical topic, but with an exhortation to caution, skepticism, and complexity.

In the past 5 years, new biomedical approaches to the definition and management of women's sexual problems have emerged and many more are in development *(7)*. Some experts view this as a great advance in women's health, whereas others see it as a worrisome example of "corporate-sponsored" incursion into medical classifications and treatments *(5)*. As of 2005, aggressive promotion of testosterone in industry-sponsored continuing medical education courses along with public relations-fueled media coverage of clinical trials on every new drug has resulted in the worrisome widespread use of inadequately tested, off-label medical treatments for women's sexual problems *(7)*. In addition, huge marketing budgets have been assigned to push over-the-counter products, such as "botanical massage oils" that promise "to alleviate sexual difficulties due to menopause or SSRI use" *(8)*. Physicians are misinformed by industry-appointed "opinion leaders" regarding the ineffectiveness for sexual problems of sex therapy, bibliotherapy, sex education, couple counseling, masturbatory training, and a whole host of nonmedical interventions. The situation calls for caution and skepticism.

THE "NORMAL" TRAP

Part of the medicalization strategy is to shift expectations regarding what constitutes normal sexual experience. I find that most patients use the word "normal" at some point in almost every consultation, as in, "Isn't it *normal* to be interested in sex more than once a month?" Or, "Isn't it *normal* to have orgasms?" Or "Is it *normal* to want to have sex when you have a new baby?" Or "Is it *normal* to watch porn on the internet every night?" I try to avoid the role of expert on sexual normality. Patients are looking as much for validation as for information, and to take a position on what is normal is mistakenly to offer overly simple answers to a couple's struggle.

It is best to find a way to discuss the source and meaning of patients' beliefs regarding what is sexually normal. A sexuality expert knows about the biopsychosocial components of sexual experience, including how people acquire and experience sexual norms. One way I do this is by expanding the discussion (e.g., if the patient dwells on hormones, I try to get around to asking something about her sex education; if the patient dwells on her partner's flaws, I try to get around to asking something about her feelings about her body, and so on).

A feminist perspective on sexual norms is grounded in diversity and acknowledges the sexual dynamics of age, class, and race values and oppressions. It is not enough to ask what *is* the patient's sexual problem, one needs to ask *why* it is a problem and how the patient learned that such a situation *would be considered* a problem. I learn more from such questions than from following up the "what is the problem" question with "how long have you had it and when did it start," as if I agreed with the patient that what she was describing was a medical condition. Ironically, such contextual and values-oriented lines of questioning have been attacked as accusing the patient that her problem is "all in her head." Recently, in an overview in *Science* of the new sex drugs for women and their controversies, urologist and drug-industry consultant Irwin Goldstein said, referring to critics of drug pushing, "They talk about medicalization. I call what they do psycholization" (ref. *7*; page 1579).

A large part of dealing with sexual problems, as I see it, is *psycho-education* to help patients develop the ability to reflect broadly on their experiences, expectations, and complaints and to develop the ability to think creatively about solutions. Needless to say, this takes time. I am not a car mechanic fixing a tie rod. An initial consultation of an hour is sometimes adequate to begin this process, but often it is not. Seeing both members of a sexual couple is essential, and the first therapeutic task is often to persuade a patient who initially comes alone to bring her partner next time and to help her devise ways to do this. This will often be a watershed moment in the couple's relationship, and it is not to be ignored.

PITFALLS OF MEDICAL MODEL THINKING

Many women want a better sex life and look for help with their sexual problems. But what, exactly, do they want help with, and what, exactly, can medical personnel offer? The prevailing medical model of sex, with its official classification nomenclature published in texts such as the *Diagnostic & Statistical Manual of Mental Disorders (DSM)* and *International Classification of Disease, 10th edition (ICD-10)*, directs professionals to a diagnostic approach that assumes a universal physical sexual response with desire, arousal, and orgasm as part of discrete sexual encounters *(9)*. All sexual complaints are assumed to fall into desire/arousal/orgasm/pain categories. The media's dissemination of this perspective is teaching people to think about and describe their sexual dissatisfactions as individual, biological, and about dysfunction, as opposed to interpersonal, complex, and about enjoyment.

In the medical model, sexual function is based on an idealized script of regular and mutually desired sexual relations requiring erection, vaginal lubrication, and mutual orgasm. The assumption that "sexual function" is coital experience where all necessary mental and physical equipment for satisfaction is inborn and functions "normally" unless impeded is the lynchpin in the contemporary medicalization of sexual life *(10)*. This reductionistic medical model contrasts with a culture- and learning-centered model, wherein the physical equipment for all human activities exists in everyone (e.g., for playing a musical instrument, participating in sports, or making love), but the activities may never be desired, and even if they are, they still require culture-based learning to shape appropriate scripts and goals. Moreover, as with other activities, sexual performance that fulfills high expectations requires training, practice, and patience, although people rarely think of sexuality that way.

I suggest that people first read a little about sex on the internet or in a bookstore before going to a doctor if they have a sexual problem. There is much misinformation on the internet and in popular books, of course, but such resources offer new vocabulary, ideas, and values clarification that can protect against too much expert-driven biomedical language, medical tests, and magical pills.

There are several clues that medical model thinking regarding women's sexual problems is not a good fit. One is the difficulty in making a discrete diagnosis. Somewhere in every article regarding "female sexual dysfunction" is an acknowledgement regarding the well-documented "comorbidity of arousal and desire disorders" (ref. *11*; page 858) It's often impossible to assess discrete elements of sexual function *(12)*. Yet medical nomenclature insists that these are separate phenomena. Another clue comes from clinical trials for "female sexual dysfunction." A panel of international experts recently suggested that because "Female subjective sexual experience is mediated to a certain extent by *expectations which are the product of prevailing societal values, familial values and partner expectations*... the definition of what constitutes a disorder may vary from one cultural subgroup to another" (ref. *13*; page 637, emphasis added). This acknowledgment of cultural variability and the priority of *meaning* in sexual experience can easily be forgotten when it comes to diagnosis and treatment within the medical model.

A 1999 *JAMA* paper on sexual dysfunction prevalence (in 18–59 year olds) indicated that approximately as many women reported that sex was not pleasurable as indicated inability to orgasm or lack of interest in sex (ref. *14*; Table 1, page 538). Are the women not experiencing pleasure *because* of desire and orgasm difficulties? Studies show that women complain more often about "contextual" factors, such as timing, technique, and tenderness, than about function *(12)*. Yet, because there are no legal drugs to prescribe for pleasure or maybe because the medical model keeps the focus on apparently objective and measurable "function," physicians rarely explore what aspects of sexual relations generate or block pleasure.

WHAT MAKES A CHAPTER ON SEXUAL PROBLEMS FEMINIST?

A feminist perspective puts women's point of view at the center of any analysis. This becomes a challenge when we see how the long history of gender, religious, and cultural oppression has constructed women's sexuality as instrumental to reproduction and secondary to men's pleasure and power *(15)*. If we do not know what women *want*, it is difficult to identify from women's point of view what constitute sexual *problems*. We cannot assume that what women want is represented in such texts as the *DSM* or the *ICD-10*.

In my clinical practice, of the four motives for noncoerced sexual activity, including procreation, physical pleasure, emotional intimacy, and to provide a service, it is the last motive, often disguised and difficult to admit, that is frequently involved in lack of sexual interest.

CASE EXAMPLE

Recently, I saw in consultation a 33-year-old unmarried woman who had lost sexual desire for her beloved boyfriend of 9 months. After an hour, we had discovered that the likely primary cause was her desperate wish to please the man so he would propose marriage, a goal she had obsessed about since mid-adolescence, and regarding which she was becoming increasingly panicky. Consequently, she was quite cut off from her own interests in sexual pleasure, and was using sex instrumentally. It sounds simple, but this college-educated, much-traveled, high-earning woman had, until seeing me, been convinced she had abnormal hormones because she was young, healthy, and "should" be interested in sex. The hardest part of the consultation was persuading her to tell me some things about herself and her relationship instead of obsessing about her biology. Such topics had not been discussed at all in her medical appointments, and it was only after several of those that a gynecologist referred her to me.

A feminist perspective that links behavior to social context acknowledges the pressure of social trends linking sexual response to social success and youthful image. As always, women want to look, feel, and perform sexually to fulfill social norms *(16)*. The norms are changing, however, as already indicated, and current norms are pressuring women to have coital orgasms and lifelong high sexual interest. In this environment, and coached by the media, women often come to physicians with their complaints. Is the health care provider's job, hearing a sexual complaint, to assess for medical conditions and, finding none, to refer patients to other resources? This might seem the sensible choice, but "assessing for medical conditions that might cause or contribute to sexual difficulties" is becoming a growth industry, entails no clear algorithm, involves a wide variety of genital tests without accepted norms (testosterone levels, vaginal balloon compliance, clitoral sensitivity, and so on), often results in ambiguous outcomes that fail to lay physical questions to rest, and are largely nonreimbursable. The decision to exclude physical factors may backfire and result in the patient becoming focused on physical issues, rather than turning to other resources, such as sexuality education or psychological counseling. The physician hearing a sexual complaint faces an important intellectual and political challenge.

AN ALTERNATIVE NONMEDICAL MODEL CLASSIFICATION SYSTEM FOR SEXUAL PROBLEMS

In 2000, a group of feminist clinicians and social scientists drafted an alternative classification system called "The New View of Women's Sexual Problems" *(17,18)*. It differs from the *DSM* and *ICD-10* model in two important ways. First, it defines sexual problems as "discontent or dissatisfaction with any emotional, physical, or relational aspect of sexual experience." There is no list of sexual problems, because a problem is defined as *anything* that is unsatisfactory. Bypassing the medical model acknowledges that we do *not* have valid scientific or health norms for sexual function, and allows us to avoid splitting hairs over whether problems with desire and arousal are "really" different conditions. It neither pathologizes those without certain features of the official sexual response cycle nor omits those whose problem is more individual or interpersonal.

Second, the "New View" proposes a detailed classification system of etiologies for all sexual problems, organized into four major categories to guide history taking and solution hunting:

1. Sexual problems caused by sociocultural, political, or economic factors.
2. Sexual problems relating to partner and relationship.
3. Sexual problems caused by psychological factors.
4. Sexual problems caused by medical factors.

Clinical use of the "New View" classification system is growing and has been elaborated in a number of recent presentations, and ongoing projects include extending it to include men's sexual problems as well as women's.

CONCLUSION: HELPING WOMEN NAVIGATE SEXUAL LIFE AND SEXUAL PROBLEMS

In response to the success of the "New View" and in response to continuing difficulties in matching women's experiences with the present conceptual models, there have been recent efforts to create an "evidence-based" conceptualization that includes both the medical "human sexual response cycle" model favored by the *DSM* and a consideration of "contextual features" *(19)*. This approach fails, it seems to me, because it attempts to reconcile fundamentally incompatible elements—a classification that rests on a definition of "normal" function and a perspective that embrace subjectivity in sexual expectations and scripts. The next few years will continue to see the feminist and medical models on women's sexual problems challenge each other. As long as the pharmaceutical industry continues to dominate medical education and training, though, most doctors will never even hear about the debate.

REFERENCES

1. Weeks J. Sexuality and its Discontents: Meaning, Myths and Modern Sexualities. Routledge & Kegan Paul, London, 1985.
2. Amaro H, Navarro AM, Conron KJ, Raj A. Cultural Influences on women's sexual health. In: Handbook of Women's Sexual and Reproductive Health (Wingood GM, DiClemente RJ, eds.). Kluwer Academic/Plenum Publishers, New York, 2002; pp. 71–92.

3. Tone A. Historical influences on women's sexual and reproductive health. In: Handbook of Women's Sexual and Reproductive Health (Wingood GM, DiClemente RJ, eds.). Kluwer Academic/Plenum Publishers, New York, 2002; pp. 7–19.
4. http://www.sexualityandu.ca/professionals/sexual/5Fdysfunction/female/contents.asp. (Last accessed 3/1/07)
5. Moynihan R. The making of a disease: female sexual dysfunction. Br Med J 2003;326: 45–47.
6. http://www2.hu-berlin.de/sexology/ECE5/critical_introduction.htm. (Last accessed 3/2/07)
7. Eserink M. Let's talk about sex—and drugs. Science 2005;308:1578–1580.
8. http://www.zestraforwomen.com/aboutzestra/uspharmacist.html. (Last accessed 3/2/07)
9. American Psychiatric Association. Diagnostic and Statistical Manual of Mental Disorders, 4th ed. Washington, DC, 1994.
10. Tiefer L. Sex is Not a Natural Act. Westview Press, Boulder, 2004.
11. Basson R, Weijmar Shultz WCM, Binik Y, et al. (2004) Women's sexual desire and arousal disorders and sexual pain. In: Sexual Medicine: Sexual Dysfunctions in Men and Women (Lue TF, Basson R, Rosen R, Giuliano F, Khoury S, Montorsi F, eds.). Paris, Health Publications, pp. 853–974.
12. Bancroft J, Loftus J, Long JS. Distress about sex: a national survey of women in heterosexual relationships. Arch Sex Behav 2003;32:193–208.
13. Heiman J, Guess MK, Connell K, et al. Standards for clinical trials in sexual dysfunction of women: research designs and outcomes assessment. In: Sexual Medicine: Sexual Dysfunctions in Men and Women (Lue TF, Basson R, Rosen R, Giuliano F, Khoury S, Montorsi F, eds.). Health Publications, Paris, 2003; pp. 633–681.
14. Laumann EO, Paik A, Rosen R. Sexual dysfunction in the United States: prevalence and predictors. JAMA 1999;281:537–544.
15. Schneider BE, Gould M. Female sexuality: looking back into the future. In: Analyzing Gender: A Handbook of Social Science Research (Hess BB, Ferree MM, eds.). Sage Publications, Newbury Park, CA, 1987; pp. 120–153.
16. Maine M. Body Wars: Making Peace with Women's Bodies. Gürze Books, Carlsbad, CA, 2000.
17. The Working Group for a New View of Women's Sexual Problems. A new view of women's sexual problems. In: A New View of Women's Sexual Problems (Kaschak E, Tiefer L, eds.). New York, The Haworth Press, 2001; pp. 1–8.
18. http://www.fsd-alert.org/manifesto.html. (Last accessed 3/2/07)
19. Basson R. Women's sexual dysfunction: revised and expanded definitions. Can Med Assoc J 2005;172(10):1327–1333.

7 Irritable Bowel Syndrome

Deborah M. Bethards, MD *and Ann Ouyang,* MBBS

Contents

INTRODUCTION AND DEFINITION

Functional gastrointestinal disorders are defined by symptoms because there are no specific disease markers available and there are no structural, mechanical, or biochemical abnormalities. These disorders are divided into seven categories based on anatomic location, as well as a pediatric grouping based on a consensus of experts *(1)* (Table 1). There can be significant overlap in these disorders in the same patient and the diagnosis is usually made by primary care physicians, gynecologists, and gastroenterologists *(2)*. This chapter will focus on the Irritable Bowel Syndrome (IBS).

IBS has been called a "biopsychosocial disorder" because there is evidence for a physiological basis for symptoms and for a true gastrointestinal sensory–motor dysfunction affecting the brain–gut axis *(3)*. This enhanced responsiveness in the brain and/or gut results in dysregulation of gut motility. Both of these biological

From: *Current Clinical Practice: Women's Health in Clinical Practice*
Edited by: Clouse and Sherif © Humana Press Inc., Totowa, NJ

Table 1
Functional Gastrointestinal Disorders[a]

Esophageal Disorders
Globus
Rumination syndrome
Functional chest pain of presumed esophageal origin
Functional heartburn
Functional dysphagia
Unspecified esophageal disorder
Gastroduodenal Disorders
Functional dyspepsia
Aerophagia
Functional vomiting
Bowel Disorders
Irritable bowel syndrome
Functional abdominal bloating
Functional constipation
Functional diarrhea
Unspecified functional bowel disorder
Functional abdominal pain
Functional abdominal pain syndrome
Unspecified abdominal pain
Functional Disorders of the Biliary Tract and the Pancreas
Gallbladder dysfunction
Sphincter of Oddi Dysfunction
Anorectal Disorders
Functional Fecal Incontinence
Functional Anorectal Pain (Levator Ani Syndrome and Proctalgia Fugax)
Pelvic floor dysfunction
Functional Pediatric Disorders

[a]From ref. *1*.

processes are modified by psychosocial factors, which result in a clinical presentation that may not respond to simple approaches. Rather than a single disease, IBS can be thought of as having multiple physiological determinants contributing to a common set of symptoms. It has been firmly established that IBS is not a psychological disorder but rather is a condition that is greatly impacted by psychosocial issues. Olden best sums up the manifestations of IBS: "The spectrum of symptoms representing IBS can present an opportunity for efficient diagnosis or mire both the physician and patient in an unsatisfying and unproductive diagnostic adventure" *(4)*.

IBS is a functional bowel disorder that is generally described to include the symptoms of abdominal pain, distention, and a change in bowel consistency and form *(5)*. The absence of a diagnostic marker for this condition has led to the development of clinical criteria to make the diagnosis. Manning et al. defined IBS by simplified symptom-based criteria in 1978; subsequently, in 1991, in Rome, Italy, international teams were convened to further develop criteria for the functional bowel disorders and these were termed Rome I and later, a revision, Rome II criteria *(2)*.

Revised Rome II criteria for the definition of IBS include the following:

At least 12 weeks or more, which do not need to be consecutive, in the preceding 12 months, of abdominal discomfort or pain that has two out of the following three features:

1. Relief with defecation.
2. Onset associated with a change in frequency of stool.
3. Onset associated with a change in the form or appearance of the stool.

Furthermore, the symptoms that cumulatively support the diagnosis of IBS according to Rome II are:

1. Abnormal stool frequency (>3/d or <3/wk).
2. Abnormal stool form (lumpy, hard, loose, watery).
3. Abnormal stool passage (straining, urgency, sense of incomplete evacuation).
4. Passage of mucus.
5. Abdominal distention or bloating.

The Rome criteria have been reported to have a positive predictive value of 98%. Most experts refer to either constipation-predominant or diarrhea-predominant IBS when describing a patient's usual presentation. The Rome criteria should be viewed as broad diagnostic guidelines; these criteria are the most helpful that we currently have available, and there is no "gold standard" test at this time.

EPIDEMIOLOGY

IBS is remarkably prevalent with reports in the literature of a prevalence of 3 to 20% of Americans; these differences in reported prevalence are probably secondary to the varying definitions of IBS (inclusion criteria) and study designs used. When combining functional dyspepsia with IBS, the functional gastrointestinal disorders may be the most common medical conditions, accounting for up to 40 to 60% of referrals to outpatient gastroenterology clinics *(6)*.

The prevalence in a large community-based sample of US women has been noted to be approx 5 to 8%, but this number is probably impacted by the actual definition of abdominal pain used. There is, however, generally thought to be a 3:1 or 4:1 female predominance, although some think that the only gender difference occurs in women with IBS and constipation *(7)*. In the US and Western cultures, more women than men seek healthcare services for symptoms of functional pain disorders, including IBS, which may result in an overrepresentation of women in these surveys *(7)*.

IBS is generally thought to be a disorder found in young and middle aged adults, usually younger than 45 years old. However, a recent review in Geriatrics in 2005 found that the prevalence may be higher in the older population than previously thought, and recommended that IBS be considered in the differential of unexplained abdominal pain in this group *(8)*.

There are varying prevalence rates noted in Caucasians vs Africa America, but this is probably related to differences in access to and patterns of seeking medical care and to which criteria are used. According to Taub *(9)*, no difference was found between these two groups if the Manning criteria were used for definition, whereas the Sandler group found a very high ratio favoring whites, using standard diagnostic criteria *(10)*. According to Camilleri et al. the prevalence rates for black and Hispanic Americans as well as Japanese and Chinese populations is the same, approximately 20%, suggesting that the worldwide prevalence is probably no different *(11)*.

IBS is the diagnosis in 28% of all patients seen in a gastroenterology office and accounts for 12% of primary care visits in the United States. It has been shown that IBS patients make twice as many doctor visits for nongastrointestinal problems as those without the diagnosis. Only approximately 25% of patients with symptoms meeting the clinical criteria for IBS actually seek medical attention, therefore, the prevalence is most likely even higher. In the eight most industrialized nations in the world, it is estimated that approx $41 million is spent annually on IBS (including direct and indirect costs) and IBS patients are more expensive to care for than those without gastrointestinal problems, most likely because of the more frequent healthcare visits and multiple studies eventually performed *(11)*. The goal of the Rome criteria is to help reduce the need for an extensive diagnostic work-up by being able to more easily make a positive diagnosis of IBS.

PATHOPHYSIOLOGY

The lifetime and short-term course of IBS are quite variable and the average severity of symptoms is usually mild to moderate, with episodes of acute exacerbation and severe symptoms.

IBS most likely develops secondary to an interplay of the following factors *(6)*:

1. Visceral hypersensitivity.
2. Motor dysfunction.

3. Psychosocial distress.
4. Postinfectious changes.
5. Luminal irritation.
6. Heredity.

Visceral Hypersensitivity

Visceral hypersensitivity refers to excessive sensing of afferent stimuli, such as volume or pressure. Visceral hyperalgesia refers to a painful stimulus resulting in a more intense response than is normal. Allodynia refers to a situation in which a previously painless sensation has now become painful.

These sensitivities have been tested in IBS patients compared with normal controls using ileal or anorectal balloon distention, reflecting the changes one would see with diarrhea and excess gas. The brains of patients with IBS are activated differently than normal controls, although there remains controversy regarding the actual location in the brain–gut axis where these differences occur. Some studies do show increased anterior cingulate or prefrontal lobe activation IBS subjects *(12)*. Interestingly, IBS patients are thought to have normal thresholds for somatic pain stimuli, which suggests that hyperalgesia in these patients is in response to stimuli from the abdominal viscera only *(11)*.

Motor Dysfunction

The second factor is related to abnormal motility in IBS patients. The enteric nervous system is composed of the myenteric plexus and the submucosal plexus; the enteric system does receive input from the brain, but can function on its own to control local motor reflexes as well as secretion. Specific motility findings described in the Consensus Report 2002 include *(11)*:

1. Increased postprandial colonic contractions.
2. Fast colonic and propagated contractions resulting in diarrhea.
3. Abnormal giant migrating contractions are seen in patients with constipation.
4. More symptomatic contractions in the rectosigmoid colon in response to normal stimuli.
5. Accelerated gut transit in diarrhea-prominent IBS.
6. Abnormal small bowel motor patterns.
7. Normal compliance and tone.

Psychosocial Stress

Psychosocial stress is the third factor implicated in the development of IBS, and one particular psychological feature seems most important: somatization. This refers to the tendency of these patients to focus on symptoms that cannot be explained and to feel as though they are suffering so much that medical attention and evaluation is needed. Only approximately 20% of patients with organic (vs functional) bowel disease present with psychological symptoms compared with 50% of those with IBS.

The major psychological features other than somatization are anxiety with or without panic, posttraumatic stress disorder, phobias, depression, paranoia, and hostility. Approximately one-half of patients with IBS are able to recall a stressful event that occurred before their symptoms began and IBS patients classically seem to have more stressful life events and feel that stress affects their symptoms adversely *(11)*.

Many of these patients deny or minimize the psychosocial factors contributing to their symptoms. A history of a previous loss that has not been accepted (e.g., stillborn child), sexual and/or physical abuse in childhood, and other unresolved traumatic life events may contribute to their illness. Hypochondriasis and stressful life events actually help to predict which patients with postinfectious IBS will develop IBS (*see* below). There is no evidence that psychosocial factors cause the symptoms of IBS, however *(11)*. Household surveys indicate that people with symptoms of IBS that do not seek medical attention (nonpatient IBS) have the same psychological profile as people without IBS. The nongastrointestinal, nonpsychiatric, comorbid disorders most associated with IBS are fibromyalgia (median of 49% have IBS), temporomandibular joint syndrome (64%), chronic fatigue syndrome (51%), and chronic pelvic pain (50%) *(13)*.

Postinfectious Changes

The information regarding a postinfectious contribution to IBS is evolving and seems to implicate an increased expression of inflammatory markers after infection, which, in turn, causes neuromuscular dysfunction. There is evidence that the duration and severity of the acute diarrheal syndrome are independent risk factors for the development of postinfectious IBS *(14)*. The postinfectious group may have a better prognosis. Some information notes residual symptoms similar to IBS after bacterial enteritis even after 6 years, especially well-described after *Campylobacter* infection, which has the highest incidence of postinfectious IBS *(15)*. Other bacteria involved are *Shigella* and *Salmonella;* persistent bowel dysfunction has been observed in an average of 25% of patients with infections with these bacteria *(6)*.

Luminal Irritation

Luminal irritation can occur in both the small bowel and the colon. Specific food intolerances were reported in the British literature to occur in 33 to 66% of IBS patients, but the evidence that the gut is truly sensitive to certain foods is limited *(6)*. The most common foods reported in Britain were wheat, dairy products, coffee, potatoes, corn, onions, beef, oats, and white wine; it is unclear whether these are food allergens or not. It is still not known whether exclusionary diets are indicated in the evaluation of patients with IBS because of a high placebo response rate. Lactose, fructose, and other sugars have also been implicated along with other osmotically active, fermentable, and poorly absorbable carbohydrates, possibly related to the overproduction of colonic hydrogen or to the known slow gas transit and reduced gas tolerance in IBS. Bile acids and short chain fatty acids can also cause luminal irritation as endogenous factors.

Heredity

Research has been limited in the area of heredity in terms of pathophysiology of IBS but a review by Levy et al. in 2003 examined families with twins. They found that having a mother or father with IBS was an independent and stronger predictor of developing IBS than having a twin with IBS. Thus, they concluded that heredity seems to contribute but "social learning… has an equal or greater influence" *(16)*.

CLINICAL PRESENTATION

As previously noted, patients with IBS present in a variety of ways. Although abdominal pain is a hallmark of this condition, some patients will complain of constipation and others of diarrhea associated with the pain, referred to as constipation-predominant vs diarrhea-predominant IBS. In women, bloating is a common complaint, but is less so in men. The amount and frequency of passing flatus in IBS is unknown and some do not think it should be regarded with the same importance as the other symptoms *(11)*. Using the previously described symptom-based Rome criteria and in the absence of "alarm symptoms," a diagnosis can usually be made by the history and physical exam with a minimum amount of testing. Currently there is still no true "gold standard" for the evaluation and characterization of IBS, and it is recommended that, because of the differences in these criteria, caution be used in deciding the prevalence of IBS. It is also assumed that the diagnosis of IBS cannot be made unless structural and biochemical problems have been excluded. This necessitates the exclusion of "alarm symptoms" or "red flags," which include the following *(4)*:

- Weight loss
- Anemia
- Occult blood in stool
- Travel history to areas with endemic parasitic diseases
- Nocturnal symptoms
- New onset after age 50 years
- Family history of colon cancer or inflammatory bowel disease
- Arthritis or dermatitis on physical exam

- Signs of malabsorption
- Signs or symptoms of thyroid dysfunction

Other symptoms strongly associated with the clinical presentation of IBS patients include fatigue, poor sleep habits, fibromyalgia, urinary symptoms, back pain, dyspareunia, and, as noted previously, they have a higher prevalence of depression and anxiety as well as somatization *(6)*.

Very little has been written regarding the physical examination of these patients because it is almost always unremarkable. However, findings of a palpable sigmoid colon that is somewhat tender as well as an increased sensitivity to air insufflation during colonoscopy/sigmoidoscopy may help support the diagnosis of IBS; these are soft findings and by no means diagnostic.

EVALUATION

The work up of patients with IBS is, at best, frustrating to the medical practitioner, whether they are primary care physicians, subspecialists, or gastroenterologists. Drossman *(17)* aptly explains this challenge by noting three explanations for this:

1. The lack of measurable biological markers.
2. "A diagnosis based solely on symptoms can be unsettling; clinicians struggle with the possibility of missing another diagnosis."
3. The effect and importance of psychosocial factors (not just stress, anxiety, and depression, but also possible true psychiatric disease) makes it difficult to develop a diagnostic approach for IBS.

Once the patient has been found to display the criteria necessary for the diagnosis of IBS and "alarm symptoms" have not been found, then the question becomes what to do, and what not to do. Olden succinctly describes the dilemma: "Pursuing all diagnostic possibilities via an extensive work-up can lead to unnecessary and costly testing. This futility, in turn, can subject the patient to unneeded expense, inconvenience, and suffering" *(18)*.

It has, for example, not been found cost-effective or necessary to do routine colonoscopies, stool for ova and parasites, or thyroid studies on these patients, but perhaps a lactose-free dietary period, to exclude lactose intolerance, is reasonable. The basic recommendation at this time includes checking a complete blood count (CBC) and chemistry panel in patients who most likely have IBS by symptom-based criteria *(4)*.

The basic work-up for diarrhea-predominant IBS should include:

1. Stool for enteric pathogens, including ova and parasites (consider checking for *Clostridium difficile* if indicated by previous infectious history or antibiotic exposure).

2. Stool for occult blood.
3. Lactose-free diet for at least 1 to 2 weeks.
4. CBC and chemistry profile.
5. Colonoscopy, if indicated by family history or other "alarm" symptoms.

The basic work-up for constipation-predominant IBS should include:

1. CBC, chemistry profile, and thyroid-stimulating hormone level.
2. Stool for occult blood.
3. Colonoscopy, if indicated by family history, age or other "alarm" symptoms.

The psychosocial evaluation of these patients should be undertaken carefully and seriously by the clinician based on the following concepts that have evolved since the 1980s regarding IBS patients *(4)*:

1. They are more likely to have anxiety, depression, and somatoform disorders.
2. They are more likely to have been physically or sexually abused as children or even as adults compared with patients with organic gastrointestinal disease.
3. It is recognized that healthcare seeking is influenced by both psychological problems and history of abuse.
4. Psychological issues and abuse history clearly influence the severity of bowel symptoms and the level of subsequent disability.

The symptoms most likely associated with IBS-related psychiatric disorders include panic disorder (palpitations, insomnia, diaphoresis, agoraphobia, and worrying behavior), depression (with anhedonia, fatigue, loss of appetite, and decreased libido) and somatization disorders, which imply multiple complaints referable to at least five organ systems *(4)*. Many clinicians may be uncomfortable discussing these issues with their patients, but it is the cornerstone of a trusting and well-constructed patient–physician relationship, especially in patients with IBS.

Naturally, if any alarm symptoms, such as rectal bleeding or weight loss are found in the initial evaluation, a logical and rigorous work-up is subsequently recommended and encouraged.

DIFFERENTIAL DIAGNOSIS

There is much discussion regarding the "overlap" of IBS symptoms with other functional gastrointestinal problems. Of the functional bowel diseases previously discussed, the most common is probably functional dyspepsia. The distinction between IBS and functional dyspepsia is best made by being aware that functional dyspepsia as a separate entity actually does occur more commonly in the upper abdomen (above the navel) and is not associated with a change in bowel movements. However, functional dyspepsia is more frequent in IBS constipation-predominant patients and those patients have more bloating and abdominal pain *(4)*.

The other most common disease entities that need to be differentiated from IBS can be summarized as follows:

1. Chronic pelvic pain syndrome including pelvic floor dyssynergia: In one study, more than 30% of the women with chronic pelvic pain had IBS, yet it was not diagnosed 40% of the time; narcotics were prescribed 35% of the time, and no IBS treatments were administered in more than 60% of the patients who actually had IBS *(18)*. These patients not infrequently undergo needless surgery.
2. Celiac sprue: This disease must be considered in all patients presenting with the possible diagnosis of IBS and an early diagnosis may be cost-effective because the treatment with a gluten-free diet is standard and very efficacious. These patients often have alarm symptoms of weight loss and anemia; they generally, but not always, have diarrhea. The lab work including tissue transglutaminase and endomysial antibodies have a positive predictive value of 90 to 100% but small bowel biopsy showing villous atrophy, which responds to a gluten-free diet, is the gold standard *(17)*.
3. Gynecological conditions: There is some suggestion that gynecological surgery itself can precipitate the onset of IBS *(19)*. Another special presentation is the menstruating woman with IBS in whom it seems that abdominal pain, bloating and stool patterns change with the menstrual cycle. There has been an effort to relate these changes to hormonal fluctuations, but this association is not yet clear. One group found no difference in the IBS symptom pattern of women with IBS, whether or not they were taking oral contraceptives, nor did there seem to be a difference in symptom baseline, except that women with diarrhea predominance had milder symptoms of all types *(20)*.
4. Inflammatory bowel disease: Endoscopic evaluation and biopsies are necessary to make this distinction and one should have a high index of suspicion if the patient has alarm symptoms (e.g., rectal bleeding, family history).
5. Bacterial overgrowth: This can mimic or worsen IBS symptoms, but the diagnostic yield in terms of testing (breath H2 test) is probably as low as 10% *(17)*. One should look for predisposing conditions, such as previous surgery and jejunal diverticulosis.
6. Functional vs slow-transit constipation: Making the distinction between these two can be difficult; better tools are needed to improve this diagnostic dilemma *(21)*. However, even though, in these conditions, abdominal pain is relieved by bowel movements (as it often is in IBS), change in bowel habits is the major symptom, not pain *(11)*.
7. Lactose intolerance: Approximately 83% of patients with both IBS and lactose intolerance had symptomatic improvement after removing lactose from their diet *(4)*.
8. Outlet constipation: Many of these patients also have a history of physical or sexual abuse. Many have concomitant IBS and pelvic floor dyssynergia.

9. Functional anorectal disorders: These include proctalgia fugax (sudden, severe paroxysmal anal pain lasting seconds to minutes) and levator ani syndrome (also referred to as "pyriformis syndrome" and "puborectalis syndrome"), which results in a dull ache in the rectum that worsens with sitting. Physical exam may reveal tenderness on palpation of the pelvic floor and levator muscle hypercontractility. Anorectal manometry may help in the diagnosis of these patients *(4)*.
10. Intestinal pseudo-obstruction: This entity is associated with abnormal abdominal X-ray findings that have the appearance of obstruction in the absence of any mechanical cause for obstruction. The etiologies include Chagas disease and paraneoplastic syndrome, as well as idiopathic causes and hereditary conditions, which are extremely rare.
11. Parasitic infections, such as *Giardia*.

Symptoms of IBS and fibromyalgia often coexist, but certainly can present separately and some think that their strong comorbidity suggests a common feature, most likely a psychological effect *(22)*.

MANAGEMENT

Treatment modalities for IBS patients can best be divided into three parts: nonpharmacological, pharmacological, and future treatment possibilities. The importance of addressing psychological issues is emphasized by Mertz, who stated "Given the psychosocial factors involved and the limited benefits of current pharmacological therapies, the treatment of IBS requires physicians to attend to the minds as well as the bodies of their patients in order to help them find relief" *(23)*.

A recommended outline of goals of diagnosis and therapy for IBS include *(6)*:

- Having an acceptably low proportion of missed nonfunctional diagnoses
- Ensuring a minimum number of patients who are younger than 45 years old undergo negative barium studies during the evaluation
- Reducing the number of work days missed
- Decreasing the number of physician office visits
- Improving the patient's quality of life

Disturbingly, there seems to be a significant increased surgical history in IBS patients. Longstreth et al. in *Gastroenterology*, 2004, found a threefold higher incidence of cholecystectomy and a twofold higher incidence of appendectomy and hysterectomy in IBS patients. There was a 50% higher incidence of back surgery in these patients *(24)*. The authors agreed that reasons for this are "unproven" but thought that there were several possible explanations: an overlap with other functional disorders that seem to predispose to surgery, onset of IBS after surgery (a possible cause of IBS) and, most likely, an inclination to perform surgery based on inaccurate diagnoses because IBS symptoms can be confusing.

A consensus report in 2002 recommends the following management plan *(9)*:

1. Establish a firm diagnosis.
2. Establish a caring physician–patient relationship.
3. Provide careful reassurance (that there is no cancer and that a normal life expectancy is predicted).
4. Explain the role of factors such as a hypersensitive gut, emotions, diet, and infections.
5. Provide dietary education, including the avoidance of sorbitol, lactose, and certain medications.
6. Medications may be tried but many have no proven benefit when compared to placebo, these include antidiarrheals, fiber and osmotic laxatives, anticholinergics, and psychotropics. The lack of benefit over placebo may be related to a very high placebo effect in clinical trials. Treatment should be aimed at the predominant symptom and reassurance should be given that new drugs are being tested.
7. Recommend psychological treatment as needed.
8. Be vigilant regarding unnecessary surgery or unknown alternative therapy.

For many patients, nonpharmacological treatment is all that is needed, but the approach should be multifaceted. Routine physical activity that the patient can readily adhere to is very important; it need not be some extreme sport, but rather walking, fast walking, or a tolerable gym work-out. The key is to encourage a focus on an activity that can be performed predictably and that does not cause the patient additional problems; this is especially important if the patient has concomitant fibromyalgia.

Generally, any dietary excess should be avoided, as well as avoiding self-defined trigger foods for each patient. Strict "exclusion diets" are not usually necessary (as true allergies are rare), can be inappropriate, and should only be conducted under a dietician's guidance. Specific triggers that might be avoided, however, include *(23)*:

1. Caffeine (in over-the-counter medications drugs, such as Excedrin®, coffee, tea, chocolate, sodas, and some frozen desserts).
2. Excessive fatty foods, which can enhance the gastro–colonic reflex.
3. Lactose, if implicated by symptoms, with a trial of avoidance.
4. Excessive fruit, sorbitol, and fructose, especially in diarrhea-predominance.
5. Beans, uncooked broccoli, cabbage, and cauliflower, especially if bloating or flatulence are special concerns.

Fiber

In those with constipation-predominance and inadequate fiber intake (recommendation is 20–30 g daily) a fiber supplement is recommended in whatever regimen is most effective and best tolerated, although supporting data are lacking *(4)*. Natural fiber (such as wheat bran, corn fiber, and psyllium seed from the ipsaghlua husk) is indigestible plant carbohydrate, which is metabolized by colonic bacteria into short chain fatty acids, gas, and fluid. The goal is to make the stool bulkier, softer, and wetter, which speeds up colonic transit time. There is evidence that fiber may decrease intracolonic pressure, either by a direct effect or by binding bile salts, resulting in less wall tension and, therefore, less pain, although conflicting evidence shows that, in normal patients, fiber has no effect on small bowel or proximal colonic emptying *(11)*.

Natural fibers can be acted on by bacteria, as noted above, resulting in gas production and worsening of bloating, and abdominal discomfort in some patients; patients should be warned that they may experience these temporary side effects. Some would recommend synthetic fibers, such as calcium carbophil (brand name examples: FiberTab®, Konsyl Fiber®, Equalactin®, or Fibercon®), which cannot be split by bacteria *(11)*.

A great deal of patience is needed when working with IBS patients to fine-tune this addition to their regimen; not all tolerate the same product and some experience worsening of symptoms with fiber supplementation. Adequate fluid intake and hydration are also important components of fiber treatment. Evidence supports the use of fiber supplementation for constipation, but there does not seem to be any beneficial effect in terms of abdominal pain or other symptoms *(11)*. In fact, in one report, no difference was found between fiber supplementation and placebo in regard to global IBS symptom improvement, and it is recommended that fiber be used to treat constipation but not IBS *per se (25)*.

Pharmacological Therapy

Generally, it is recommended that medication not be used unless absolutely necessary because not all IBS patients need pharmacological intervention. When medication is used, experts recommend it be administered only on an as-needed basis. Clearly, available treatments do not address underlying pathology, which is still poorly understood.

ANTIDIARRHEAL MEDICATIONS

There are two available treatments most often recommended for diarrhea-predominant IBS. Loperamide (Imodium®; 2 to 4 mg, up to four times a day) improves symptoms of diarrhea, fecal soiling, and urgency, but not pain and bloating. It is the preferred opiate (rather than codeine or diphenoxylate) because it does not cross the blood–brain barrier. There are no long-term safety or efficacy data available. Despite its usefulness in relieving diarrhea in some patients, loperamide is no different than placebo in relieving "global"

IBS symptoms *(25)*. The second drug that can be used is cholestyramine, but it is only effective if bile acid excess is the problem; one scoop or packet is administered with meals. A third drug, a combination diphenoxylate hydrochloride and atropine sulfate (Lomotil®), may be used, but patients should be warned of the possible anticholinergic side effects of dry mouth, dizziness, and drowsiness.

Treatment for Constipation

Aside from the fiber supplements, lactulose may also be tried (1–2 tbsp twice daily), or 70% Sorbitol (1 tbsp twice daily); both may cause bloating. Miralax, polyethylene glycol (GoLYTELY®) can be used. Also, see information regarding tegaserod (in "Serotonin Receptor Modulators").

Antispasmodics and Smooth Muscle Relaxants

Many drugs are under investigation in the United States and Europe, but only a few are approved in the United States. These drugs are generally used intermittently to treat acute pain, distention, or bloating. There is no clear evidence yet that they are efficacious, but they may be helpful by reducing the duration and magnitude of the abnormal colonic response *(26)*. The most commonly used antispasmodic is dicyclomine (Bentyl®), which seems to be effective through its anticholinergic effects, but loses that effectiveness with chronic use. Dicyclomine may be prescribed at doses as high as 20 to 40 mg four times daily as needed, although lower doses are more commonly used. Hyoscyamine is a smooth muscle relaxant usually dosed at 0.125 to 0.25 mg (by mouth or sublingually) four times a day as needed. Librax® (brand name for the combination of clidinium and chlordiazepoxide) is also helpful, but should be avoided because of the possible habituation to the benzodiazepine component (clidinium alone is no longer available).

Tricyclic Antidepressants

These antidepressants may have analgesic effects as well as effects on gut sensation and motility. They have been mostly studied in IBS patients who have abdominal pain and diarrhea. These drugs are used on a continuous basis and are reserved for those with continuous or frequently recurring symptoms; it make take as long as 3 to 4 months to provide relief of symptoms *(11)*. Tricyclic antidepressants are better than placebo at relieving global IBS symptoms as well as abdominal pain by ameliorating the enhanced pain perception that these patients have *(25)*. The most commonly prescribed tricyclic depressants are amitryptiline, doxepin, desimpramine, and nortriptyline. Adverse effects include dry mouth, constipation, bladder and sexual dysfunction, and dizziness; blurred vision and drowsiness can occur but usually resolve with time.

SELECTIVE SEROTONIN-REUPTAKE INHIBITORS (SSRI'S)

The selective serotonin reuptake inhibitor group of drugs has not yet proven very effective in IBS but can be tried in patients with IBS who have worse symptoms despite other treatments.

SEROTONIN RECEPTOR MODULATORS

Serotonin (5-hydroxytryptamine or 5-HT), found primarily in the enterochromaffin cells, seems to be the most important neurotransmitter in the enteric nervous system in visceral (gut) sensitization. Serotonin is released with mechanical or chemical stimulation and mediates bowel contraction and relaxation, sensations of pain and nausea, and intestinal secretion. The observation that IBS patients release more serotonin into the blood postprandially formed the basis that visceral hypersensitivity may be mediated with serotonin agonists and antagonists. The five serotonin receptor modulators include:

Serotonin-3 Receptor Antagonists. Serotonin-3 receptors are activated by serotonin that is released in response to mucosal stimulation; their activation results in increased intestinal secretion, motility, and sensation. The antagonists to this pathway, thus, result in a reduced gastrocolic reflex, a slowed colonic transit time, and increased colon compliance as well as diminished sensitivity of the colon to distention, resulting in a decrease in urgency and diarrhea *(23)*. Alosetron (Lotronex®) is currently the only available drug in this group and is recommended in diarrhea-predominant IBS. Alosetron (1 mg twice daily) has been shown to decrease abdominal pain and fecal urgency and to improve quality of life; constipation occurs in 22 to 39% of patients. One in 700 patients were found to develop ischemic colitis (although this remains controversial) from the drug and, therefore, it was withdrawn and then re-introduced with strict guidelines *(23)*. It was originally recommended only for use in women with severe diarrhea-predominant IBS, but recent reports show a beneficial response in men also.

Partial Serotonin-4 Receptor Agonists. Peristalsis is activated by stimulation of the serotonin-4 receptors resulting in an increase in gastric emptying as well as small bowel and colonic motility. These drugs are similar to the prokinetic drug, cisapride, now removed from the market. Tegaserod (Zelnorm®) is the only Food and Drug Administration (FDA)-approved drug for use in constipation-predominant IBS (6 mg twice daily) and seems to benefit women more than men. All four trials of tegaserod have shown statistically significant improvement in global IBS scores compared with placebo *(24)*. Tegaserod does not cross the blood–brain barrier; the side effect profile is minimal, consisting of transient diarrhea in approx 10% of patients. It is FDA-approved at this time for 12 weeks of therapy *(23)*. However, tegaserod wash voluntarily removed from the market in 2007 due to safety concerns.

Full Serotonin-4 Receptor Agonists. This group of drugs seems promising but needs further investigation. The best known is prucalopride for constipation-predominant IBS.

NEWER THERAPIES

Newer therapies being investigated for IBS include the k-opioid agonist, fedotozine, other serotonergic agents, neurokinin, and other serotonin-3 and serotonin-4 drugs, as well as probiotics and Chinese herbal therapies *(11)*.

Hypnosis, Cognitive Behavioral Therapy. Psychotherapy, StressLRelaxation Management and Biofeedback

Despite the prominence of psychological factors in IBS and experimental evidence of efficacy, psychological treatment is now only used in approximately 10% of IBS patients presenting to primary care physicians and gastroenterologists. Lack of adequate insurance coverage for mental health issues is the major obstacle to treatment. The psychological methods for treating IBS are especially helpful when other modalities fail or when psychological factors are paramount, but not when psychiatric disease *per se* is identified *(8)*. Psychological intervention is not needed in all patients. The mechanism probably involves modifying the patient's cognition regarding symptoms as well as helping to decrease the stress associated with the physical symptoms *(27,28)*.

Data on the efficacy of hypnotherapy for IBS is limited by small studies and few numbers of expert hypnotherapists. The largest study to date, in 2002, included 250 patients and the findings have been replicated in many other studies since then *(28)*. Findings included a significant improvement in severity of diarrhea and pain, anxiety, depression, use of medication, frequency of office visits and quality of life.

Cognitive behavioral therapy seems to be most promising in women with functional bowel disorders, but patients with somatization disorder are less likely to respond to any therapy *(27)*. Psychotherapy seems to help patients not by affecting their symptoms of pain but rather by improving their overall quality of life by placing their symptoms in perspective.

Other Nonpharmucological Treatments

One double-blind, placebo controlled trial demonstrated improvement in IBS symptoms with herbal treatment compared to controls *(29)*. However, more data are needed to understand what types and combinations of herbs may be helpful in IBS *(29)*. Peppermint oil has also been tried, but its use is limited by increased acid reflux symptoms (through relaxation of the lower esophageal sphincter); it may, however, have some antispasmodic effects *(23)*.

Gastroenterology Referral

Appropriate and timely referral to a gastroenterologist is important and should be explored if any "red flags" arise early in the primary care physician's evaluation. Otherwise, the primary care physician truly has an important role in diagnosing IBS and providing initial treatment trials and reassurance to their patients without embarking on an expensive and frustrating work-up. Patients with IBS become quite concerned regarding their symptoms and need the gentle guidance of a physician who knows them and has preferably worked with them for a while. Sometimes, the most difficult thing to do is to avoid expensive and useless testing in these patients. Approximately 15 to 20% of IBS patients eventually do get referred to a gastroenterologist, and these are usually refractory patients who often have a higher prevalence and severity of psychopathology *(30)*.

QUALITY OF LIFE AND FINANCIAL ISSUES IN IBS

IBS is associated with a significantly impaired quality of life and disability *(31)*. The consequent morbidities associated with IBS are best measured by quality of life, work- and social-related impairments, and health-seeking behavior or use of healthcare *(27)*.

Up to 40% of IBS patients tend to avoid social activities, travel, and even work because of fear of fecal incontinence, flatulence, bloating, vomiting, and abdominal pain. They may also avoid sexual activity and family activities because of these fears as well as having disturbed sleep patterns and anxiety. Patients usually rate the severity of their IBS on the basis of their quality of life, which is clearly determined by what activities they feel able to participate in and subsequently accomplish; these patients feel they are less productive at work and at home *(32)*.

The financial burden for IBS is significant. In the United States, average work days lost per year for functional gastrointestinal disorders is 14.8 days compared with 8.7 days in control subjects *(6)*. For IBS specifically, the numbers are 13 days compared with 4 days *(11)*.

In a US survey performed over 2 years and reported in 2003, patients with IBS had a statistically higher number of outpatient doctor visits (medical, surgical, and emergency room), radiological procedures, laboratory work, and outpatient prescriptions, resulting in substantially higher healthcare costs than patients without IBS; the severity of abdominal pain seemed to be the most predictive factor of healthcare usage and cost because of time spent in bed, reduced quality of life, and absence from work *(33)*.

SUMMARY

IBS, part of a greater group of illnesses classified as Functional Gastrointestinal Disorders, is one of the most common illnesses encountered by primary care physicians. Patients with IBS have significant impairments in work productivity as well as quality of life issues, such as fatigue, generalized body pain, and a distorted perception of their health, which interrupts activities of daily living *(31)*. The classification of legitimate symptom criteria has enabled the medical community to better understand and diagnose IBS. As primary care physicians become more comfortable treating IBS, they may be better able to manage patient expectations and to avoid unnecessary and expensive testing. Treatment for IBS is limited, but many potential therapies are undergoing investigation.

REFERENCES

1. Drossman DA (ed.). Rome II: The Functional Gastrointestinal Disorders. 2nd ed., 2000.
2. Chey WD, Olden K, Carter E, et al. Utility of the Rome I and II criteria for irritable bowel syndrome in U.S. women. Am J Gastroenterol 2002;97:2803–2811.
3. Camilleri M. Management of the irritable bowel syndrome. Gastroenterology 2001;120: 652–668.
4. Olden KW. Diagnosis of the irritable bowel syndrome. Gastroenterology 2002;122:1701–1714.
5. Gonsalkorale WM, Houghton LA, Whorwell PJ. Hypnotherapy in irritable bowel syndrome: a large-scale audit of a clinical service with examination of factors influencing responsiveness. Am J Gastroenterol 2002;97:954–961.
6. Jones J, Boorman J, Cann P, et al. British Society of Gastroenterology guidelines for the management of the irritable bowel syndrome. Gut 2000;47(Suppl II):ii1–ii19.
7. Chang L, Heitkemper MM. Gender differences in irritable bowel syndrome. Gastroenterology 2002;123:1686–1701.
8. Ehrenpreis ED. Irritable bowel syndrome. 10–20% of older adults have symptoms consistent with diagnosis. Geriatrics 2005;60(1):25–28.
9. Taub E, Cuevas JL, Cook EW, et al. Irritable bowel syndrome defined by factor analysis gender and race comparisons. Digestive Diseases and Science 1995;40:2647–2655.
10. Sandler R. Epidemiology of irritable bowel syndrome in the United Stated. Gastroenterology 1990;99:409–415.
11. Camilleri M, Heading RC, Thompson WG. Consensus report: clinical perspectives, mechanisms, diagnosis and management of irritable bowel syndrome. Aliment Pharmacol Ther 2002;16:1407–1430.
12. Naliboff BD, Berman S, Chang L, et al. Sex-related difference sin IBS patients: central processing of visceral stimuli. Gastroenterology 2003;124:1738–1748.
13. Whitehead WE, Palsson O, Jones KR. Systematic review of the comorbidity of irritable bowel syndrome with other disorders: what are the causes and implications? Gastroenterology 2002;122:1140–1156.
14. Ji S, Park H, Lee D, et al. Post-infectious irritable bowel syndrome in patients with Shigella infection. J Gastroenterol Hepatol 2005;20:381–386.
15. Spiller RC. Neuropatholgy of IBS? Gastroenterology 2002;123:2144–2147.
16. Levy RL, Jones KR, Whitehead WE, et al. Irritable bowel syndrome in twins: heredity and social learning both contribute to etiology. Gastroenterology 2001;121:799–804.

17. Drossman DA. Irritable bowel syndrome: how far do you go in the workup? Gastroenterology 2001;121:1512–1515.
18. Williams RE, Hartmann KE, Sandler RS, et al. Recognition and treatment of irritable bowel syndrome among women with chronic pelvic pain. Am J Obstet Gynecol 2005;192: 761–767.
19. Talley NJ. Unnecessary abdominal and back surgery in irritable bowel syndrome: time to stem the flood now? Gastroenterology 2004;126:1899–1903.
20. Heitkemper MM, Cain KC, Jarrett ME, et al. Symptoms across the menstrual cycle in women with irritable bowel syndrome. The American Journal of Gastroenterology 2003;98:420–430.
21. Talley NJ. Differentiating functional constipation from constipation-predominant irritable bowel syndrome:management implications. Rev Gastroenterol Disord 2005;5:1–9.
22. Chang L, Berman S, Mayer EA, et al. Brain responses to visceral and somatic stimuli in patients with irritable bowel syndrome with and without fibromyalgia. Am J Gastroenterol 2003;98:1354–1361.
23. Mertz HR. Irritable bowel syndrome. New Engl J Med 2003;349:2136–2146.
24. Longstreth GF, Yao JF. Irritable bowel syndrome and surgery: a multivariate analysis. Gastroenterology 2004;126:1665–1673.
25. Brandt LJ, Bjorkman D, Fennerty B, et al. Systematic review on the management of irritable bowel syndrome in North America. Am J Gastroenterol 2002;97(Suppl):S7–S26.
26. Sullivan MA, Snape WJ Jr. Colonic myoelectrical activity in irritable bowel syndrome. Effect of eating and anticholinergics. N Engl J Med 1978;298:878–883.
27. Clouse RE. Managing functional bowel disorders from the top down: lessons from a well-designed treatment trial. Gastroenterology 2003;125:249–252.
28. Palsson OS, Whitehead WE. The growing case for hypnosis as adjunctive therapy for functional gastrointestinal disorders. Gastroenterology 2002;123:2132–2135.
29. Bensoussan A, Talley NJ, Hing M, et al. Treatment of irritable bowel syndrome with chinese herbal medicine. JAMA 1998;280:1585–1589.
30. Longstreth GF, Burchette RJ. Family practitioners' attitudes and knowledge about irritable bowel syndrome: effect of a trial of physician education. Fam Pract 2003;20:670–674.
31. Grainek IM, Hays RD, Kilbourne A, et al. The impact of irritable bowel syndrome on health-related quality of life. Gastroenterology 2000;119:654–660.
32. Gore M, Frech F, Tai KS, et al. Burden of illness in patients with irritable bowel syndrome with constipation. Am J Gastroenterol 2003;98(Suppl):S219.
33. Longstreth GF, Wilson A, Knight K, et al. Irritable bowel syndrome, health care use, and costs: a U.S. managed care perspective. Am J Gastroenterol 2003;98:600–607.

8 Urinary Incontinence

Harriette M. Scarpero, MD
and Tamara G. Bavendam, MD

Contents

From: *Current Clinical Practice: Women's Health in Clinical Practice*
Edited by: Clouse and Sherif © Humana Press Inc., Totowa, NJ

INTRODUCTION

Urinary incontinence (UI) is the condition of involuntary urine loss. This loss may be of varying degree, from a minimal drop of urine to severe high-volume leakage that soils clothing and furniture. Interestingly, the degree of bother associated with UI does not always correlate with the severity of the leakage. However, UI often has a substantial effect on an individual's perception of well-being, body image, and quality of life (QOL).

According to population studies, 20 to 50% of women in the United States experience at least some urine leakage *(1)*. The percentage of women with more severe leakage is estimated at 7 to 10% *(2)*. The actual prevalence of urinary incontinence in women is not known. Most women who experience urinary incontinence never seek or receive treatment. Existing national databases capture only the minority of incontinent women who are treated for incontinence. The economic impact of urinary incontinence is better understood. According to the recently published Urologic Diseases in America Project, urinary incontinence in women was the chief reason for more than one million office visits in the year 2000, at a cost of 452 million dollars *(3)*.

The tremendous social and economic impact of incontinence is reflected in the vast number of television and print advertisements for incontinence products and pharmacological agents. Despite the public's recognition of the disorder, embarrassment and fear can still inhibit a woman from discussing incontinence with her physician. Some women mistakenly think that urinary incontinence is a normal consequence of childbirth or aging. With the prodigious growth of information and treatment options for UI in the past decade, primary care providers are called on to screen for UI. Their medical training may not have fully prepared them for the task. Traditional medical training has been quite compartmentalized, and the pelvic compartment has been largely left to urologists and gynecologists. Primary care training is often deficient in instruction regarding pelvic anatomy and lower urinary tract (LUT) function. The purpose of this chapter is to provide the basic practical information necessary to perform initial incontinence evaluations, institute treatment, and identify when to refer incontinent patients to specialists.

THE ANATOMY OF CONTINENCE

UI occurs when the bladder pressure exceeds the pressure of the bladder outlet mechanism. The inability of the bladder outlet mechanism to maintain continence may be caused by anatomic factors, functional factors, or more commonly, a combination of the two. The bladder outlet mechanism in a woman is composed of the muscles and ligaments of the pelvic floor as well as the urethral muscle and mucosa. The entity of the "pelvic floor" includes the pelvic viscera, the peritoneum overlying it, endopelvic fascia, levator ani muscles, coccygeus, obturator internus, piriformis, and perineal membrane *(4)*. The muscles, associated fascia and ligaments, and the fascial attachments of the viscera work in concert to support the contents of the abdominopelvic cavity. The load carried by the pelvic floor is shared by all of its components. Damage to the pelvic muscles by injury, disease, or surgery increases the load on the fascia and vice versa.

The muscles of the pelvic floor consist of a group of muscles collectively known as the levator ani and the coccygeus. The levator ani are known separately as the pubococcygeus, iliococcygeus, and puborectalis (Fig. 1). The levator ani muscle shares in the mechanisms of defecation and urination as well as visceral support. Levator dysfunction as a result of nerve damage in uncomplicated vaginal delivery may lead to loss of pelvic organ support, as well as constipation or fecal and urinary incontinence. The innervation of the levator muscles has classically been attributed to the pudendal nerve, but recent detailed pelvic dissections of female cadavers found evidence that the levator ani were innervated by a nerve that originates from the third to fifth sacral foramina, termed the "levator ani nerve" *(5)*. Pelvic fascia, known as endopelvic fascia, can be subdivided further into the pubourethral ligaments, urethropelvic ligaments, pubocervical fascia, and the uterosacral ligament complex (Fig. 2). These subdivisions help to distinguish the importance of the fascia for specific support roles. The pubourethral ligaments are the fascial support of the mid-urethra to the inner surface of the inferior pubis. They support and stabilize the urethra and anterior vaginal wall. The external sphincter is located just distal to these ligaments. Laxity of these ligaments is partially responsible for stress urinary incontinence (SUI) as described by the integral theory *(6)*. The urethra is also supported on both sides by levator fascia. Proximally, this lateral urethral support is termed the urethropelvic ligaments. The urethropelvic ligaments are the endopelvic fascia that fuses the periurethral fascia to the arcus tendineus. It is the major support for the bladder neck and proximal urethra. These specialized areas of the endopelvic fascia are contiguous and not truly distinct structures.

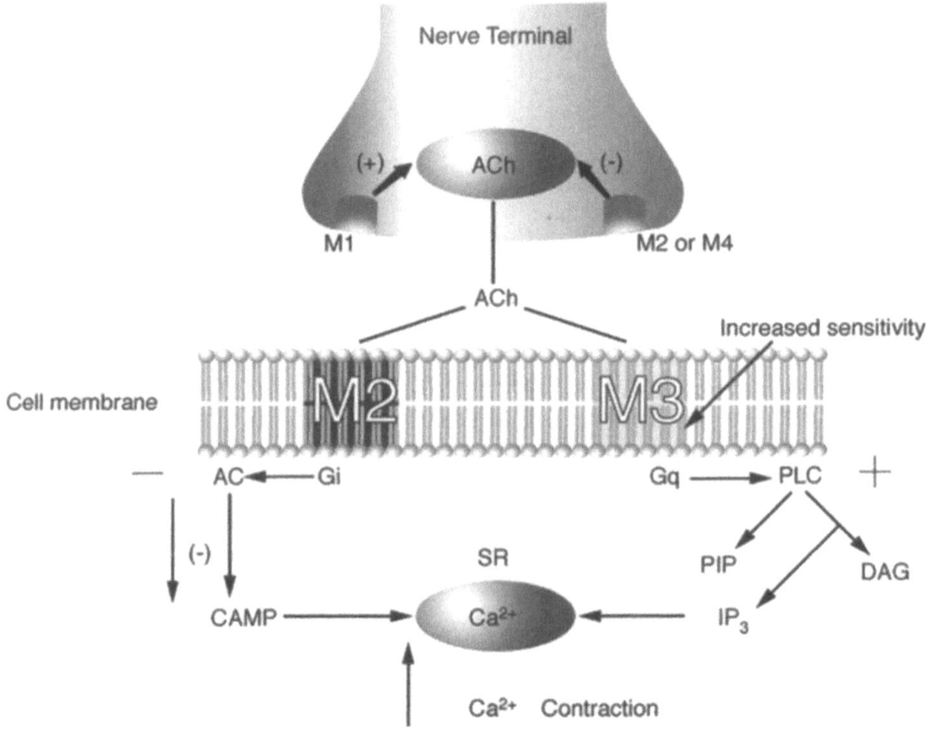

Fig. 1. Muscles of the levator ani and levator hiatuses: (**A**) urethra, (**B**) urogenital hiatus, (**C**) rectal hiatus, (**D**) pubococcygeus, (**E**) Iliococcygeus, and (**F**) coccygeus. Adapted from ref. *(59)*.

Urethral support is not determined by fascia alone. The pelvic muscles also are responsible. The fascial attachments responsible for urethral support are that of the pubourethral ligaments, periurethral tissue, and anterior vaginal wall to arcus tendineus fascia pelvis (paravaginal fascial attachment). The muscular component is the connection of periurethral tissues to the levator ani muscle. When these attachments are intact, continence is maintained. During increased abdominal pressure, the urethra is compressed against this firm supportive layer, as explained by the "Hammock Theory" of continence *(7)*. Weakening of these supports can lead to anterior wall relaxation and diminishment of the occlusive action of the vaginal support. It may be possible, as well, that aging and hormonal changes associated with menopause may alter the composition and strength of connective tissue *(8–11)*.

Urethral anatomy and its functional anatomic components are another important determinant of continence and are known as the intrinsic urethral

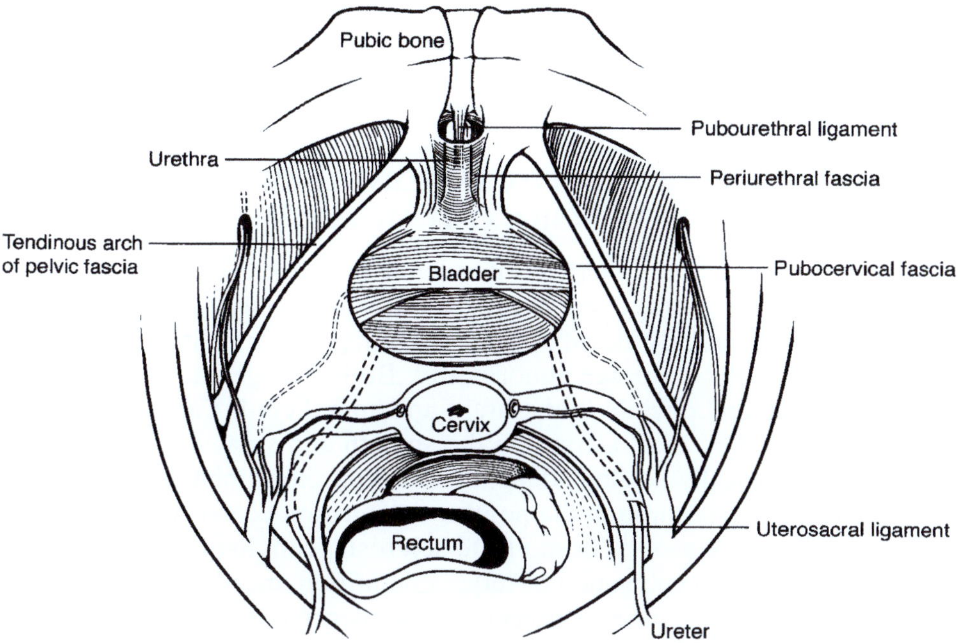

Fig. 2. Anatomy of the pelvis from a transabdominal perspective. Adapted from ref. *(60)*.

closure mechanism. The urethra is composed of a transitional epithelial mucosa with numerous infoldings that, in the normal state, provide excellent coaptation. A spongy vascular network lies beneath the mucosa and is surrounded by a thin layer of periurethral tissue. Smooth and striated muscle also surround the urethra and provide inwardly directed forces with the submucosal layer to strengthen coaptation. Damage to any of these functional components can result in intrinsic sphincteric deficiency (ISD) and clinical UI. Additionally, a minimal functional urethral length is necessary for continence. A distinction must be made between anatomic and functional urethral length. Anatomic length refers to the distance between the internal meatus and external urethral meatus. The functional urethral length refers to the portion of the urethra in which urethral pressure exceeds bladder pressure.

In summary, female continence is maintained by the interplay of several anatomic and functional mechanisms. With increases in intra-abdominal pressure, the abdominal pressure is passively transmitted to the proximal urethra, followed by an active contraction of the striated external sphincter. The suburethral supportive layer of periurethral fascia, anterior vaginal wall, and levator ani muscles acts as a backboard of support, against which, the urethra is compressed during increases in intra-abdominal pressure. Reflex contraction of the levator muscles directly increases mid-urethral pressure. Addition of voluntary contractions of levator and obturator muscles increases tension on the urethropelvic ligaments, which exacts the same effect.

BRIEF OVERVIEW OF THE INNERVATION OF THE LUT AND NEUROPHYSIOLOGY OF MICTURITION

LUT function may be simplified into two distinct and exclusive operations: low-pressure urine storage and coordinated urine emptying. Urinary tract disorders may be similarly classified as either storage abnormalities or emptying abnormalities. UI is a storage abnormality. Both storage and emptying are controlled by neural circuits in the brain and spinal cord. They are possibly further influenced by local activity in the smooth and striated muscles of the LUT. In neurologically healthy adults, there is conscious inhibitory control of the micturition reflex through the pontine micturition center. Disease states, such as stroke, Parkinson's, or multiple sclerosis, can disrupt the voluntary control and result in precipitation of reflex micturition, manifested clinically as bladder overactivity and urinary urgency incontinence (UUI).

Emptying or micturition is a parasympathetic mediated action primarily via the muscarinic receptor subtype M_3. The nerves responsible for micturition pass through the S2–S4 segments of the spinal cord. The pelvic nerve supplies parasympathetic input via acetylcholine to the bladder for detrusor contraction. Somatic innervation to the external sphincter is provided by the pudendal nerve via the action of acetylcholine at nicotinic receptors. The hypogastric nerve (T10–T12) carries sympathetic input responsible for bladder relaxation and exerts its effect through β-adrenergic receptors (β_3) at the detrusor and α_1 receptors in the bladder neck and proximal urethra. Micturition is accomplished by disinhibition of the pontine micturition center, sphincter relaxation, and acetylcholine stimulation of detrusor muscarinic receptors, which induces contraction. Five distinct subtypes of muscarinic receptors (M_1–M_5) exist in the LUT *(12)*. Although M_2 receptors are the predominant subtype within the detrusor, M_3 seems to be directly responsible for detrusor contraction *(13)*. The action and significance of M_2 in the detrusor is not known, but it may indirectly contribute to contraction by inhibiting detrusor relaxation and may have a prominent role in contraction under pathological conditions.

INCONTINENCE TERMINOLOGY

Four types of UI are distinguished: stress, urgency, mixed, and overflow. SUI is the involuntary loss of urine with activities that increase intra-abdominal pressure, such as coughing, sneezing, and walking. Prevailing theories of continence hold that the etiology of SUI is not purely anatomic. All women who leak likely have some degree of intrinsic sphincter deficiency, a functional deficit, because not all women with anatomic defects leak. On the other hand, it is possible to have pure ISD, as in the woman with a fixed immobile urethra with leakage.

UUI is the involuntary loss of urine preceded by a strong uncontrollable urge to urinate. Urgency can occur with a sensory or motor dysfunction. In sensory urgency, the woman experiences an intense desire to urinate without an involuntary detrusor contraction. She may experience such an intense urge that she must "let go" of urine to relieve the sensation. Urgency associated with an involuntary phasic contraction of the detrusor that cannot be suppressed may result in precipitous voiding. In women without a known neurological lesion, the uninhibited contractions are termed idiopathic detrusor overactivity. In cases of women with a neurological disease, the uninhibited detrusor contractions are termed neurogenic detrusor overactivity. The exact mechanisms causing UUI are not fully understood, and most cases are deemed idiopathic.

Mixed incontinence describes the condition of both SUI and UUI. Mixed incontinence presents a therapeutic challenge for the clinician because the two types of incontinence are treated differently. Women with mixed incontinence are at high risk for worsening of the urgency component after surgery for SUI. These patients require a thorough urodynamic assessment before considering invasive therapy to confirm the diagnosis and establish the more predominant type. Even with this information, women with mixed incontinence remain a difficult population to treat.

Overflow incontinence is leakage secondary to the inability to void completely. When the bladder capacity is great enough to produce a bladder pressure in excess of the outlet pressure, leakage will occur until pressure in the bladder is less than the outlet. Overflow incontinence may be observed in the diabetic patient who has impaired sensation and detrusor contraction as a result of diabetic neuropathy. It may also be seen in the contracted, fibrotic irradiated bladder, in which the bladder pressure increases dramatically with filling as a result of loss of elasticity and impaired compliance or in bladder outlet obstruction. Outlet obstruction in women occurs most commonly after surgeries to correct SUI.

Some clinicians also recognize "spontaneous" leakage, in which the woman is not aware of any inciting factors for her leakage. This type of leakage may be caused by very low outlet resistance, so that leak is essentially gravitational, requiring almost imperceptible activities. It may alternatively be related to an uninhibited contraction in a person with impaired bladder sensation, so that they are unaware of any urge associated with leak. Small-volume spontaneous leakage that is vague and rarely more than dampness in underwear or small pad, may be watery vaginal secretions—physiological or pathological. Leakage may also be related to extra-urethral causes, such as vesicovaginal fistula, or ectopic ureter. However, leakage in these cases is usually of a much larger volume as it bypasses the sphincter mechanism. Fistulas are most commonly a consequence of hysterectomy but related to obstructed labor outside of the Western world. Ectopic ureters are congenital and typically present in childhood with recurrent urinary tract infections (UTIs) and incontinence.

EVALUATION

Urinary incontinence is a disorder of urine storage; however, it is important to catalog the extent of all storage and emptying symptoms that the woman may be experiencing. The health care provider (HCP) should inquire about urinary frequency and quantify how many times the woman voids in a 24-hour period. Separately, the number of times she gets up at night to void (nocturia) should be recorded. Nocturia may represent a normal physiological increase in urine production at night or may be related to detrusor overactivity. The patient's fluid intake during the day and the timing of her fluid intake should be estimated. This information is important because urinary frequency and high urine production may be caused by an excessive fluid intake. If she drinks a significant amount at night or routinely consumes alcohol or caffeine at night, the diuresis may be self-imposed. It is also helpful to ask whether the patient with nocturia is waking with an urge to void or waking for other reasons and then choosing to void while she is up. Many elderly women have sleep disturbances rather than LUT problems as the source of their nocturia. Urgency may be associated with frequency, and the severity of urgency may be gauged by asking whether the patient is able to delay voiding and for how long? Finally, the incontinence should be investigated for its nature, causative factors, severity, and duration. Does the woman have any coping behaviors, such as self-imposed frequency or fluid restriction to prevent her bladder from getting full? The nature of UI can be determined by asking under what circumstances she leaks. Is it with activity, urge, both, or spontaneous? If with activity, what is the least amount of activity required to make her leak? UUI can be hard for some women to recognize. For those women who may not be able to easily associate their leakage with urgency, the HCP should listen for classic scenarios of UUI in her history, such as leakage while doing dishes or as she puts her key in the door when she arrives home. The duration of the incontinence may be revealing of any transient and reversible causes for it (Table 1). Did the patient just begin to experience leakage recently, concurrent with a change in medication? In most cases, women describe UI as having been progressive over time. It may have

Table 1
Transient/ Reversible Causes of Urinary Incontinence

Delirium
Infection (Urinary tract infection)
Atrophic changes of the genital tract
Pharmacological agents
Psychological/psychiatric factors
Excess urine production
Restricted mobility
Stool impaction

been mild after the birth of her first child but escalated quickly after subsequent births or after menopause. The severity of UI is assessed in the history by several methods. First, the woman's pad usage is commonly given as a measure of the leakage severity. A patient who uses three pads a day would be considered as having worse incontinence than the patient who used one pad per day. However, not all pads are the same, and women have different levels of tolerance for wet pads. Therefore, it is more helpful to determine whether she is wearing thick or thin pads and whether the pads are damp or saturated when they are changed. The degree of bother from UI can be assessed by asking her to quantify her bother on an escalating scale of 1 to 10.

Emptying symptoms, such as hesitation, straining to void, intermittent or slow stream, and a feeling of incomplete emptying are essential to document in the history. Impaired voiding may be the source of storage symptoms, particularly UI. Any other urological symptoms or complaints should be documented as part of a genitourinary review of symptoms. For instance, does the woman have any pelvic pain, dyspareunia, hematuria, pyuria, history of UTIs, history of urolithiasis, or history of urological or gynecological malignancy? UI is the most common disorder of the pelvic floor, but the HCP should screen for other pelvic floor disorders, such as constipation, diarrhea, fecal soilage, a history of splinting to defecate, or evidence of a vaginal bulge.

Has the woman ever sought help for her UI before? What was her previous experience with that HCP? Some women have been told that nothing could be done for her problem or, conversely, that the only option was surgery. She may have undergone painful and unnecessary procedures for LUT symptoms, such as urethral dilations, by well-intentioned but misinformed HCPs in the past. Negative experiences may have kept her from seeking further options. It is helpful to document any previous treatment for her UI and her response to each treatment. Has she tried pelvic floor exercises (Kegel's) in a dedicated fashion? Has she been administered a trial of medication? What agent was used and for how long? Did she have any adverse reaction to medication for UI? Has she had any previous surgery for UI?

The remainder of the history is the same as would be performed for a new patient with any complaint, but special emphasis is placed on certain areas.

MEDICAL HISTORY

Many medical conditions may have repercussions for the LUT. Diabetes can contribute to urinary urgency, frequency, impaired bladder sensation, and impaired emptying. Congestive heart failure and venous insufficiency may contribute significantly to nocturia because fluid in dependent portions is mobilized while recumbent, leading to increased urine production at night. Neurological diseases, such as cerebrovascular accidents, Parkinson's, multiple sclerosis, spinal cord injury, and neuropathies may all affect the LUT as well. Generally, an incontinent, young, premenopausal, nulliparous woman without any other risk factors for UI should be considered at risk for an occult neurological disorder *(14)*. LUT symptoms of incontinence and/or retention accompanied by any neurological sign or symptom such as visual disturbance, numbness or tingling in an extremity, or lack of coordination should prompt the HCP to refer for neurological consultation.

SURGICAL HISTORY

Any history of previous pelvic surgery should be identified. Hysterectomy and oophorectomy may contribute to hormonal changes and pelvic organ prolapse. UI in the patient with a previous anti-incontinence surgery may signify a failed surgery, leakage caused by detrusor overactivity, or overflow incontinence secondary to iatrogenic obstruction. A history of radical pelvic surgery, as for gynecological malignancy, suggests possible nerve damage to the pelvic floor and LUT.

FAMILY HISTORY

Connective tissue diseases, some of which are familial, are a risk factor for UI and pelvic organ prolapse *(15)*. It is, therefore, helpful to document whether such diseases run in the family and whether there are other incontinent women in her immediate family. Any neurological diseases in the woman's immediate family should also be documented.

SOCIAL HISTORY

Whether cigarette smoking in women is linked to SUI and UUI is not clear, but some investigators support this claim *(16)*. Heavy alcohol or illicit drug use

Table 2
Drugs That Affect the Lower Urinary Tract

Potentiate Urinary Retention	*Potentiate Urinary Incontinence*
Psychotropics	ACE Inhibitors
Antidepressants	α-adrenergic blockers
Antipsychotics	Alcohol
Sedative/hypnotics	Caffeine
Calcium channel blockers	Diuretics
Anticholinergics	
α-adrenergic agonists	
β-agonists	
Narcotics	

may also promote incontinence by altering cerebral control and antidiuretic hormone production.

MEDICATIONS

A complete list of prescription and over-the-counter medications is necessary, because many classes of drugs have effects on the LUT (Table 2). Diuretics, particularly in the elderly, can promote frequency, urgency, and UI by increasing the urine output. α-blockers taken for hypertension may promote UI by decreasing outlet resistance. Anticholinergics and drugs with anticholinergic effects, such as many antidepressants, in women with poor emptying may develop worsening of their emptying and overflow incontinence. Sedative hypnotics may impair a woman's ability to sense when her bladder is full and impair her ability to get to the bathroom, leading to enuresis.

OBSTETRICS AND GYNECOLOGY HISTORY

The woman's hormonal status should be documented. UI is more common in the postmenopausal woman. Premenopausal women may note that leakage is worse just before menses. As a woman enters the perimenopausal phase, she may begin to experience changes in the LUT, such as frequency, urgency, and/or incontinence for the first time. Additional questions that have relevance to pelvic floor dysfunction include: How many pregnancies and births has she had? Did she deliver vaginally or by Caesarean section? Was her delivery complicated by tears and to what extent? How large was her largest baby? Pregnancy alone, as well as vaginal delivery, are significant risk factors for pelvic floor disorders and specifically, UI. SUI occurs in 32 to 85% of pregnant women and peaks in the third trimester; however, the majority will have resolution

Table 3
Findings in the Woman's History That Indicated a Need for Referral to a Female Urologist or Urogynecologist

1. Continuous incontinence
2. Urinary retention, significant voiding symptoms, or documented incomplete emptying
3. Spontaneous loss of urine or bedwetting
4. History of neurological disease, injury, or surgery associated with urinary incontinence
5. History of repeated urethral dilation or internal urethrotomy
6. History of previous incontinence surgery that either failed or made the problem worse
7. History of radical pelvic surgery
8. History of pelvic radiation

of SUI within 3 months of delivery *(17)*. Because of the high rate of spontaneous resolution, SUI during pregnancy or in the immediate postpartum is best treated conservatively. Multiparas may be at higher risk for persistence of SUI in the postpartum, although whether obstetrical pelvic floor damage is cumulative is controversial *(18,19)*. Injury to the levator ani and pudendal nerve are the most likely obstetrical injuries leading to UI. The risk of pudendal nerve injury is increased by forceps delivery, increased duration of the second stage of labor, third-degree perineal tear, large infant size, and multiparity *(20)*. Another obstetrical risk factor for UI is episiotomy, therefore, episiotomy is no longer part of a routine vaginal delivery. Current opinion is that episiotomies are associated with a greater risk of perineal trauma and diminished rate of perineal recovery compared with an intact perineum *(21,22)*. Pelvic radiation may have grave consequences for bladder function. The long-term effects of radiation include bladder ischemia and resultant fibrosis or fistula. Radiation cystitis can lead to urinary incontinence caused by loss of reservoir compliance and decreased outlet resistance. This is a functional problem diagnosed best by a urodynamic study. Women with a history of pelvic radiation should be referred to a urologist.

As part of a thorough UI evaluation, an attempt should be made to determine the impact that the UI has on the patient's quality of life (QOL). UI is a QOL issue, and treatment choices are dependent on how bothered she is by her condition. The collection of health-related QOL (HRQOL) data in urinary incontinence has become as important to evaluation and treatment as objective measures, such as pad tests and urodynamics. Questionnaires can be a helpful way to describe the impact of symptoms on QOL. Two commonly used validated instruments specific for UI are the Urogenital Distress Inventory and the Incontinence Impact Questionnaire *(23)*. Both have been condensed into short forms that are more convenient for clinical use. They may also be useful as a semi-objective way of assessing response to treatment. Another useful instrument for LUT symptoms in general is the American Urological Association Symptom Index (AUASI). Although not validated in women, scores have been shown to correlate highly with degree of bother in women *(24)*. This seven-item instrument provides more information regarding emptying symptoms than the short forms of the Urogenital Distress Inventory and Incontinence Impact Questionnaire, and may be a helpful adjunct questionnaire.

PHYSICAL EXAM

The physical exam is focused on the abdomen and pelvis, but an abbreviated neurological assessment is also routinely included. With the woman seated on the exam table, her back is examined for evidence of scars indicating neurological surgery, spinal curvature, spinal pain, tenderness or stiffness suggesting arthritis or degenerative joint disease, or sacral dimple or tuft suggesting occult spinal dysraphism. Deep tendon reflexes can be checked as well as sensation and strength in her lower extremities as a screening of the lumbosacral nerve roots. Alterations in normal function by this simple screening may prompt further neurological evaluation/consultation.

In a recumbent position, the abdomen is examined for evidence of scars indicating previous abdominal or pelvic surgery that may have been overlooked in the history. Palpation of the abdomen may reveal any organomegaly, masses, or ascites that may influence intra-abdominal pressure and, thus, impact continence. The inguinal canal is palpated for evidence of adenopathy.

A pelvic exam may or may not be out of the scope of the primary care provider's standard practice. The following description of a detailed pelvic exam is more consistent with what would be expected from evaluation by a specialist. The patient is asked to move into the dorsal lithotomy position for the pelvic exam. First inspection includes documentation of skin changes on the perineum and inner thighs. Severely incontinent women often have erythematous and chaffed perineal skin caused by constant wetness and irritation from continence pads. Vulvar skin may also appear whitish or erythematous, because of hypoestrogenism or vulvar dystrophies. Perineal sensation can be assessed at this time with both the soft and firm ends of a cotton swab. Although not necessary in healthy patients, those with known or suspected neurological conditions should have a bulbocavernous reflex checked. This reflex can be elicited by tapping the clitoris with a cotton swab. An intact reflex produces contraction of the bulbocavernosus muscles and an anal wink. Evidence of constant urine leakage from the vagina in this position may indicate an extra-urethral source that needs further radiological evaluation, looking for fistula or ectopic ureter.

While still in lithotomy, the introitus is inspected at rest and with Valsalva to identify any vaginal bulge indicative of pelvic organ prolapse. A simple supine stress test can be performed before the speculum exam by spreading the labia to visualize the urethral meatus and asking the woman to cough or Valsalva. Urine leakage per meatus with cough or Valsalva suggests SUI; however, this test is not 100% specific for SUI. In some cases, leakage may be caused by stress-induced detrusor overactivity that only urodynamics could distinguish. In women with significant prolapse of the bladder (known as cystocele or anterior compartment prolapse), SUI may not be evident until the prolapse is reduced; therefore, the supine stress test may need to be repeated after reduction by a packing, pessary, or speculum. Evidence of SUI after reduction is known as occult SUI. The speculum exam is made easier by separating the two halves of a Graves speculum. The anterior blade is put aside and the lower blade is used for inspection of the pelvic floor. The lower blade of the speculum is used to retract the posterior vaginal wall for better visualization of the anterior wall. The vaginal walls are examined for evidence of mucosal atrophy, such as dry, thin tissue with loss of normal rugation. The urethra is palpated for any mass or tenderness. The bladder is palpated bimanually and any distention or tenderness is noted. The patient is again asked to Valsalva and any descensus of the anterior vaginal wall is documented and graded. Several different grading systems exist *(25,26)*. Descensus of the anterior vaginal wall with movement of the urethral meatus during Valsalva is known as hypermobility. It signifies some degree of lack of anatomic support. Traditionally a Q-tip test has been used to gauge the degree of hypermobility; however, a Q-tip placed in the urethra is likely to be painful *(27,28)*. The presence of urethrovesical junction mobility can be determined by examination during Valsalva and a Q-tip test is not necessary. The pelvic floor musculature can be assessed for strength and sensation by palpation of the levator ani laterally. Palpation of these muscles while the patient performs a Kegel exercise helps determine the strength of the patient's pelvic floor muscles as well as her ability to isolate the pubococcygeus. Inability to isolate the proper muscles or lack of strength in the muscles signifies a need for special attention during future pelvic floor exercise treatment regimens. Women with complaints of pelvic pain frequently have very tense levator muscles on one or both sides.

The posterior compartment of the pelvic floor must be assessed. The lower blade is flipped and used to retract the anterior wall for determination of any rectal prolapse (rectocele or posterior compartment prolapse). A gentle rectal exam is performed to rule out a rectal mass and assess the integrity of the rectovaginal septum, and check for normal rectal tone. Before completing the exam, if UI has not been demonstrated with the patient in lithotomy, or if there is evidence of pelvic organ prolapse, the woman should be examined in the standing position. The patient is asked to elevate one foot on a step which separates her legs for better visualization of the perineum. She is then asked to cough or Valsalva to elicit leakage. In this upright position, any prolapse is graded at rest and with Valsalva as well.

LABORATORY TESTS

A urinalysis is an integral part of any urological evaluation. In the woman complaining of UI, the urinalysis should be performed to exclude a UTI or hematuria. Dipstick positive results for leukocyte esterase and blood, suggestive of UTI, should be confirmed by microscopic examination of a centrifuged specimen. If microscopic findings are consistent with a large number of white blood cells and bacteria, a urine culture should be obtained. Infection is a common transient cause of UI, or it may be a reason for UI exacerbation. A finding of greater than three to five red blood cells per high power field is considered significant enough to prompt a full hematuria workup, including a urine cytology, a contrasted upper tract study (CT scan with contrast or intravenous pyelogram), and a cystoscopy. Hematuria may be the first or only presentation of urothelial malignancies; although malignancy is a rare source for irritative LUT symptoms and associated UUI. A urine pregnancy test should be considered in the woman of childbearing age, not using reliable birth control, because urinary frequency and incontinence are common in pregnancy.

VOIDING DIARIES

Voiding diaries are an inexpensive and easy way of obtaining baseline data on a patient's voiding patterns in her own environment. The information obtained may provide insights into behavioral factors that could be responsible for UI. No standardization exists for what information should be recorded, and patient compliance is an issue with any diary. In most cases, the voiding diary should include the time of micturition, time and type of incontinence, and voided volume in a 24-hour period. In addition, the patient should quantify her fluid intake as closely as possible and record the time at which she is drinking. Recording the type of beverage can help point out if she is a heavy consumer of bladder irritants, such as caffeine and alcohol. Review of the voiding diary provides an assessment of the patient's day and night time frequency, a quantification of how much she drinks a day, and an estimate of her functional bladder capacity, which is the largest amount of urine her bladder will comfortably hold. Comparing voiding diaries before and after initiation of treatment may be used to assess response.

PAD TEST

A pad test is a semi-objective measurement of urine loss. Used pads are weighed and compared with the dry weight of an identical pad. Simply asking a woman how many pads she uses per day is not a reliable way of determining the severity of UI, because not all pads are equal and every woman has a different tolerance for when to change a pad. For example, some women change a pad every time they go to the bathroom whether it is wet or not, whereas others wait until a pad is saturated to change it. The patient who uses only two pads per day but finds them saturated when she changes then may have worse UI than the woman who uses five pads but finds them only damp. Pad tests may be 1 hour or 24 hours in duration, and, similar to voiding diaries, compliance is improved with the shorter task.

UROFLOW/FREE FLOW

The uninstrumented uroflow is an office test that screens for voiding phase abnormalities. A cystometrogram alone, which examines only the filling phase, can miss abnormalities in the voiding phase that may be contributing to the storage problem or impacting the success of treatment *(29)*. The uroflow may be particularly helpful in the patient with voiding symptoms, such as hesitancy, straining, or a feeling of incomplete emptying. Although a uroflow can detect impairment in flow and emptying, it cannot distinguish between obstruction and impaired detrusor contractility. It may be most useful as a quick screen to detect those who need further urodynamic investigation. It is also a good benchmark against which to compare an instrumented flow known as a pressure-flow study. Abnormalities in the instrumented flow may be related to artifact introduced by the urethral catheter. If the interpreting physician has an uninstrumented flow with which to compare, she may more readily identify a true voiding abnormality and avoid overinterpreting artifact.

URODYNAMICS

Multichannel urodynamics refers to a sophisticated study of bladder function. It may be divided into two separate but related phases: storage (cystometrogram) and emptying (pressure–flow). It is used to assess detrusor activity and contractility, sensation, capacity, compliance, force and duration of contraction, flow, and ability to empty. It is the only tool that can diagnose the underlying pathophysiology of the UI. If performed with simultaneous fluoroscopy, relevant anatomic features, such as the site of bladder outlet obstruction, presence of vesicoureteral reflux, bladder diverticula, and the integrity of the sphincter are identified. Most urologists and urogynecologists perform multichannel urodynamics before any procedure for SUI and in all complicated UI cases, such as those with a history of surgery, radiation, or neurological disease.

CYSTOSCOPY

Cystoscopy is not necessary for the evaluation of uncomplicated UI unless the patient has associated hematuria, defined as at least 3 to 5 red blood cells per high powered field, or pyuria in the absence of infection. The urologist or urogynecologist may opt to perform cystoscopy in a case of failed incontinence surgery or recurrent UI.

TREATMENT

Treatment options vary from noninvasive to surgical intervention. Some of the factors that influence treatment choice are the nature of the UI, the amount of bother it causes, whether previous treatment has been instituted, and how successful it was. Most importantly, a woman should be given all of her options, so that she may make a truly informed decision. Conservative treatment that uses noninvasive modalities first is a safe and logical approach that can be initiated by the primary care physician as well as the specialist.

BEHAVIORAL MODIFICATION

Behavioral therapy includes education, keeping voiding diaries and charts, the development of timed voiding and bladder training regimens, physiotherapy with or without biofeedback, and reinforcement. Behavioral therapies have been shown to work for both SUI and UUI. In a recent study, 52.5% of women with SUI who were given a book on modifying their behavior had a positive response and improvement in their SUI *(30)*. This result likely represents the best response to behavioral modification in a highly motivated population. The power of behavioral modification is also reflected in the significant placebo effect noted in most overactive bladder drug studies. It is not truly a placebo effect but the effect of patients becoming more aware of their condition and altering behaviors based on keeping periodic voiding diaries.

PELVIC MUSCLE EXERCISES

Pelvic muscle exercises (PME) are a viable option in neurologically intact patients who are highly motivated for treatment of SUI or UUI. It may be used alone or as an adjunct to other treatment such as pharmacotherapy. Also known as “Kegel exercises” after Dr. Arnold Kegel, the obstetrician–gynecologist who first introduced them, they are a series of levator ani contractions. How PME effect their change on LUT function is not clearly understood, but success depends on the patient first being able to isolate the pelvic floor muscles and the existence of pelvic floor contractility. The goal of PME is to isolate the pelvic floor muscles and produce repeated high intensity contractions of the levator ani muscle fibers. The levator ani is composed of both slow and fast twitch fibers. The majority of levator ani is slow-twitch muscle fibers (Type I) which produce a slower more sustained contraction of less force. These fibers assist in muscle endurance, and contraction of them over time helps maintain pelvic support and urethral closure pressure. Fast twitch fibers (Type II) are key for sudden increases in intra-abdominal pressure and urethral closure. Exercising these muscle fibers contributes to muscle strength. The proportion of Type II fibers decreases with inactivity, aging, and innervation damage.

PME are useful for rehabilitation of muscles with both low tone (weak/atrophic) and high tone. Patients with low tone are usually bothered by problems or UI, fecal incontinence, or pelvic organ prolapse. The high-tone pelvic floor is seen in patients with spastic pelvic floor muscles and chronic pelvic pain. PME are used to enhance muscle relaxation in these patients.

Some patients have difficulty isolating the pubococcygeus and may require the aid of a physical therapist or advanced practice clinician with special expertise in the treatment of the pelvic floor to learn how to identify the muscles. The correct technique is to "draw in" and "lift up" the muscles around the vagina and anal sphincter. PME performed incorrectly will be of no benefit but are not likely to be harmful. The patient should be cautioned, however, not to perform the exercises while urinating. Although starting and stopping the urine stream does use the same muscles, it can set up poor voiding habits and impair emptying. An optimal PME regimen would have the patient do exercises three times a day for 10 to 15 minutes each time. Results with exercises are generally not seen for approx 8 weeks, and the main obstacle to this treatment is lack of patient compliance.

Biofeedback using EMG is a way by which the patient is immediately made aware of her pelvic floor muscle function. It can measure strength, endurance, and contractility of the muscle. Muscle training with biofeedback can improve muscle relaxation and strengthen weak pelvic muscles. Additional reinforcement is provided by the clinician who monitors the exercise and provides verbal feedback.

Vaginal weights are another form of biofeedback technique applied to the treatment of SUI. Use of the weights is very easy to learn and requires no supervision. The weights are plastic cone shaped vaginal inserts. The patient inserts the lightest weight first and retains it during activity for up to 15 minutes. She then attempts to retain heavier weights until she reaches a weight that she cannot retain. In theory, the vaginal weights provide sensory feedback to prompt the pelvic floor muscles to contract, preventing extrusion of the weight.

The application of low-grade electrical stimulation (ES) via skin electrodes to the pelvic floor muscles to produce a passive contraction can be added to PME regimens. It is used both for contraction of the pelvic floor muscles and to inhibit unwanted detrusor contractions. The addition of biofeedback with ES can help provide awareness of the passive contraction. Originally, this modality required daily trips to the therapist's office, but the ease of use has been improved with the introduction of a battery-operated home unit. Results of ES vary, and its benefit in UI is controversial.

BARRIER METHODS

Pessaries and other intravaginal devices can be used as first line treatment for SUI, mixed urinary incontinence, and associated pelvic organ prolapse. They are particularly helpful in elderly or unhealthy women who may not be candidates for surgery. Women who leak with only a certain activity such as jogging or dancing may opt for the use of an incontinence pessary during those activities rather than undergoing surgery. Pessaries prevent UI by supporting the bladder neck and preventing urethral mobility rather than occluding the urethra. Incontinence pessaries should not have a negative effect on voiding, and in cases of severe prolapse, the use of a pessary may actually improve voiding.

Tampons are practical, inexpensive, and easy devices that have been shown to be of some help in women with a mild degree of SUI. In some cases, even a contraceptive diaphragm can improve bladder neck support and prevent SUI. The Continence Ring is a pessary created specifically for the management of SUI. A small knob on the ring is positioned at the bladder neck to provide support and prevent leak. Pessaries must be fitted to the individual woman's vaginal capacity and conformations. The fitting process is largely by trial and error, necessitating a great deal of time and patience on the part of both the woman and the practitioner. The pessary should fit snugly but not be uncomfortable. It needs to be removed and cleaned regularly. If the patient is unable to do this herself, she will need to have her HCP do this in the office every 6 weeks. Concomitant use of estrogen cream in the postmenopausal woman is helpful to keep the tissue healthy and resilient. Contraindications to pessary use include severely atrophic vaginal tissues, inability to remove the pessary and lack of reliability to present to the office for routine changes, undiagnosed vaginal bleeding or discharge, or vaginal or cervical cancer.

External adhesive foam pads (Miniguard®, Uromed®, or Softpatch®) have been developed as a barrier method for SUI. The pad is placed between the labia, over the urethral meatus, to create a seal and prevent leakage. It can be worn up to 5 hours a day and through the night. The pad is removed for urination, and a new one is placed after voiding. Disposable urethral suction caps (CapSure®, or FemAssist®) that fit over the meatus are another option. FemSoft™ is a small disposable tube with a balloon on one end that works as an occlusive intraurethral plug to prevent UI. It also requires fitting to determine the optimal size by measurement of the urethra. The tube is inserted into the urethra with a reusable syringe. When the woman desires to urinate, she deflates the balloon on the tube by pulling a string on the device, and the entire device is removed. Like any foreign body in the urinary tract, this device carries a higher risk of infection and irritation than the external barrier methods, but a multicenter study of 150 women found statistically significant reductions in daily incontinence episodes and pad weight tests at a mean of 15 months of follow-up. Significant improvements in QOL were also observed, and adverse events were mild and transient *(31)*.

PHARMACOTHERAPY

SUI is a medical condition rarely treated pharmacologically. Currently, no Food and Drug Administration (FDA)-approved drug exists for SUI, and the medications commonly used to treat it are used off-label. Imipramine, α-adrenergic agonists, and estrogens have been tried with anecdotal success. Investigation into the use of β-adrenergic antagonists, β-adrenergic agonists, and combined serotonin (5-HT) and norepinephrine (NE) reuptake inhibitors is ongoing. Conversely, pharmacotherapy is the mainstay of treatment for UUI, and the most effective agents are antimuscarinics. The market has virtually exploded with new antimuscarinics within the last year.

Duloxetine is a balanced dual 5-HT and NE reuptake inhibitor that is currently FDA-approved for depression and diabetic neuropathy (Cymbalta®) and has been investigated for a SUI indication. It is the most exciting new development in the pharmacotherapy of SUI in recent decades, but, recently, the manufacturer withdrew its application to the FDA. Currently duloxetine is not approved for the treatment of SUI, and the FDA is evaluating additional data.

Duloxetine, a centrally acting agent, affects SUI by blocking the reuptake of 5-HT and NE in Onuf's nucleus, where the pudendal motor neurons are located in the spinal cord. When higher levels of 5-HT and NE exist, there is an increased activity on a greater number of postsynaptic receptors, a greater activation of pudendal nerve motor neurons, and increased urethral sphincter tone. Duloxetine has shown little or no inhibition of dopamine reuptake or affinity for histaminergic, dopaminergic, adrenergic, or cholinergic receptors; therefore, it should produce few side effects.

In Phase III studies undertaken in North America, 683 women with SUI and complaining of at least seven weekly episodes of SUI were enrolled. They were randomized to either 80 mg/d duloxetine or placebo for 12 weeks. Women receiving duloxetine showed statistically significant reductions of incontinent episode frequency versus placebo (50% vs 27%; $p < 0.001$). Even women with severe or high-grade SUI showed equivalent improvement, indicating that duloxetine was effective in SUI of all degrees. Improvements in QOL were statistically significant in the total population of women with severe SUI (+11 vs +6.8; $p < 0.001$). Improvements were associated with significant increases in voiding intervals, indicating that the response was not caused by voiding more frequently. A full 10.5% of duloxetine-treated patients and 5.9% of placebo-treated patients became completely dry *(32)*.

The most common side effect from the drug and the most common cause of discontinuation of studies with it is nausea, reported by 22.7% of patients in one study. The nausea was considered mild-to-moderately severe in 87% and 74% of those affected who completed the study.

Estrogens have been supported for the treatment of both SUI and UUI in the past, but its effectiveness for these disorders is controversial. A recent meta-analysis of estrogens for the treatment of LUT symptoms concluded that the literature does not support estrogen as a treatment for UI. It may be helpful for the symptom of urgency, and in a topical vaginally administered form, it is clearly helpful for the prevention of recurrent UTIs in postmenopausal women *(33)*. Recently published findings of the Women's Health Initiative support a higher risk of UI in women receiving conjugated equine estrogen alone and conjugated equine estrogen with medroxyprogesterone acetate *(34)*. The topic of estrogen replacement remains an issue fraught with unclear and often contradictory conclusions.

The vagina is an estrogen-sensitive organ. Estrogen receptors have also been identified in the female bladder trigone and urethra *(35,36)*. Hypo-estrogenization of the vaginal tissues contributes to vaginal irritation manifested as atrophic vaginitis. When these changes are seen in the vagina, similar irritation is likely occurring in the urinary tract. A low-dose topical estrogen used two to three times a week may help lessen these bothersome problems with little systemic absorption. In the patient who cannot use estrogens in any form or chooses not to, a nonprescription mucosal protectant preparation, such as Replens®, can be used for vaginal irritation and dryness.

Imipramine hydrochloride is a tricyclic antidepressant that has both systemic anticholinergic effects and a possible α-adrenergic effect at the bladder outlet. It also inhibits the reuptake of NE and 5-HT, which may be another mechanism by which it could increase outlet resistance. A few small open-label studies have shown improvement in women with SUI using a 75 mg daily dose; however, to date, no randomized controlled trials of imipramine exist *(37,38)*.

α-adrenergic agonists have been used for their ability to increase tone at the bladder outlet and reduce SUI. Ephedrine and pseudoephedrine have shown improvement in UI in women with minimal to moderate SUI, but little effect is observed in those with a greater degree of leakage *(39,40)*. Use of these agents is significantly hampered by their nonselective nature. Side effects of increased blood pressure, anxiety, headache, tremor, palpitations, and dysrhythmias make them undesirable and unsafe in some patients. Phenylpropanolamine and agents with phenylpropanolamine as an ingredient were removed from the market because of dangerous cardiovascular side effects.

Antimuscarinics for the treatment of UUI are standard first-line treatment in patients with significant bother from the condition. The rationale for their use is that muscarinic receptor subtype M_3 is responsible for detrusor contraction, and M_2 may also play a role, particularly in some pathological conditions *(41,42)*. All currently available antimuscarinics have a significant effect at the M_3 receptor and varied degrees of effect at other muscarinic receptors subtypes. None of the available agents is completely uroselective and, therefore, these medications have side effects caused by their action on muscarinic receptors outside of the urinary tract. The most common side effects of dry mouth, constipation, and blurry vision are caused by the effect of the drug at the salivary gland, bowel, and ciliary muscle, respectively. Newer drug-delivery systems seen in the long-acting and transdermal preparations have helped improve the side effect profile. The choice of antimuscarinic to treat UUI is based on the individual patient's needs and concerns, and the physician's familiarity and comfort with a particular agent.

MINIMALLY INVASIVE AND SURGICAL OPTIONS FOR URINARY INCONTINENCE

Bulking Agents for SUI

Bulking agents are minimally invasive, temporary options for the treatment of SUI. Originally described for the treatment of ISD, use has been expanded to include patients with hypermobility and to salvage a recurrent incontinence after sling procedures or urethrolysis *(43–45)*. These materials are injected with transurethral or periurethral method during cystourethroscopy to coapt the mucosa of the proximal urethra and increase outlet resistance. One of the major advantages of this modality is that they can be injected as an office procedure with minimal discomfort and little risk of complication. The risk of permanent urinary retention is almost negligible and rates of de novo detrusor overactivity are less than or equal to that with surgery. Disadvantages are that one injection may not be enough to obtain dryness, so it is often repeated the following month. Lack of significant improvement after three successive injections generally signals that further injections of the same agent will be futile. Additionally studies suggest that bulking agents need to be re-injected over time.

Two FDA-approved bulking agents are available for use today: Contigen® and Durasphere™. Contigen® (Bard, Inc., Covington, GA) is a glutaraldehyde cross-linked bovine collagen that causes no inflammatory reaction and becomes colonized by host fibroblasts after injection. Patients must be skin tested 30 days before injection to prove that the patient is not allergic. Injection of Contigen® is easy in experienced hands and well tolerated by the patient. Its effect is not permanent and repeat injections will be necessary. Durasphere™ (Carbon Medical Technologies, Inc., St. Paul, MN) is composed of non-absorbable pyrolytic zirconium oxide beads in a carrier gel. It is a reasonable first-option bulking agent and also offers an option for the patient with an allergy to Contigen®. An advantage of this material is that no skin test is needed before its administration. Durasphere™ injection requires a larger bore needle than collagen, and there is a greater learning curve for the successful injection of this material than for collagen. However, it is still a viable option for office administration.

Success rates of bulking agents vary widely from study to study, and our ability to interpret the results is hampered by differences in the definitions of cure and dry used and lack of long-term results. Overall, short-and intermediate-term results with both agents support dry rates of 25%, improvement rates of 50%, and failure rates of 25%. Patient satisfaction with bulking agents is highly dependent on them having the correct expectations of improvement rather than cure.

SURGERY FOR SUI

Current consensus of the American Urologic Association is that retropubic suspensions and autologous fascial sling procedures are the most effective procedures for long-term success. Both procedures show cure rates of approximately 85% at 4 years *(46)*. Data at 10 years and beyond, in some cases, shows cure rates similar to the short-term rates. The classic pubovaginal sling requires the harvest of autologous fascia for sling material, but modifications, such as alternative sling materials, bone anchor suspension, and mid-urethral slings have been developed to reduce operating time, surgical morbidity, and post-operative complication. The term "sling procedure" can now mean a variety of different procedures. Numerous alternative biological materials (allografts and xenografts) are commercially available and obviate the need to harvest autologous fascia. Use of these tissues poses new questions and concerns regarding biocompatibility, reaction, or integration with host tissue, and disease transmission. Allografts and xenografts are meant to function as scaffolding for the ingrowth of native tissue that ultimately will replace the graft, but recent data questions the permanence of some materials.

Autologous fascia is an attractive sling material because it is cost effective, available, and biocompatible by definition. Rectus fascia and fascia lata are the autologous sling materials of choice. Regardless of the material used, the pubovaginal sling attempts to restore sufficient outlet resistance to prevent SUI without compromising normal voiding or producing voiding dysfunction. Historically, the pubovaginal sling was reserved for SUI caused by ISD or previous surgical failure, but its use has expanded to include all forms of SUI. The evolution of our theories of the pathophysiology of SUI has extended the use of pubovaginal slings to all types of SUI. The pubovaginal sling, therefore, may be applied universally in SUI. The choice of what anti-incontinence procedure to perform and by what technique is still based on a variety of factors: the patient's wishes, patient's characteristics, surgeon's experience, and surgeon's comfort level with a particular technique.

Complications of slings include harvest site infection, seroma or hematoma formation, herniation, or pain at the site. Transient obstructive symptoms are quite common. Urinary retention requiring urethrolysis, which is the surgical "loosening" of a previous suspension procedure if it considered too tight, occurs in 1 to 2% of cases. No cases of rejection have been reported with autologous materials, and the few reported cases of erosion were likely caused by excessive sling tension or overly aggressive periurethral dissection *(47)*. The classic autologous fascial sling can be relied on to provide a cure rate of 84% or better. Sling surgery with most alternative biological materials produces short-term success rates comparable to autologous fascia. Rates of postoperative voiding dysfunction and urinary retention also seem similar. Allografts and xenografts undoubtedly shorten operative times and obviate the morbidity of fascial harvest, but these shortcuts may be costly in the long term. Current literature points to higher risks of early failure and immunogenicity leading to rejection and poor tissue healing *(48–51)*. DNA of unclear transmissibility has been isolated in several sling products, including cadaveric fascia lata (CFL), cadaveric dermis, and bovine pericardium *(52)*. Patients must be counseled preoperatively and informed consent must include information regarding the sling material to be used.

Synthetic mid-urethral slings, such as the tension-free vaginal tape reconstitute tension in the pubourethral ligaments and increase resistance in the urethra. Placed under no tension, the sling works by physically kinking the urethra during strain. Mid-urethral slings have now become the most common surgical procedure performed for SUI. Long-term outcomes in SUI demonstrate 84.7% of women are objectively and subjectively cured of stress leakage and another 10.6% are improved *(53)*. In patients with mixed symptoms, 85% are cured of stress and urge symptoms *(54)*. The outcomes in patients with ISD were not as favorable.

The cure rate in this group was only 74%, with 12% improved *(55)*. The failure rate was 14%, with risk factors for failure identified as age older than 70 years, a very low resting urethral pressure, and an immobile urethra.

SURGERY FOR UUI

Invasive therapies for UUI are reserved for those patients who fail to respond to pharmacological agents. Sacral nerve stimulation via the InterStim™ device (Medtronic, Inc., Minneapolis, MN) is an FDA-approved modality for the treatment of refractory urgency, frequency, UUI, and nonobstructive urinary retention. The exact mechanism by which it works is not understood, but it is based on the finding that ES of the sacral nerve root can reduce inappropriate neural activity and inhibit the overactive detrusor muscle. The implantable InterStim™ device includes a neurostimulator, an extension cable, and a quadripolar stimulating electrode that is implanted into the S3 sacral foramen. Optimal lead placement will produce a bellowing of the pelvic floor muscles in response to acute stimulation, and a sensation of pulling in the rectum or vagina in the woman. After placement of the "test" lead, the patient has control over the voltage amplitude to maintain a comfortable level of stimulation. Voiding diaries are kept for 3 to 7 days and compared with preimplantation diaries. Most patients will be able to detect a positive response within only a few days. If she responds well to the test phase, the permanent stimulation generator is implanted. Results of a multicenter randomized controlled trial demonstrated that 77% of those randomized to neurostimulation had no heavy leakage episodes compared with 8% in the control group, and 47% of those treated became fully dry at 6 months *(56)*. A treatment benefit has been shown up to a mean of 30.8 months *(56)*. Complications of this procedure include pain at the neurostimulator or lead site, new pain, lead migration, infection, or mechanical malfunction. Surgical revision or explant may be necessary to resolve certain adverse events. No reports of permanent injury have been published.

Although still investigational and not FDA-approved for use in overactive bladder, there is a growing body of experience with the use of botulinum toxin A for the treatment of neurogenic and non-neurogenic detrusor overactivity. Botulinum A toxin is a presynaptic neuromuscular blocking agent that produces a selective and reversible muscle weakness for up to 6 months when injected intramuscularly *(57)*. The technique most commonly used requires 300 U of Botox®. Aliquots of 0.1 mL, containing 10 U of Botox® are injected into the detrusor using a cystoscopic injection needle *(58)*. The procedure is performed as an outpatient, and in most cases can be performed with local anesthesia. The effect lasts approximately 6 months, and repeated injections can be performed. The incidence of adverse events with injection into the bladder is low. Rare cases of systemic side effects, such as generalized muscle weakness lasting 2 to 4 weeks have been reported *(58)*. Potentially, the detrusor muscle could be decompensated, necessitating intermittent catheterization to empty. Contraindications to Botox® therapy for detrusor overactivity include myasthenia gravis, Eaton-Lambert syndrome, pregnancy, and breast feeding *(58)*.

Although rarely necessary in the neurologically intact patient with an anatomically normal bladder, bladder augmentation by enterocystoplasty or detrusor myomectomy are other options for refractory UUI. These major abdominal procedures essentially accomplish the same goal to disrupt the native detrusor for the prevention of involuntary contractions. Voluntary detrusor contractions may also be disrupted, so patients must be willing to catheterize postoperatively. Failure to comply with catheterization could result in bladder perforation.

CONCLUSIONS

Urinary incontinence is a treatable disorder with significant negative impact on a patient's QOL, as well as serious economic burden to society. HCPs entrusted with the care of women should screen for UI, be familiar with the fundamentals of the UI evaluation, and be able to identify high-risk patients who should be referred to a urologist or urogynecologist.

Treatment options are varied and may be dependent on the type of incontinence present. It is crucial, however, that a patient be informed of all of her options: noninvasive to surgical. The patient's degree of bother is one of the most important determinants of treatment.

REFERENCES

1. Thom D. Variation in estimates of urinary incontinence prevalence in the community: effects of differences in definition, population characteristics, and study type. J Am Geriatr Soc 1998;46:473.
2. Hunskaar S, Burgio K, Clark A, et al. Epidemiology of fecal and urinary incontinence and pelvic organ prolapse. In: Incontinence. 3rd International Consultation on Incontinence, 3rd ed. Edited by P. Abrams, L. Cardozo, S. Khoury and A. Wein. Plymouth: Health Publication, Ltd. 2004.
3. Thom DH, Nygaard IE, Calhoun EA. Urologic Diseases in America Project: Urinary Incontinence in Women – National Trends in Hospitalization, Office Visits, Treatment and Economic Impact. J Urol 2005;173:1295–1301.
4. Wei JT, DeLancey JOL. Functional anatomy of the pelvic floor and lower urinary tract. Clin Obstet-Gynecol 2004;47(1):3–17.
5. Barber MD, Bremer RE, Thor KB, et al. Innervation of the female levator ani muscles. Am J Obstet Gynecol 2002;187:64–71.
6. Petros PE, Ulmsten U. An integral theory and its method for the diagnosis and management of female urinary incontinence. Scand J Urol Nephrol Suppl 1993;153:1–93.
7. DeLancey JO. Structural support of the urethra as it relates to stress urinary incontinence: the hammock hypothesis. Am J Obstet Gynecol 1994;170(6):1713–1720.

8. Ulmsten U. Connective tissue factors in the aetiology of female pelvic disorders. Am Med 1990;22(6):403.
9. Falconer C, Ekman-Ordeberg G, Blomgren B, et al. Paraurethral connective tissue in stress-incontinent women after menopause. Acta Obstet Gynecol Scand 1998;77(1):95–100.
10. Falconer C, Edman-Ordeberg G, Ulmsten U, et al. Changes in paraurethral connective tissue at menopause are counteracted by estrogen. Maturitas 1996;24(3):197–204.
11. Goepel C, Hefler L, Methfessel HD, et al. Periurethral connective tissue status of post-menopausal women with genital prolapse with and without stress incontinence. Acta Obstet Gynecol Scand 2003;82:659–664.
12. Caulfield MP, Birdsall NJM. International union of pharmacology. XVII. Classification of muscarinic acetylcholine receptors. Pharmacological Reviews 1998;50:279–290.
13. Chess-Williams R: Muscarinic receptors of the urinary bladder: detrusor, urothelial and prejunctional. Autonomic & Autacoid Pharmacology 2002;22:133–145.
14. Rosenblum N, Scarpero HM, Nitti VW. Voiding Dysfunction in young, multiparous women: symptoms and urodynamic findings. Int Urogynecol J Pelvic Floor Dysfunct 2004;15(6): 373–377.
15. Cauley ME, Schaffer J: Urinary incontinence and pelvic organ prolapse in women with Marfan or Ehlers Danlos syndrome. Am J Obstet Gynecol 2000;182(5):1021–1023.
16. Bump RMD. Cigarette smoking and urinary incontinence in women. Am J Obstet Gynecol 1992;167(5):1213–1218.
17. Viktrup L, Lose G, Rolff M, et al. The symptom of stress incontinence caused by pregnancy or delivery in primiparas. Obstet Gynecol 1992;79:945–949.
18. Stanton SL, Kerr-Wilson R, Harris VG. The incidence of urological symptoms in normal pregnancy. Br J Obstet Gynaecol 1980;87:897–900.
19. Meyer S, Schreyer A, DeGrandi P, et al. The effects of birth on urinary continence mechanisms and other pelvic floor characteristics. Obstet Gynecol 1998;92:613–618.
20. Allen RE, Hosker GL, Smith ARB, et al. Pelvic floor damage in childbirth : a neurophysiological study. Br J Obstet Gynaecol 1990;97:770–779.
21. Klein MC, Gauthier RJ, Robbins JM, et al. Relationship of episiotomy to perineal trauma and morbidity, sexual dysfunction, and pelvic floor relaxation. Am J Obstet Gynecol 1994;171:591–598
22. Rockner G, Jonasson A, Olund A. The effect of mediolateral episiotomy at delivery on pelvic floor muscle strength evaluated with vaginal cones. Acta Obstet Gynecol Scand 1991;70:51–54.
23. Uebersax JS, Wyman JF, Shumaker SA, et al. Short forms to assess life quality and symptom distress for urinary incontinence impact in women: the incontinence impact questionnaire and the urogenital distress inventory. Neurourol and Urodyn 1995;14:131–139.
24. Scarpero HM, Fiske J, Xue X, et al. American Urological Association Symptom Index for lower urinary tract symptoms in women: correlation with degree of bother and impact on quality of life. Urol 2003;61(6):1118–1122.
25. Muir TW, Stepp KJ, Barber MD. Adoption of the pelvic organ prolapse quantification system in peer-reviewed literature. Am J Obstet Gynecol 2003;189(6):1632–1635.
26. Bump RC, Mattiasson A, Bo K, et al. The standardization of terminology of female pelvic organ prolapse and pelvic floor dysfunction. Am J Obstet Gynecol 1996;175:10–17.
27. Crystle CD, Charme LS, Copeland WE. Q-tip test in stress urinary incontinence. Obstet Gynecol 1971;38:313–315.
28. Bergman A, McCarthy TA, Ballard CA, et al. Role of the Q-tip test in evaluating stress urinary incontinence. J Reprod Med 1987;32:273–275.
29. Carlson KV, Fiske J, Nitti VW. Value of routine evaluation of the voiding phase when performing urodynamic testing in women with lower urinary tract symptoms. J Urol 2000;164(5):1614–1618.

30. Goode PS, Burgio KL, Locher JL, et al. Effect of behavioral training with or without pelvic floor electrical stimulation on stress incontinence in women: a randomized controlled trial. JAMA 2003;290(3):345–352.
31. Sirls LT, Foote JE, Kaufman JM. Long-term results of the FemSoft™ urethral insert for the management of female stress urinary incontinence. Int Urogynecol J Pelvic Floor Dysfunct 2002;13:88–95.
32. Dmochowski RR, Miklos JR, Norton PA, et al. Duloxetine versus placebo for the treatment of North American women with stress urinary incontinence. J Urol 2003;170(4 Pt 1): 1259–1263.
33. Hextall A. Oestrogens and lower urinary tract function. Maturitas 2000;36(2):83–92.
34. Hendrix SL, Cochrane BB, Nygaard IE, et al. Effects of estrogen with and without progestin on urinary incontinence. JAMA 2005;293(8):935–948.
35. Wolf H, Wandt H, Jonal W: Immunohistochemical evidence of estrogen and progesterone receptors in the female lower urinary tract and comparison with the vagina. Gynecol Obstet Invest 1991;32(4):227–231.
36. Wilson PD, Barker G, Barnard RJ, et al. Steroid hormone receptors in the female lower urinary tract. Urol Int 1984;39(1):5–8.
37. Lin HH, Shen BC, Lo MC, et al: Comparison of treatment outcomes for imipramine for female genuine stress incontinence. Br J Obstet Gynaecol 1999;106:1089–1092.
38. Gilja I, Radej M, Kovacic M, et al. Conservative treatment of female stress incontinence with imipramine. Urol 1984;132:909–911.
39. Diokno A, Taub M. Ephedrine in treatment of urinary incontinence. Urol 1975;5:624–627.
40. Awad S, Downie J, Kiruluta J. Alpha adrenergic agents in urinary disorders of the proximal urethra: Part I. Sphincteric incontinence. Br J Urol 1978;50:332–336.
41. Yamaguchi O, Shishido K, Tamura K, et al. Evaluation of MRNAs encoding muscarinic receptor subtypes in human detrusor muscle. J Urol 1996;156:1208–1213.
42. Yamanishi T, Yasuda K, Chapple CR, et al. The role of M_2 muscarinic receptors in mediating contraction of the pig urinary bladder in vitro. Br J Pharmacol 2000;131: 1482–1488.
43. Herschorn S, Radomski SB. Collagen injections for genuine stress urinary incontinence: patient selection and durability. Int Urogynecol J 1997;8:18–24.
44. Steele AC, Kohli N, Karram MM. Periurethral collagen injection for stress incontinence with and without urethral hypermobility. Obstet Gynecol 2000;95:327–331.
45. Goldman HB, Rackley RR, Appell RA. The efficacy of urethrolysis without re-suspension for iatrogenic urethral obstruction. J Urol 1999;161:196–198.
46. Leach GE, Dmochowski RR, Appell RA, et al. Female Stress Urinary Incontinence Clinical Guidelines Panel Summary Report on the surgical management of female stress urinary incontinence. The American Urological Assoc. J of Urol 1997;158:875–880.
47. Webster TM, Gerridzen RG. Urethral erosion following autologous rectus fascial sling. Can J Urol 2003;10:2068–2069.
48. Fitzgerald MP, Mollenhauer J, Brubaker L. Failure of allograft suburethral slings. BJU Int 1999;84:785–788.
49. Carbone JM, Kavaler E, Hu J, et al. Pubovaginal sling using cadaveric fascia and bone anchors: disappointing early results. J Urol 2001;165:1605–1611.
50. O'Reilly KJ, Govier FE. Intermediate term failure of pubovaginal slings using cadaveric fascia lata: a case series. J Urol 2002;167:1356–1358.
51. Owens DC, Winters JC. Pubovaginal sling using Duraderm graft: intermediate follow-up and patient satisfaction. Neurourol Urodynam 2004;23:115–118.
52. Choe JM, Bell T. Genetic Material is present in cadaveric dermis and cadaveric fascia lata. J Urol 2001;166(1):122–124.

53. Nilsson GG, Kuuva N, Falconer C, et al. Long-term results of the tension-free vaginal tape (TVT) procedure for surgical treatment of female stress urinary incontinence. Int Urogynecol J Pelvic Floor Dysfunct 2001;12(suppl 2):55–58.
54. Rezapour M, Ulmsten U. Tension-free vaginal tape (TVT) in women with mixed urinary incontinence: a long-term follow-up. Int Urogynecol J 2001;12(suppl 2):515–518.
55. Rezapour M, Falconer C, Ulmsten U. Tension-free vaginal tape (TVT) in stress incontinent women with intrinsic sphincter deficiency (ISD): a long-term follow-up. Int Urogynecol J 2001;12(suppl 2):512–514.
56. Schmidt RA, Jonas V, Oleson KA, et al. Sacral nerve stimulation for treatment of refractory urinary urge incontinence. Sacral Nerve Stimulation Study Group. J Urol 1999;162: 352–357.
57. Stohrer M, Schurch B, Kramer G, et al. Botulinum-A toxin for treating detrusor hyperreflexia in spinal cord injured patients: a new alternative to anticholinergic drugs? Preliminary results. J Urol 2000;164(3 Pt 1):692–697.
58. Rackley R, Abdelmalak J. Urologic Applications of Botulinum toxin therapy for voiding dysfunction. Curr Urol Rep 2004;5:381–387.
59. Benzl JS: Anatomy and physiology. In: Female Pelvic Floor Disorders (Benson JT, ed.). Norton Medical Books, New York, 1992.
60. DeLancey JOL, Richardson AC. Anatomy of genital support. In: Female Pelvic Floor Disorders (Benson JT, ed.). Norton Medical Books, New York, 1992.

9 Diabetes in Women

Ronald A. Codario, MD

CONTENTS

BACKGROUND

The current epidemic of obesity and the increase in type II diabetes have had a profound effect on health care in women in the United States. Alarmingly, there has been a 70% increase in type II diabetes among women between the age groups of 30 and 39 from 1990 to 1998. It is estimated that nearly 2 million reproductive age women in the United States have type II diabetes with about 30% of these cases as yet undiagnosed *(1)*.

The common risk factors for the development of type II diabetes include: sedentary life style, diets rich in saturated fat, trans fat and excessive calories, inherited factors, and obesity (BMI>25 kg/m^2) *(2)*. In the United States alone, over 50% of women of 20 years of age or more are overweight. Close to 60% of these engage in little or no physical activity. This excess body weight contributes

From: *Current Clinical Practice: Women's Health in Clinical Practice*
Edited by: Clouse and Sherif © Humana Press Inc., Totowa, NJ

significantly to insulin resistance, subsequent impaired glucose tolerance and ultimately increased risk for developing diabetes, and other health problems.

Type II diabetes is primarily a vasculopathic disease that begins decades before its clinical diagnosis with the macrovascular complications beginning in the pre-diabetic stage characterized by those group of risk factors termed the metabolic syndrome. It is important for primary care physicians to understand, recognize, and treat this condition to prevent the development of type II diabetes.

The National Cholesterol Education Program (NCEP) ATP-3 guidelines *(3)* list three or more of the following as diagnostic of metabolic syndrome: waist circumference equal to or greater than 40 in. in men, equal to or greater than 36 in. in women, triglycerides equal to or greater than 150 mg/dL, HDL cholesterol less than 40 mg/dL in men, less than 50 mg/dL in women, systolic blood pressure equal to or greater than 130 mmHg or diastolic blood pressure equal to or greater than 85 mmHg, and a fasting blood sugar equal to or greater than 100 mg/dL.

The Diabetes Prevention Project *(4)* randomized 3234 non-diabetic individuals, 25 years of age or older, with impaired glucose tolerance and fasting glucoses between 95 and 125 mg/dL to a placebo, a life style modification program, a goal of 7% weight loss, and 150-min physical activity weekly or metformin 850 mg twice daily. In this study, 68% of the participants were women, with 45% being members of minority groups. Life style intervention reduced the incidence of type II diabetes by 58% when compared with placebo, while the metformin intervention resulted in a 31% reduction in development of type II diabetes.

Clearly, therapeutic life style changes can have a major impact; not only in treating this condition, but also preventing progression to type II diabetes. The NCEP ATP-3 criteria may not be consistently predictive in all ethnic and gender groups with differences existing among whites, African-Americans and Hispanic-Americans. The prevalence of the metabolic syndrome is significantly higher in Mexican-American females at 27%, while in African-American and white women the incidence is approximately the same 20–23% *(5)*.

Among males age of 45–65 years, the incidence is 8.3 per 100 persons in whites, 14.1 for African-Americans, and 13.7 for Hispanics. However, in females, age of 45–65 years, the rate is 6.7 for whites, 16.6 for African-Americans, and 13.2 for Hispanics. With aging, however, come more significant disparities *(6)*.

The incidence of diabetes between the ages of 65–74 years in males is 16.4 for whites, 23.0 for African-Americans, and 23.5 for Hispanics; while the rates in females are 12.8 for whites, 25.4 for African-Americans, and 23.8 for Hispanics. Alarmingly, there has been increase of 33% in the overall prevalence of diabetes in the past 30 years, while the rate has tripled in African-Americans *(7)*. In 1999, the diabetes age adjusted death rate per 100,000 was 18.4 among

Asian-Americans, 22.8 among white-Americans, 33.6 among Hispanic-Americans, 50.1 among African-Americans, and 50.3 among Native-Americans *(8)*.

This disparity is even more striking in cardiovascular disease, where African-Americans are dying at the rate of 336.5 per 100,000 versus whites at approx 263 per 100,000.

Data from the Third National Health and Nutrition Examination Survey indicated that the prevalence of type II diabetes is higher among non-Hispanic black women and Mexican-American women than non-Hispanic white women with 4–6% of United States women older than 50 having undiagnosed diabetes *(9)*. This disease affects approx 10% of women older than 65 years of age and 20% older than 80 years of age.

DIAGNOSTIC CRITERIA

Anyone of the following three abnormalities is diagnostic of type II diabetes: fasting plasma glucose equal to or greater than 126 mg/dL, random plasma glucose equal to or greater than 200 mg/dL, 2-h plasma glucose equal to or greater than 200 mg/dL during an oral glucose tolerance test consisting of 75-g glucose *(10)*.

In the late 1990s, diabetes began being classified according to the underlying metabolic problems both in type I and in type II. Patients with type I diabetes have autoimmune destruction of the pancreatic β-cells producing little or no insulin. This is associated with the presence of anti-insulin antibodies as well as auto-antibodies to other components of the insulin-producing system, like glutamic acid decarboxylase, pancreatic islet cells, and tyrosine phosphatase. Although the onset of type I diabetes can occur at any age, it is more prevalent in children and requires insulin treatment for survival *(11)*.

Type II diabetes is characterized by the triple disturbance of insulin resistance, delay in first phase insulin secretion due to β-cell dysfunction and increase in hepatic gluconeogenesis and glycogenolysis *(12)*. Glucose regulation is determined by a complex interaction of various hormones: amylin and insulin, supplied by the pancreatic β cells; glucagon, secreted by the pancreatic α cells; and gastrointestinal peptides (incretins), including glucose-dependent insulinotropic polypeptide (gastric inhibitory peptide or GIP) and glucagon-like peptide-1 (GLP-1) *(13)*. GLP-1 is released from the L cells of the small intestine after eating, stimulating insulin secretion, reducing glucagon levels, and delaying gastric emptying *(14)*. GLP-1 is then rapidly metabolized by dipeptidyl peptidase IV (DPP-IV).

Although type II diabetes is more common in adults, it is increasing at an alarming rate in children and adolescents. Although impaired insulin secretion and insulin resistance precede the development of postprandial hyperglycemia in the type II diabetic phenotype, insulin resistance is more prominent in the

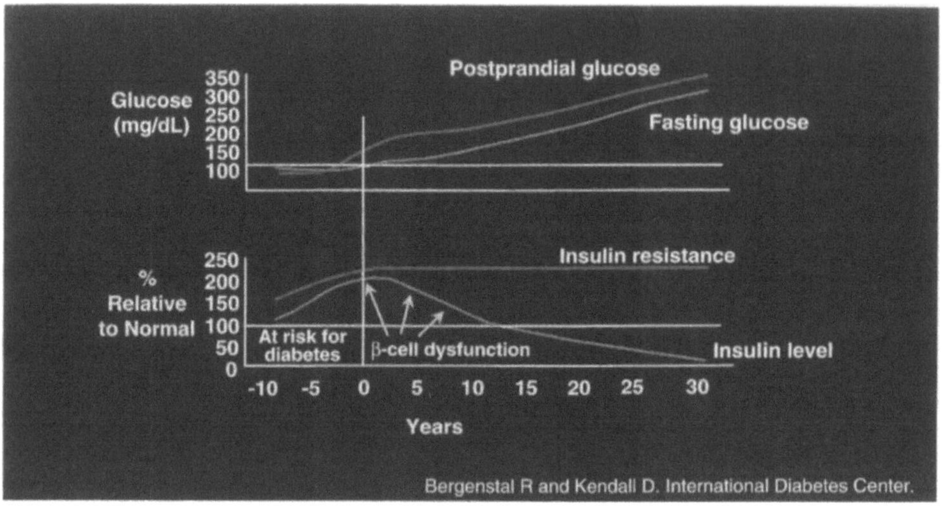

Fig. 1. Natural history of type II diabetes.

pre-diabetic state and plays an important role in the pathogenesis of macrovascular disease. Insulin resistance represents the earliest manifestation of type II diabetes and can occur as much as 5–10 years before postprandial glucoses elevate to the abnormal range (>140 mg/dL) and 10–15 years before reaching the diabetic range (>200 mg/dL) (Fig. 1).

Some individuals fall into a mixed category termed "1.5 diabetes" also known as latent autoimmune diabetes of adults (LADA). These individuals are usually treated with oral medications and diet, but end-up requiring insulin due to an autoimmune impairment of insulin and are sometimes referred to as "double diabetics", because they demonstrate the insulin-resistant characteristics of type II diabetes with the autoimmune destruction of β cells seen in type I diabetes *(15)*. Many of these individuals are overweight and require insulin within 5–10 years of the diagnosis. Individuals with latent autoimmune diabetes are at higher risk for developing other autoimmune diseases and possessing auto-antibodies to thyroid and adrenal cells. In these individuals with LADA, the maintenance of tight blood glucose control may help slow the destruction of β cells, delaying the dependency on insulin and decreasing the risk of diabetic complications.

SCREENING

Early diagnosis is critical to prevent and delay the macro- and microvascular complications of this disease. Macrovascular disease begins with impaired glucose tolerance, while microvascular disease begins with the onset of type II diabetes. The American Diabetes Association recommends screening for diabetic women with one or more of the following risk factors: (1) obesity (BMI>25 kg/m^2), (2) minority ethnicity (Hispanic-American, Asian-American, Pacific Islander, Native American, and African-American, (3) family history of diabetes, (4) sedentary life style, (5) pre-eclampsia, (6) gestational diabetes mellitus, (7) large for gestational age at birth, delivering a child equal to or greater than 9 pounds, (8) cigarette smoking, (9) high-saturated fat diet, (10) polycystic ovary syndrome, (11) dysmetabolic syndrome, also known as syndrome X or metabolic syndrome *(16)*.

The most reliable method for detecting type II diabetes in the average patient is the 2-h glucose tolerance test using 75-g oral glucose solution administered following a 12-h fast. Individuals with fasting plasma glucoses equal to or greater than 126 mg/dL or a 2-h glucose value greater than 200 mg/dL are classified as being diabetic. It is important to remember that screening for fasting plasma glucose alone at a cut off value of 126 mg/dL can only be approx 50% sensitive in identifying type II diabetes *(17)*. Hence the 2-h glucose tolerance test can diagnose diabetes earlier. Screening intervals depend on the number and type of risk factors an individual patient may develop over a period of time.

PREVENTION OF TYPE II DIABETES

Several large-scale clinical trials have been performed to evaluate the prevention of type II diabetes in women at high risk. In addition to the previously cited Diabetes Prevention Program Study, a Finnish trial randomized 522 obese women and men with BMI's exceeding 31 kg/m^2 to either intense training and dietary restriction to a less intense training program *(18)*. The mean rate reduction was 7% in the intensive group when compared with 1% in the non-intensive group after 3.5 years, with a 58% reduction in the relative risk of type II diabetes in the weight loss group.

The Diabetes Prevention Program showed that therapeutic life style changes resulted in 58% risk reduction when compared with 31% risk reduction with metformin *(19)*. The Troglitazone in the Prevention of Diabetes Study looked at obese women with a history of gestational diabetes mellitus treated with short-term troglitazone after delivery and then followed for 2 years *(20)*. This trial was subsequently discontinued when troglitazone was removed from the market but resumed with pioglitazone. Here, the data were impressive, indicating significant reduction in the risk of developing diabetes when these patients were placed on a thiazolidinedione. Hence, diet and exercise can play a critical role in the prevention of type II diabetes in women at risk for developing the disease.

GESTATIONAL DIABETES

Glucose intolerance, with the onset or first recognition during pregnancy, is referred to as gestational diabetes. Approximately 200,000 cases of each year or 7% of all pregnancies are complicated by this condition *(21)*. It is customary to perform risk assessment testing during the first prenatal visit. Patients with family history of diabetes, marked obesity, previous history of gestational diabetes, and glucosuria are considered high risk and should receive glucose testing as soon as possible and retested if necessary at the 24th to the 28th week of pregnancy.

Patients considered at low risk that do not require glucose testing are younger than 25 years of age, normal weight before pregnancy, no known diabetes in first degree relatives, no history of abnormal glucose tolerance test or poor obstetric outcomes, or no ethnic predisposition *(22)*.

Initial screening for this condition consists of plasma glucose measurement 1 h after the administration of a 50 g oral glucose load. If 1-h glucose is equal to or greater than 140 mg/dL than an oral glucose tolerance test should be performed using 75 g of glucose. Under these circumstances (75 g glucose load), a 1-h glucose equal to or greater than 180 mg/dL or a 2-h glucose equal to or greater than 155 mg/dL establishes a diagnosis of gestational diabetes *(23)*.

It is important to diagnose gestational diabetes in women since there is an increased risk of fetal macrosomia, neonatal hypoglycemia, polycythemia, hypocalcemia, jaundice, and intrauterine fetal death along with maternal hypertension and increased need for caesarean deliveries with this condition and with women who are diabetic before becoming pregnant *(24)*. In addition, women that manifest gestational diabetes are at increased risk for development of type II diabetes after pregnancy with a 50% incidence 10 years after delivery. These women should all undergo oral glucose tolerance test 6 weeks after delivery *(25)*. Thiazolidinedione therapy, weight loss, dietary changes, and exercise are all important to decrease the risk of developing type II diabetes.

MANAGEMENT OF TYPE I DIABETES

Daily insulin production in normal individuals ranges from 24 to 36 U, with insulin being secreted on a constant basis into the portal circulation *(26)*. Many variables can effect the daily insulin requirement, including hormonal, physical, psychological, dietary, exercise, and stress, but, in general, patients with type I diabetes generally require 0.5–1 U/kg of body weight daily. It is important to understand that daily insulin dose must be increased to compensate for stress in patients with diabetes, since stress is responsible for increased production of growth hormone, catecholamines, and cortisol.

Table 1
Onset, Peak and Duration of Various Insulins[a]

Insulin	*Onset (min)*	*Peak (hr)*	*Effective Duration (hr)*	*Maximum Duration (hr)*
Bolus insulin				
Aspart (NovoLog)	5–10	1–3	3–5	4–6
Lispro (Humalo)	15	0.5–1.5	2–4	4–6
Glulisine (Apidra)	5–10	0.5–1.5	2–4	4–6
Regular (Humulin R) (Novolin R)	30–60	2–3	3–4	6–10
Inhaled insulin (Exubera)	10–20	0.5–1.0	2–3	3–4
Basal insulin				
NPH (Humulin N) (Novolin N)	2–4	4–10	10–16	14–18
Lente (insulin zinc suspension)	3–4	4–12	12–18	16–20
Ultralente (extended insulin zinc suspension)	6–10	none	18–20	20–24
Glargine (Lantus)	1–2	peakless	24	24
Detemir (Levemir)	2–3	6–10	14–18	16–22

Source: Feinglos MN, Bethel MA. Emerging care for type 2 diabetes: using insulin to each lower glycemic goals. Cleve Clin J Med 2005;72(9):791–799.

Production of these substances enhances insulin resistance and promotes hyperglycemia.

The characteristics of the various insulin preparations are listed in Table 1.

An important principal of optimizing therapy in patients with type I diabetes is to closely mimic the physiologic needs of the patient. This can be accomplished when the daily insulin dose consists of a 50:50 ratio of pre-meal (bolus) insulin to reduce postprandial hyperglycemia and basal insulin to suppress hepatic glucose production. This can be achieved with the use of an insulin pump for continuous subcutaneous insulin infusion or multiple daily injections of short-acting insulin, or the combination of short-acting analog insulin and the long-acting analog insulin, glargine, which provides basal insulin with once daily administration, lacks a peak action and provides smooth continuous delivery similar to continuous β-cell insulin secretion.

Other alternative approaches include using intermediate acting insulin (NPH) at bedtime with short-acting insulin administered before each meal or giving mixed insulins twice daily, once before breakfast, and once before supper.

Traditionally two-thirds of the daily dose of mixed insulin is administered in the morning with the remaining one-third at night.

Due to its peakless nature, insulin glargine given once a day along with the administration of short-acting analog insulins either before or after a meal seems to be the more popular approach.

When short-acting insulin analogs are given prior to a meal, the dose of the short-acting insulin can be adjusted according to the carbohydrates being ingested allowing 1 U short-acting insulin per 10–15 g carbohydrate. A more practical post-meal approach can be used with self-monitoring of blood glucose (SMBG) 1 h after each meal followed by the administration of 2-U short-acting insulin for every 50 mg/dL over 150 mg/dL. Hence, if the glucose is between 150 and 200 mg/dL, then 2-U insulin are used, between 201 and 250 mg/dL: 4 U, between 251 and 300 mg/dL: 6 U, between 301 and 350 mg/dL: 8 U, and between 351 and 400 mg/dL: 10 U *(27)*.

Although the post-meal or postprandial use of analog insulins may not be as physiologic as the pre-meal administration, many patients find this approach more convenient. It can be very effective as long as the patient is compulsive with postprandial SMBG.

Pramlintide is a soluble, non-aggregating amylin analog given by subcutaneous injection at mealtime. This regulates postmeal glucose levels by suppressing postprandial glucagon elevations in diabetics and delaying gastric emptying. This agent allows exogenous insulin therapy to match physiologic needs improving the regulation of gluconeogenesis and prandial glucose influx. This injectable is now approved for use in type 1 and type II diabetics *(28)*.

Inhaled insulin availability has now provided another unique way of delivering bolus insulin for needle phobic patients. The FDA device currently available delivers 40% of the dose of powdered human insulin deep into the lungs with 10% of this total dose being bioavailable *(29)*. Those patients with type I or type II diabetes who received a combination of regular insulin and NPH two to three times daily or a combination of inhaled insulin and ultralente at night, the HbA1c did not change significantly between the two treatment groups *(30)*. Hypoglycemia was lower in the ultralente and inhaled insulin group. Adding inhaled insulin three times daily to an oral regimen was more effective over a 12–24-wk period than adding a second oral agent taken once or twice daily *(31)*.

Inhaled insulin use is not indicated for those patients with asthma or chronic obstructive lung disease, since insulin absorption can be unpredictable in these patients, especially with concomitant bronchodilator use *(32)*.

Maintenance of the inhaler requires weekly cleaning, while the internal valve that crushes the insulin pellet must be replaced two weeks.

Continuous subcutaneous insulin infusion has the advantage of delivering both basal and bolus insulin, permitting the patient to determine exactly how much insulin is required before a meal and delivering exactly that amount. This method provides flexibility of dosing because the constant, smooth delivery, using only rapid acting insulin, reduces the variation in insulin absorption and targets only one area for injection. Analog insulins are ideal for this purpose, decreasing the risk of hypoglycemia, and eliminating depot sequestration seen with increasing doses of subcutaneous human insulin.

Hence it is important for the physician to become familiar with the duration of action of the various insulins and other injectables while tailoring the regimen according to the patient's individual needs.

Islet cell transplantation in type I diabetics simulates donors by means of a complex purification process extracting the islets of Langerhans *(33)*. Under this procedure, cells can be injected percutaneously directly into the liver through the portal vein through radiographic guidance. Therefore, it is necessary for patients to take anti-rejection medication. These medications, of course, can increase the risk of infection, nephrotoxicity, mouth ulceration, hyperlipidemia, and lymphoma.

Therapeutic life style changes play a critical role in the management of the female patient with type I diabetes. Physicians should communicate to the patient, the basic concepts of insulin therapy and the importance of balancing exercise and diet. Because these patients are entirely dependent on exogenous insulin, the meals must match the time course of the selected insulin regimen. Patients must learn to adjust the insulin doses for periods of physical activity.

Irregular consumption of and long delays before meals should be avoided to decrease the risk of hypoglycemia. Portion control is important in order to attenuate weight gain. If hypoglycemia occurs, the patient should avoid over-compensating by consuming excess carbohydrates.

Exercise can significantly reduce overall insulin requirements, improving insulin sensitivity, reducing cardiovascular complications, and enhancing overall health. When extremities are used for insulin administration, exercise can rapidly reduce blood glucose levels due to increased muscle glucose utilization *(34)*. The continuous presence of exogenous insulin can cause glucose levels to fall precipitously during exercise. Hence, patients should constantly carry with them a rapidly utilizable source of glucose.

MANAGEMENT OF TYPE II DIABETES

Many clinical trials have emphasized the importance of tight glycemic control in reducing the complications of type II diabetes *(35)*. Tight control requires aggressive, effective use of oral agents, and early initiation of insulin therapy to achieve glycemic goals. Type II diabetes results from multigenic, heterogeneous, and complex interrelated causes *(36)*. In distinction to type I diabetes, which is characterized by severe insulin deficiency, this disease manifests itself by increased hepatic glucose production, enhanced insulin resistance, and impaired insulin secretion.

Fasting glucose levels depend upon both hepatic glycogenolysis and gluconeogenesis, basal insulin levels, insulin sensitivity, and the duration and level of the previous prandial glucose. Post-meal glucose levels are affected by pre-meal glucose, first phase insulin release, and insulin sensitivity *(37)*. Excessive hepatic glucose production during the sleeping hours between 12 midnight and 8 am may be responsible for the majority of incremental increases in day long hyperglycemia. Insulin resistance and impaired insulin secretion are more prominent in the pre-diabetic state and play an important role in the pathogenesis of macrovascular disease in the type II diabetic, preceding the development of postprandial hyperglycemia *(38)*.

Hence, in the management of the patient with type II diabetes, careful attention should be given to addressing the three disturbances that underlie the condition (hepatic glucose production, insulin resistance, and impaired insulin release). Insulin resistance can be worsened by several factors, including estrogens, nicotinic acid, oral contraceptives, phenothiazines, anti-psychotic medications (olanzapine, risperidone, clozapine, quetiapine, ziprasidone, and aripiprazol) corticosteroids, sedentary life style, aging, genetic factors, and obesity *(39)*.

When normal plasma glucose concentrations are exceeded by 50 to 100 mg/dL for as long as 24 h, downregulation of the glucose transport system results in muscle enhancement of insulin resistance and diminished response to therapy *(40)*.

Agents that are effective in reducing fasting hyperglycemia include the long acting and intermediate insulins and their analogs, sulfonylureas, biguanides (metformin), thiazolidinediones (rosiglitasone and pioglitasone), incretin analogs or mimetics (exenatide), and the DPP-IV inhibitors (sitagliptin and vildagliptin). The thiazolidinediones have been shown to play an important role in delaying and preventing the development of type II diabetes. New agents like the incretin analogs and DPP-IV inhibitors can also preserve β-cell function *(41)*.

Agents that are effective in primarily reducing postprandial hyperglycemia include the short-acting insulins and their analogs, meglitinides (repaglinide), D-phenylalanine derivatives (nateglinide), α-glucosidase inhibitors (acarbose and miglitol), as well as the DPP-IV inhibitors and incretin analogs.

Exenatide is a synthetic version of exendin-4, a naturally occurring component of Gila monster saliva *(42)*. This analog of GLP-1 binds to the GLP-1 receptor, exhibiting dose-dependent and glucose-dependent enhancement of insulin secretion, while slowing gastric emptying, suppressing glucagon release, and promoting weight loss, with open label extension studies showing sustained lowering of A1C of approx 1.0% and continuous weight reduction averaging 12 pounds at the 2-year period *(43)*. Its glucose lowering effects are partially independent of its insulinotropic activity since blood glucose can be reduced in C-peptide negative type I diabetics, as well as insulin requiring type II diabetics *(44)*. This product has been approved for type II diabetics who are also being treated with a sulfonylurea, metformin or both. Exenatide not affected by DPP-IV inhibitors.

The DPP-IV is a serine protease, that is widely distributed throughout the body *(45)*.It cleaves *N*-terminal amino acids and deactivates bioactive peptides, including the incretins GLP-1 and GIP. DPP-IV deactivates GLP-I by greater than 50% in 1–2 min and deactivates GIP by greater than 50% in about 7 min *(46)*.

Two DPP-IV inhibitors are available in this class: sitagliptin and vildagliptin–both available as oral agents.

Sitagliptin showed a 0.77% decrease in A1C over a 12-week period of time with no weight gain when compared with placebo in a randomized trial in 743 patients when compared with a 1.0% drop in A1C and 1.1 kg weight gain with glipizide at study end *(47)*.

Vildagliptin, given once daily for 12 weeks to 107 patients with type II diabetes receiving metformin monotherapy, showed a 0.6% drop in A1C, with an additional 1.1% grater reduction in A1C when compared with metformin alone in a 40-week study extension *(48)*.

The DPP-IV inhibitors seem to work best with A1C's less than 8.0 *(49)*.

Mildly elevated fasting plasma glucose levels with glycosylated hemoglobin A1C's less than 8% can also respond to insulin sensitizers (thiazolidinedione/metformin) or a sulfonylurea as initial monotherapy in conjunction with diet and exercise. In the female patient who presents with fasting glucoses between 160 and 180 mg/dL and A1C levels between 8 and 9%, combination therapy with an insulin sensitizer (metformin or thiazolidinedione) and an insulin secretagog (sulfonylurea, repaglinide, and nateglinide) is usually necessary *(50)*.

Fixed drug combinations containing a secretagog and a sensitizer are ideal for this purpose, starting with the lowest dose and titrating upward. In addition, a sensitizer combination is also available (metformin and rosiglitazone). This can be used with or without a secretagog for synergistic glycemic control. It is important to understand that repaglinide and nateglinide have approval for combination therapy with sensitizers (metformin and/or thiazolidinediones) and should not be used with a sulfonylurea.

An attractive combination is metformin and a sulfonylurea, providing additive glucose and lipid lowering effects as well as addressing insulin sensitivity and secretion. The fixed metformin/glyburide or metformin/glipizide agent can be given with meals or once a day. This fixed dose combination should not be used for fasting blood glucoses less than 150 mg/dL due to an increased risk of hypoglycemia.

Metformin, alone or in combination, is not indicated when the serum creatinine is greater than 1.4 mg/dL in women or if the creatinine clearance is less than 60 ml/min and is also not indicated in patients with congestive heart failure or those patients prone to metabolic or respiratory acidosis or significant hepatic disease. It should be withheld for at least 24 h before any dye studies are attempted and re-started after normal renal function is assured *(51)*.

When a thiazolidinedione (rosiglitazone or pioglitazone) is added to metformin, there is a synergistic decline in the A1C concentration from 0.8 to 1%. Synergistic effects on triglyceride lowering and enhanced increases in HDL are seen when pioglitazone is combined with metformin *(52)*. The combination of a thiazolidinedione and a biguanide are popular since the former agent enhances insulin sensitivity in the muscles, while the latter agent inhibits hepatic gluconeogenesis and increases hepatic insulin sensitivity.

Combination therapy with repaglinide and metformin has also been shown to be additive with reduction of A1C values of 1.4% when these two drugs are used in combination when compared with 0.4% with repaglinide alone and 0.3% with metformin alone *(53)*. Repaglinide is metabolized through the cytochrome P450-3A4 enzyme system and should be avoided in elderly, malnourished, or debilitated patients and with caution and at reduced doses in patients with renal insufficiency. Repaglinide is ideally suited for those patients who have postprandial hyperglycemia as the predominant abnormality causing type II diabetes.

Nateglinide, metabolized by cytochrome P450-3A4 and 2C9, is indicated for combination therapy with metformin and is ideal for the elderly female patient with postprandial hyperglycemia as the predominant abnormality. When used in combination with metformin or a thiazolidinedione, synergistic lowering of A1C can be achieved *(54)*.

The α-glucosidase inhibitors, acarbose and miglitol, have been approved for monotherapy in combination with sulfonylureas, insulin, and metformin. These agents act by reversibly inhibiting membrane bound intestinal α-glucoside hydrolase enzymes and should be taken with the first bite of food with each meal. Membrane bound intestinal α-glucosidase inhibitors hydrolyze the conversion of oligosaccharides and disaccharides to glucose and other monosaccharides in the brush border of the small intestine. These products delay glucose absorption, subsequently lowering postprandial glucose *(55)*.

In some instances, triple oral agent therapy can be used to address all three deficiencies in type II diabetes as long as the agents used have synergistic actions. This can be accomplished by a secretagog with both sensitizers. When hypoglycemia develops with the combination of oral agents that contain a secretagog and a sensitizer, it is the secretagog that should be stopped first.

In general, oral agent combinations are desirable and very effective since fewer than 25% of patients with type II diabetes that present to primary care offices with fasting glucoses in the range of 200–240 mg/dL will be able to reach a target A1C level of less than 7%, even if treated with maximum doses of a sensitizer or a sulfonylurea *(56)*. Even those that initially get a good response to a single agent will subsequently need a second or third agent in the future due to the progressive nature of the disease.

For patients with fasting glucoses in excess of 180–200 mg/dL with A1C's exceeding 9%, the addition of an intermediate bedtime (NPH) or once daily long acting insulin (glargine) in addition to combination therapy with a secretagog and/or sensitizers may be necessary. Ultimately, the majority of patients with type II diabetes will require insulin either alone or in combination with other oral agents or other insulins.

Any individuals who present with gestational diabetes, latent autoimmune diabetes, fasting blood glucoses in excess of 280 mg/dL with ketonuria or ketonemia or become pregnant while on oral agents are candidates for insulin therapy.

For those patients that have not reached goal with combination therapy, bedtime insulin along with the continuation of the oral agents effectively reduces elevated fasting glucose levels, requires less insulin, and minimizes weight gain. Another attractive combination is the addition of once a day, glargine insulin for smooth continuous basal insulin delivery. Glargine insulin, when given at bedtime, along with oral agents during the day, has been shown to be just as effective as bedtime NPH insulin and daytime oral agents in reducing A1C and fasting plasma glucose levels with low rates of hypoglycemia.

In any combinations involving thiazoldinediones and insulin, weight gain can be a significant problem and caution should be exercised due to the potential for increasing edema and congestive heart failure. If thiazoldinediones are to be used with insulin for synergistic glycemic and lipid-lowering effects, the lowest dose of each agent should be used to attenuate fluid retention and weight gain *(57)*.

When adding insulin to a oral agent, oral agents should be kept at the same dose to decrease insulin requirements. Whether NPH insulin is added at bedtime or glargine insulin once daily, the doses of insulin should be adjusted slowly, increasing by 2 U if fasting blood sugar is equal to or greater than 120 mg/dL, 4 U if equal to or greater than 140 mg/dL, and 6 U if the fasting blood glucose is equal to or greater than 180 mg/dL. These insulin adjustments should be made every 1–2 weeks depending upon the patients needs *(58)*.

NUTRICEUTICALS AND HERBS

The nutriceutical, chromium picolinate, exerts effects at the cellular level by influencing the phosphorylation of tyrosine kinase, which enhances glucose uptake and metabolism in the skeletal muscle along with increasing glucose transporter activity. This may decrease insulin resistance *(59)*. Daily intake of 1500–4000 mg of EPA (eicosapentanoic acid) and 1000–2000 mg of DHA (docosahexanoic acid)ω -3 fatty acids have been shown to improve insulin sensitivity in skeletal muscle reducing fasting glucose and improving lipids. Clinical trials are underway with various doses of chromium up to 1000 mcg twice daily to determine its efficacy and safety. Similar claims have been made for cinnamon, but more data are necessary to evaluate its efficacy.

Some notable herbal medicines used in the treatment of diabetes are the following *(60)*:

1. Panax Ginseng (1–3 g) can slow the absorption and digestion of carbohydrates, but can also inhibit warfarin and should not be taken by patients on this drug.
2. Garlic (*Allium sativum*) contains allicin, which can enhance insulin activity through its effects on receptor sites. Recommended doses would be 4-g fresh garlic daily or 200–400 mg in the encapsulated form.
3. Cactus (*Opuntia streptacantha*) is used in Mexico as a food additive for diabetics. Effects on glucose are due to soluble fiber and pectin content.
4. Gumar (*Gymnema sylvestre*) stimulates insulin secretion from the pancreas without affecting insulin sensitivity. It may also decrease glucose absorption in the intestine. The dose used is 400–600 mg daily.
5. Onion (*Allium cepa*) allegedly works in the same manner as garlic at a dose of 400 mg daily.
6. Fenugreek (*Trigonella foenum graecum*). The seeds of this medicinal plant contain trigonelline and nicotinic acid which reportedly can lower glucose, cholesterol, and triglycerides and raise HDL.
7. Bitter Melon (*Momordica charantia*) contains a substance called polypeptide P, which reportedly has an insulin-like activity. This is available as a liquid and given in a capsule form, with one to two capsules (5–15 cc of liquid) three times daily being the suggested dose.

It is important to understand that none of these has the endorsement of The American Diabetic Association and lack clinical-based evidence to support their use.

COMPLICATIONS OF DIABETES

Microvascular: these include retinopathy, nephropathy, and neuropathy.

Diabetic retinopathy is the leading cause of non-congenital blindness among adults affecting over 5 million Americans. Each year 5000 Americans are diagnosed with new legal blindness, 80,000 possess macular edema, and 63,000 are diagnosed with proliferative diabetic retinopathy *(61)*. In the diabetic, changes in retinal blood flow can occur after several years of having the condition. This causes retinal ischemia promoting proliferation of new blood vessels which are friable and more prone to leak resulting in fibrosis and scarring. The three phases of diabetic retinopathy are non-proliferative, preproliferative, and proliferative. Primary and secondary prevention includes blood pressure, lipid and glycemic control, and regularly scheduled examinations by an ophthalmologist. The Early Treatment Retinopathy Study showed that aspirin had no effect on the progression of retinopathy, but was not shown to be contraindicated in patients with diabetic retinopathy when required for cardiovascular disease *(62)*. Early evaluation by an ophthalmologist at the time of diagnosis of diabetes is important, even if the patient is not having any visual abnormalities, since early non-proliferative retinopathy can be treated with laser photocoagulation therapy.

Diabetic nephropathy is the most common cause of end-stage renal disease in the United States especially among African-Americans, Hispanic, and Native Americans, with up to one-third of patients with type I or type II diabetes developing some degree of nephropathy. This disease is particularly aggressive in those patients with type I diabetes. Early detection and aggressive intervention in diabetic nephropathy can prevent or even delay progression of the disorder with tight control of blood pressure and glucose with administration of angiotensin receptor blockers playing a critical role in prevention.

With this in mind, a screening urinalysis should be done upon diagnosis of diabetes and annually in all patients. The American Diabetes Association position statement on diabetic nephropathy states that microalbuminuria is present if the microalbumin/creatinine ratio exceeds 30 mcg/mg creatinine in a spot urine or greater than 30 mg of albumin in a 24-h collection, or greater than 20 mcg of albumin per minute in a 4-h timed specimen *(63)*. The threshold for clinical albuminuria is reached at 300 mcg/mg creatinine. The classification of a patient should be based on at least two or three abnormal results on specimens collected within a 3–6 month period of time. In patients with type II diabetes, the three stages of nephropathy have been described *(64)*. Stage I is indicated by a progression from normal urinary albumin excretion rate to microalbuminuria. Stage II, which is characterized by a progression from microalbuminuria to macroalbuminuria, with more than 300 mg/day of urinary protein and stage III with nephrotic syndrome and end-stage renal disease. The National Kidney Foundation divides chronic kidney disease into five stages by the glomerular filtration rate (GFR) *(65)*.

Stage 1 – Kidney damage with normal or increased GFR>90 ml/min.
Stage 2 – Kidney damage with mild decrease in GFR: 60–89.
Stage 3 – Moderate decrease in GFR: 30–59.
Stage 4 – Severe decrease in GFR: 15–29.
Stage 5 – Kidney failure – GFR<15 or dialysis.

Glomerular filtration rates usually decreased by 4–22 ml/min per year once diabetic nephropathy develops. Changes at the cellular level include renal and glomerular hypertrophy, glomerular basement membrane thickening, and mesangial expansion leading to subsequent tubulo-interstitial fibrosis and glomerular sclerosis. The development of proteinuria is usually preceded by changes in renal function characterized by hyperperfusion, hyperfiltration, and increased capillary permeability to macromolecules. The National Kidney Foundation currently recommends a blood pressure goal of less than 125/75 mmHg for diabetic patients with nephropathy with losartan at 100 mg and irbesartan at 300 mg once a day having the official FDA approval for this indication *(66)*. In general, patients with type II diabetes and overt nephropathy should have a protein intake of 0.8 g/kg of body weight daily. However, once the glomerular filtration rate begins to decrease, restriction of protein intake to 0.6 g/kg per day may have an effect on slowing this decrease in some patients. It is always advisable to have the input of a registered dietitian well versed in diabetes before embarking on a protein restricted meal regimen.

Diabetic neuropathies: Diabetic neuropathies can be characterized as focal or diffuse polyneuropathies, either sensory or autonomic *(67)*. The focal or mononeuropathies are not necessarily specific for diabetes with the primary symptom usually being one of local discomfort characterized by abnormal conduction of a single nerve, the brachial lumbosacral plexus, or multiple peripheral nerves. Focal neurological abnormalities such as lateral femoral cutaneous nerve palsy are more commonly seen in middle aged patients or patients that present with some type of sensory motor polyneuropathy. In addition, diabetic motor neuropathies can involve the third, fourth, or sixth cranial nerves, causing ocular palsies, the femoral nerve causing foot drop, the ulnar nerve characterized by wrist drop and the median nerve associated with carpal tunnel syndrome and weakness in apposition of the thumb. Sometimes these conditions can resolve spontaneously within weeks *(68)*.

Mononeuritis multiplex is characterized by more than one nerve being involved simultaneously. In addition, patients with long standing diabetes can develop atrophy, pain, and fasciculation of limb girdle muscles also referred to as diabetic amyotrophy.

The diffuse polyneuropathy syndromes of diabetes can be either peripheral, sensory or cardiovascular/autonomic. The peripheral sensory neuropathies can vary in their presentations, involving the upper and lower extremities, but usually affect the lower extremities first. Sensory neuropathies are usually characterized by abnormalities in vibratory sensation, pinprick, light touch, proprioception, or position sense *(69)*.

Painful neuropathy is an exceptionally difficult symptom to treat, with pain relief sometimes being provided by anti-inflammatory medications, carbamazepine, various anti-epileptic medications, tricyclic anti-depressants, narcotic and non-narcotic analgesics, and topical capsaicin. These conditions can get considerably worse with uncontrolled diabetes or with smoking.

Patients with cardiovascular autonomic neuropathy can present with orthostatic hypotension, variation in heart rate and tachy/bradyarrhythmias, gastrointestinal autonomic neuropathy (usually causing diarrhea), and gastroparesis which can be heralded by nausea, vomiting, early satiety, and symptoms of gastroesophageal reflux. Diabetic diarrhea, usually a nocturnal disorder, can occur at anytime of the day and can be especially difficult and stubborn to treat *(70)*.

Increased age and longer duration of diabetes increase the risk for neuropathy. Lipid levels, BMI, smoking, and hypertension are all modifiable risk factors for diabetic neuropathy. Thus far, since treatments for diabetic neuropathy have proven to be minimally (if at all) effective, prevention represents the best therapeutic strategy to prevent or slow progression.

Both the DCCT trial and the UKPDS trials have shown the importance of tight glycemic control in preventing microvascular disease and with the benefits of treatment not being confined to a threshold at 6.5%, but a continuum, with reductions below 6.5% continuing to demonstrate benefit *(71)*.

Macrovascular Disease

In the United States, more than 9 million women have diabetes with 10% in the type I category *(72)*. The association of diabetes with risk in women is very significant that this disease erases any protective female advantage for coronary heart disease. Initial reports in the Framingham study in 1979 demonstrated that men and women had a similar risk for coronary heart disease *(73)*. It is significant to note, however, that the risk for coronary heart disease in women with diabetes is five times the risk when compared with women without diabetes. Regrettably, the prevalence of coronary heart disease mortality in women is also increasing. A review in the Journal of the American Medical Association in 1998 reported a 36% decline in coronary heart disease mortality in non-diabetic men when compared with a 27% decline in women *(74)*. However, in diabetic women, there was an increase in coronary heart disease of 23%.

Not only are women with diabetes at a greater risk for coronary heart disease, but they also experience more adverse outcomes after experiencing an acute cardiovascular event. Both early (28 days) and late (2 years) mortality are greater in women than in men with diabetes *(75)*.

Various interrelating factors contribute to the acceleration of coronary heart disease risk in diabetic women. These include low social and economic status, higher rates of depression, central obesity, more severe elevations in circulating lipids, and blood pressure along with a greater tendency for poor glycemic control *(76)*. Wide fluctuations in range of glucose are a significant contributing factor for macro- and microvascular disease complications in women with diabetes. Various factors can influence glycemic control in women, including menstrual irregularity, insulin sensitivity, pregnancy, variability in glucose control throughout the perimenopausal period, a higher frequency of eating disorders, and use of hormonal contraception.

Low HDL cholesterol and high triglycerides clearly have a greater adverse impact on risk for vascular disease in women when compared with men *(77)*. In addition, elevations in both systolic and diastolic blood pressure occur more frequently in diabetic women when compared with men independent of body fat distribution, fasting insulin, age, or body weight.

The presence of hypertension increasingly aggravates the risk for vascular complications in diabetes *(78)*. In the United States, the majority of women with type II diabetes are overweight with weight gain increasing the risk for type II diabetes and coronary heart disease in women. Greater adverse metabolic risk profiles are associated with a waist-to-hip ratio greater than 0.76. This correlates even greater than the presence of gynecoid or peripheral obesity *(79)*. In addition, women with diabetes have a higher prevalence of depression and are more likely to be of a lower social economic status than individuals without diabetes.

The American Diabetes Association currently recommends that all women greater than 45 years of age be screened with a fasting glucose test on a regular basis preferably yearly *(80)*. Individuals at high risk, who should be screened more frequently and at an earlier age, include: those with a history of gestational diabetes, positive family history, members of racial or ethnic groups with high prevalence rates, or obesity.

Those individuals with signs and symptoms consistent with the existence of polycystic ovary syndrome (acne, hirsutism, infertility, and irregular menses) are also at greater risk. This syndrome affects 5% of pre-menopausal women, 20% of whom have either overtly abnormal glucose tolerance or impaired glucose tolerance. Over 40% of these women are obese when presenting to their physicians *(81)*.

The Diabetes Prevention Program stressed the importance of weight reduction and exercise to reduce the likelihood of developing diabetes and to improve overall glucose tolerance *(82)*. The use of metformin was effective to a lesser degree in women with a BMI greater than 35 kg/m^2.

Hence, all primary care providers should encourage their female patients to avoid sedentary behavior, restrict fat intake, and obesity. Institution of a regular exercise program consisting of 35 min of physical activity three to four times weekly has been associated with improved glucose tolerance and weight reduction in conjunction with a prudent dietary program.

Clinical trials have clearly demonstrated that it is not the intensity of exercise but the duration that is important *(83)*. In addition, multiple short periods of exercise in the form of brisk walking also produce beneficial cardiorespiratory fitness and weight loss. Since diabetes is a coronary artery disease risk equivalent, medical management must stress reduction of all risk factors including glycemic, lipid, and hypertension control, along with the inhibition of platelet aggregation.

Three recent randomized controlled clinical trials have shown that hormone replacement therapy carries no benefit either in primary or secondary prevention of cardiovascular disease. An increase in overall cardiovascular disease events and combined endpoints in the Women's Health Initiative study *(84)* prompted early discontinuation, while a greater frequency of recurrent cardiovascular disease events in the Heart and Estrogen/Progestin Replacement Study (HERS) trial *(85)* in patients that were randomized to hormone replacement therapy when compared with placebo during the first year highlighted the risks of hormone replacement therapy. In addition, in the Women's Angiographic Vitamin and Estrogen or WAVE trial *(86)*, cardiovascular benefits were not demonstrated with hormone replacement therapy in postmenopausal women with established coronary disease but rather an increase in cardiovascular events.

In the HERS trial, hormone replacement therapy did reduce the incidence of diabetes by 35%. However, despite this observation, hormone replacement therapy is not recommended for any woman with or without diabetes as part of a therapeutic strategy for the primary or secondary prevention of coronary heart disease *(87)*.

It should also be noted that diabetic patients that have had a myocardial infarction increase their risk of a second infarction by 45%. Data from Molberg, published in Circulation in 1999 from the Diabetes Mellitus, Insulin Glucose Infusion in Acute Myocardial Infarction trial revealed that 232 women admitted to the hospital with acute myocardial infarction improved survival up to 3.4 years after discharge with the early institution of intensive insulin therapy *(88)*. In this study, admission blood glucose levels were the strongest predictor of a fatal outcome. It has also been established that β blockers improve long-term survival and decrease the risk of recurrent myocardial infarction both in diabetic and in non-diabetic individuals *(89)*.

In 1999, Chen reported statistically significant differences in 1 year mortality for insulin and non-insulin–dependent diabetic patients given β blockers when compared with those not given β blockers after sustaining a myocardial infarction *(90)*. In the Glycemic Effects in Diabetes Mellitus trial, the α/β blocker carvedilol was shown to be superior to metoprolol in terms of its lipid and microalbuminuric lowering effects in diabetic patients *(91)*.

Screening for Coronary Heart Disease

According to the ADA Consensus Development Conference, stress testing should be performed in any individuals with diabetes who meet one of the following criteria *(92)*: (1) resting electrocardiogram suggestive of ischemia or infarction, (2) peripheral or carotid occlusive disease, (3) typical or atypical cardiac symptoms, (4) equal to or greater than 35 years of age, planning a vigorous exercise program, (5) two or more risk factors in addition to diabetes, including total cholesterol greater than 240 mg/dL, HDL cholesterol less than 35 mg/dL, LDL cholesterol greater than 160 mg/dL, blood pressure greater than 140/90 mmHg, smoking, positive test for micro- or macroalbuminuria, and family history of premature coronary disease. It is important to note that women have a higher rate of false/positive exercise stress tests than men and a negative exercise stress test also has a lower negative predictive value. Hence, perfusion imaging, in combination with exercise testing, improves the accuracy in women. Symptoms of coronary artery disease in women tend to be different than men with shortness of breath and fatigue being more prevalent that chest discomfort *(93)*. The clinician should have a high index of suspicion in the diabetic female to enhance discovery of underlying ischemic heart disease.

Other Complications of Diabetes in Women

The genitourinary tract is significantly affected by diabetes in women *(94)*. Acute urinary tract infections have a positive correlation with increased glucose levels. The female patient is more prone to lower urinary tract infections with diabetes as a result of recurrent vaginitis, diabetic microangiopathy, renal vascular disease, impaired leukocyte function, and diabetic neuropathy associated with neurogenic bladder or urinary retention *(95)*.

Asymptomatic bacteriuria and structural abnormalities of the urinary tract are more common in women with diabetes and are more likely to be associated with significant upper urinary tract disease. Due to the risk of ascending infection, non-pregnant women with diabetes, as well as pregnant patients, should be treated for asymptomatic bacteriuria. Symptomatic pyelonephritis is four to five times more common in diabetic women versus their non-diabetic counterparts. In addition, cystourethroceles and rectoceles are more common in women with diabetes as a result of vascular compromise and/or recurrent vaginitis *(96)*. Female patients should be educated about the importance of frequent voiding and complete emptying of the bladder with appropriate attention to even minor symptoms of a urological disorder.

Infections

The most common infections in female patients with diabetes are urinary tract, respiratory tract and skin *(97)*. Colonization and overgrowth of organisms can present a significant problem in the female patient with group D streptococcal infections being more common in diabetic women. Anaerobic infections are much more likely, predisposing the patient to abscess formation, emphesematous complications, and necrotizing soft tissue infections due to defects in polymorphonuclear leukocytes and vascular compromise *(98)*. Localized soft tissue infection in the form of furuncles, impetigo, carbuncles, and cellulitis due to staph and β-hemolytic strep are also commonly found in diabetic women. Vulvar abscesses in diabetics must be considered necrotizing fasciitis until proven otherwise. Any vulvar abscesses, cellulitis or postoperative wound infections need to be aggressively evaluated and treated *(99)*.

GYNECOLOGICAL ABNORMALITIES

Recently, there has been a trend toward a higher incidence of condylomata acuminata in patients with diabetes, but few definitive perspective data exist as of this time *(100)*. In addition, it is believed that human papilloma virus may also be more prevalent in women with diabetes *(101)*. Vulvovaginal candidiasis is also increased in the diabetic women. Hyperglycemia increases the risk of candidiasis, in addition to high estrogen states, use of antibiotics and systemic glucocorticoids. Hence, proper patient education about the appropriate undergarments and avoidance of tight clothes, such as pantyhose, should be considered.

In a study of women with diabetes with and without symptoms of vulvovaginal candidiasis, candida glabrata was isolated most frequently (50% of cases) followed by candida albicans (35%) *(102)*. The best in-office test for diagnosing vulvovaginal candidiasis is microscopy, but this can lack accuracy, missing up to 50% of cases, especially with candida glabrata, which tend to lack hyphae formation.

Hence, the obtaining of proper cultures, not only in investigating recurrent infections, but also in treatment failures, is important in managing this condition. Fortunately, topical imidazoles and triazoles are associated with cure rates of about 85–90%, although candida glabrata and candida tropicalis are less sensitive to standard imidazol antifungals *(103)*. Oral anti-mycotic agents can also be used for these infections. In type I diabetics, menarche age is increased by approx 1 year, with irregular menses common especially in the face of uncontrolled diabetes. The prevalence of menstrual irregularities in the diabetic population can be twice that of controlled subjects. Cyclical changes occur in insulin and glucose requirements during the menstrual cycle with variations of insulin dosages to achieve glycemic control occasionally demonstrating inconsistent results.

Risk Reduction in the Female Diabetic

Only a comprehensive program of overall risk reduction can achieve optimal results in diabetic women. This includes careful attention to hypertension, dyslipidemia, hyperglycemia, and platelet aggregation. Antihypertensive therapy with an angiotensin-converting enzyme (ACE) inhibitor or angiotensin receptor blocker is indicated for patients with diabetes and blood pressures greater than

130/80 mmHg or microalbuminuria *(104)*. The Heart Outcomes Prevention Evaluation Study trial demonstrated the efficacy of ramipril in reducing the risk for myocardial infarction, stroke, overall cardiovascular mortality and morbidity, and revascularization in individuals with diabetes greater than 55 years of age *(105)*. Women of child bearing age, who are not using contraception, should be warned about the harmful effects to developing fetuses of ACE inhibitor or angiotensin receptor blocker use and should discontinue these agents immediately when the patient becomes pregnant. For lipid control, a target LDL cholesterol should be less than 100 mg/dL with HDL's greater than 55 mg/dL in diabetic women.

Data from several large lipid lowering trials indicate the benefits of statin therapy in diabetic women with coronary disease *(106)*. There are relative risk reductions from 24% to 34% in non-diabetic women and 19% to 42% in the presence of diabetes. Hemoglobin A1C should be less than 6.5% with postprandial sugars less than 140 mg/dL and fasting sugars less than 100 mg/dL. It is to be understood that the pursuit of the optimal A1C represents a continuum goal below 6.5%—not a threshold at this value.

The UKPDS demonstrated a 14% reduction in the risk for coronary heart disease for each 1% reduction in A1C, even below 6.5% *(107)*. In addition, an independent association in women has been described between A1C and the prevalence of coronary heart disease.

Aspirin therapy is indicated for diabetic individuals greater than 21 years of age to attenuate vasoconstriction and inhibit platelet aggregation *(108)*. The current recommendation is 160–325 mg of aspirin daily for type II diabetics unless contraindicated by recent gastrointestinal bleeding, bleeding tendencies, or allergies. In the Hypertension Optimal Treatment trial, 75 mg of aspirin daily reduced pooled cardiovascular risk by 15% and myocardial infarction by 36% *(109)*. In diabetic patients that have had a myocardial infarction or stroke, low doses can be as effective as high doses and can reduce cardiovascular events by as much as 25%.

In those patients that are allergic to aspirin, clopidogrel (Plavix) my be substituted. The Clopidogrel versus Aspirin in Patients at Risk for Ischemic Events trial, showed clopidogrel to be equally effective as 325 mg of aspirin in reducing the risk of vascular death, ischemic stroke, or myocardial infarction *(110)*. Subanalysis of the diabetic cohort in this trial showed clopidogrel to be particularly effective in patients with peripheral vascular disease.

The importance of addressing all four risk factors in the diabetic was shown in the Steno-II trial which enrolled 160 patients with type II diabetes and microalbuminuria *(111)*. Patients with an average age of 55 years were placed into an intensive therapy group and a conventional therapy group. The intensive group all received ACE inhibitors, dietary intervention, aspirin, more than 30 minutes of exercise weekly, tight glucose control with A1C's less than 6.5, blood pressures less than 130/80 mmHg, total cholesterol less than 175 mg/dL, and triglycerides less than 150 mg/dL in addition to smoke cessation.

Outcomes in the intensive strategy group were consistently better than the conventionally managed group with primary outcomes of composite cardiovascular death, non-fatal myocardial infarction, coronary revascularization, non-fatal stroke, amputation or peripheral vascular surgery reduced by 53% in the intensive strategy group, with neuropathy being reduced by 61%, retinopathy by 58%, and autonomic neuropathy by 3%.

SUMMARY

Early detection of diabetes in women is essential to prevent serious complications, with improved mortality and morbidity accomplished by aggressively controlling the multiple risk factors underlying the disease. It is only with this aggressive multifaceted approach that better survival and improved life quality can be achieved.

REFERENCES

1. Vinicor F. Diabetes and Women's Health Across the Life Stages: A Public Health Perspective. Centers for Disease Control, US Department of Health and Human Services, Atlanta; 2002.
2. Narayan KM, Boyle JP, Thompson TJ, Sorenson SW, Williamson DF. Lifetime risk for diabetes mellitus in the United States. JAMA 2003;290(14):1884–1890.
3. Executive Summary of the Third Report of The National Cholesterol Education Program (NCEP) expert panel on detection, evaluation, and treatment of high blood cholesterol in adults (Adult Treatment Panel III). JAMA 2001;285(19):2486–2497.
4. Knowler WC, Barrett-Connor E, Fowler SE. Reduction in the incidence of type 2 diabetes with lifestyle intervention or metformin. N Engl J Med 2002;346(6):393–403.
5. Ford ES, Giles WH, Dietz WH. Prevalence of the metabolic syndrome among US adults: findings from the third National Health and Nutrition Examination Survey. JAMA 2002: 287:356–359.
6. Isomaa B, Almgren P. Tuomi T, Cardiovascular morbidity and mortality associated with the metabolic syndrome. Diabetes Care 2001;24:2486–2497.
7. Jack L, Boseman L, Vinicor F. Aging Americans and diabetes. A public health and clinical response. Geriatrics 2004;59:14–17.
8. Smedley BD, Stith AY, Nelson AR. Unequal Treatment: Confronting Racial and Ethnic Disparities in Health Care. National Academic Press, Washington, DC; 2003.
9. Harris MI, Flegal KM, Cowie CC. Prevalence of diabetes, impaired fasting glucose, and impaired glucose tolerence in US adults. The Third National Health and Nutrition Examination Survey. Diabetes Care 1998;21:136–144.
10. American Diabetes Association. Standards of medical care in diabetes. Diabetes Care 2004;27(Suppl. 1):S15–S35.
11. Pietropaolo M, LeRoith D. Pathogenesis of diabetes: our current understanding. Clin Cornerstone 2001;4:1–16.
12. Ramlo-Halsted BA, Edelman SV. The natural history of type 2 diabetes. Implications for clinical practice. Prim Care 1999;26:771–789.

13. Dungan KM, Buse JB. Glucagon-like peptide 1 based therapies for type 2 diabetes. Clin Diabetes 2005;23:56.
14. Salehi M, D'Alessio D. New therapies for type 2 diabetes based on glucagon-like peptide1. Cleve Clin Med 2006;72(4):382–388.
15. Codario R. Type 2 Diabetes, Pre-Diabetes, and the Metabolic Syndrome: The Primary Care Guide to Diagnosis and Management. Humana Press, Clifton, NJ; 2005, p. 14.
16. American Diabetes Association. Standards of medical care in diabetes. Diabetes Care 2004;27(Suppl. 1):S15–S35.
17. Genuth S, Alberti KG, Bennett P. Follow up report on the diagnosis of diabetes mellitus. Diabetes Care 2003;26:3160–3167.
18. Tuomilehto J, Lindstrom J, Eriksson JG. Prevention of type 2 diabetes mellitus by changes in lifestyle among subjects with impaired glucose tolerance. N Engl J Med 2001;344: 1343–1350.
19. Kanaya AM, Narayan KM. Prevention of type 2 diabetes: data from recent trials. Prim Care 2003;30:511–526.
20. Buchanan TA, Xiang AH, Peters RK. Prevention of type 2 diabetes by treatment of insulin resistance: comparison of early vs. late intervention in the TRIPOD study. Diabetes 2002; 51(Suppl. 2):A35.
21. Moses RG. The recurrence rate of gestational diabetes in subsequent pregnancies. Diabetes Care 1996;19(12):1348–1350.
22. Dornhorst A, Rossi M. Risk and prevention of type 2 diabetes in women with gestational diabetes. Diabetes Care 1998;21(Suppl. 2):B43–B49.
23. Report of the Expert Committee on the Diagnosis and Classification of Diabetes Mellitus. Diabetes Care 2000;23(Suppl. 1):S4–S19.
24. Jovanovic L, Pettit DJ. Gestational diabetes mellitus. JAMA 2001;286:2516–2518.
25. Kim C, Newton KM, Knopp RH. Gestational diabetes and the incidence of type 2 diabetes: a systematic review. Diabetes Care 2002;25:1862–1868.
26. Pietropaolo M, LeRoith D. Pathogenesis of diabetes: our current understanding. Clin Cornerstone 2001;4:1–16.
27. Codario R. Type 2 Diabetes, Pre-Diabetes, and the Metabolic Syndrome. The Primary Guide to Diagnosis and Management. Humana Press, Clifton, NJ;2005, p. 101.
28. Schmitz O, Rungby B. Amylin agaonists: a novel approach in the treatment of diabetes. Diabetes 2004;53(Suppl. 3):S233.
29. McMahon G, Arky R. Inhaled insulin for diabetes mellitus. N Engl J Med 2007:497–502.
30. Patton JS, BukarJ, Nagarian S. Inhaled insulin. ADV Drug Deliv Rev 1999;35:235–247.
31. DeFronzo RA, Bergenstahl RM, Cefalu WT. Efficacy of inhaled insulin in patients with type 2 diabetes not controlled with diet and exercise. Diabetes Care 2005;28: 1922–1928.
32. Becker RH, Sha S, Frick AD, Fountaine RJ. The effect of smoking cessation and subsequent resumption on absorption of inhaled insulin. Diabetes Care 2006;29:277–282.
33. Ryan EA, Lakey JR, Paty BW, Imes S, Korbutt GS, Kneteman NM. Successful islet transplantation: continued insulin reserve provides long term glycemic control. Diabetes. 2002; 51:2148–2157 (PMID: 12086945).
34. Pierce NS. Diabetes and exercise. Br J Sports Med 1999;33:161–173.
35. Palumbo PJ. Glycemic control, mealtime glucose excursions and diabetic complications in type 2 diabetes mellitus. Mayo Clin Proc 2001;76:609–618.
36. DeFronzo RA. Pathogenesis of type 2 diabetes: metabolic and molecular implications for indentifying diabetes genes. Diabetes Rev 1997;5:177–269.
37. Henry RR. Glucose control and insulin resistance in non-insulin dependent diabetes mellitus. Ann Intern Med 1996;124:97–103.

38. Grundy SM. 2002 Obesity, metabolic syndrome, and coronary atherosclerosis. Circulation 2002;105:2696–2698.
39. Codario R. Type 2 Diabetes, Pre-Diabetes, and the Metabolic Syndrome: The Primary Care Guide. Humana Press, Clifton, NJ; 2005, p. 17.
40. LeRoith D. Beta cell dysfunction and insulin resistance in type 2 diabetes: role of metabolic and genetic abnormalities. Am J Med 2002;113(Suppl. 6A):3S–11S.
41. Hoogwerf B. Exenatide and pramlintide: new glucose lowering agents for trating diabetes mellitus. Cleve Clin J Med 2006;73(6):477–484.
42. Nielsen LL, Baron AD. Pharmacology of exenatide for the treatment of type 2 diabetes. Curr Opin Investig Drugs 2003;4:401–405.
43. Nielsen LL, Young AA, Parkes DG. Pharmacology of exenatide: a potential therapeutic for improved glycemic control of type 2 diabetes. Regul Pept 2004;117:77–88.
44. Parkes D, Jodka C, Smith P. Pharmacokinetic actions of exendin-4 in the rat: comparison with glucagon-like peptide-1. Drug Dev Res 2001;53:260.
45. Ahren B, Gomis R, Standl E. Twelve and fifty two week efficacy of the dipeptidyl peptidase IV inhibitor LAF237 in metformin-treated patients with type 2 diabetes. Diabetes Care 2004;27:2874.
46. Scott R, Herman G, Zhao P. Twelve week efficacy and tolerability of MK-0431, a dipeptidyl peptidase IV inhibitor, in the treatment of type 2 diabetes. Abstract Book, Diabetes Association 65th Scientific Sessions 2005;41-O.
47. Salehi M, D'Alessio D. New therapies for type 2 diabetes based on glucagon like peptide-1. Cleve Clin J Med 2006;73(4):382–388.
48. Nauck MA, Meininger G, Sheng D, Terranella L, Stein PP. Efficacy and safety of the dipeptidyl peptidase-4 inhibitor, sitagliptin, compared with the sulfonylurea, glipizide, in patients with type 2 diabetes inadequately controlled on metformin alone. Diab, Obes Metab 2007;9:194–205.
49. Aschner P, Kipnes MS, Lunjceford JK, Sanchez M, Mickel C, Williams-Herman DE. Effect of the dipeptidyl peptidase-4 inhibitor sitagliptin monotherapy on glycemic control in patients with type 2 diabetes. Diabetes Care 2006;29:2632–2638.
50. Codario R. A guide to combination therapy in type 2 diabetes. Patient Care 2003;37:16–24.
51. DeFronzo RA. Pharmacologic therapy for type 2 diabetes mellitus. Ann Intern Med 1999; 133:73–74.
52. Egan J, Rubin C, Mathisen A. Pioglitazone 027 Study Group: combination therapy with pioglitazone and metformin in patients with type 2 diabetes. Diabetes 1999;48:A117.
53. Moses R, Slobodniuk R, Boyages S. Effect of replaglinide addition to metformin monotherapy on glycemic control in patients with type 2 diabetes. Diabetes Care 1999;22:119–124.
54. Raskin P, McGill J, Hale P. Replaglinide/rosiglitazone combination therapy of type 2 diabetes. American Diabetes Association 61st Scientific Session. Abstract 516-P. Diabetes 2001;50(Suppl. 2):4.
55. Izucchi SE. Oral antihyperglycemic therapy for type 2 diabetes: scientific review. J Am Med Assoc 2002;287:360–372.
56. Dailey GE. Improving oral pharmacologic treatment and management of type 2 diabetes. Manag Care 2004;13:41–47.
57. Yki-Jarvinen H, Ryysy L, Nikkila K. Comparison of bedtime insulin regimens in patients with type 2 diabetes mellitus: a randomized controlled study. Ann Int Med 1999;130:389–396.
58. Dressler A, Yki-Jarvinen H, Ziemen M. Less hypoglycemia and better post dinner glucose control with bedtime insulin glargine compared with bedtime NPH insulin during insulin combination therapy in type 2 diabetes. Diabetes Care 2000;23:1130–1136.
59. Gulland J. Growing evidence supports role of chromium in prevention treatment of diabetes. Hollistic Primary Care 2003;4:8.

60. Yeh GY, Eisenberg DM, Kaptchuk TJ. Philips RS. Systematic review of herbs and dietary supplements for glycemic control in diabetes. Diabetes Care 2003;26:1277–1294.
61. American Diabetes Association. Diabetic retinopathy. Diabetes Care 2002;26(Suppl. 1): S99–S102.
62. Davis MD, Fisher MR, Gangnon RE. Risk factors for high risk proliferative diabetic retinopathy and severe visual loss: early treatment diabetic retinopathy Report#18. Invest Ophthalmol Vis Sci 1998;39:233–252.
63. American Diabetes Association. Diabetic nephropathy. Diabetes Care 2003;26(Suppl. 1): S94–S98.
64. Mogensen CE, Vestbo E, Poulsen PL. Micoralbuminuria and potential confounders. A review and some oservations on variability of urinary albumin excretion. Diabetes Care 1995;18:572–581.
65. The National Kidney Foundation Kidney Disease Outcome Quality Initiative. Clinical practice guidelines for chronic kidney disease: evaluation, classification, and stratification. Am J Kidney Dis 2002;39(Suppl. 1):S1–S266.
66. Bakris GL, Williams M, Dworkin L. Preserving renal function in adults with hypertension and diabetes: a consensus approach. National Kidney Foundation Hypertension and Diabetes Executive Committees Working Group. Am J Kidney Dis 2000;41(Suppl. 1): S22–S25.
67. Sinnreich M, Taylor BV, Dyck JB. Diabetic neuropathies. Neurologist 2005;11:63–79.
68. Gominak S, Parry GJ. Diabetic neuropathy. Adv Neurol 2002;99:99–109.
69. Simmons Z, Feldman EL. Update on diabetic neuropathy. Curr Opin Neurol 2002;15:595–603.
70. Verne GN, Sninsky CA. Diabetes and the gastrointestinal tract. Gastroenterol Clin North Am 1998;27:861–874.
71. Davidson JA. Rationale for more aggressive guidelines for diabetes control. Endocr Pract. 2002;8(Suppl. 1):13–14.
72. Pietropaolo M, LeRoith D. Pathogenesis of diabetes: our current understanding. Clin Cornerstone 2001;4:1–16.
73. Gu K, Cowie CC, Harris MI. Diabetes and decline in heart disease mortality in US adults. JAMA 1999;281;1291–1297.
74. Downs JR, Clearfield M, Weis S. Primary prevention of acute coronary events with lovastatin in men and women with average cholesterol levels. JAMA 1998;279:1615–1622.
75. Assmann G, Carmena R, Cullen P. Coronary heart disease: reducing the risk: a worldwide view. International Task Force for the Prevention of Coronary Disease. Circulation 1999; 100:1930–1938.
76. Wilson PW. Diabetes mellitus and coronary heart disease. Am J Kidney Dis 1998;32: S89–S100.
77. Gaede P, Vedel P, Larsen N. Multifactorial intervention and cardiovascular disease in patients with type 2 diabetes. N Engl J Med 2003;348:383–393.
78. Tight blood pressure control and risk of macrovascular and mcirovascular complications in type 2 diabetes: UKPDS 38. UK Prospective Diabetes Study Group. BMJ 1998;317: 703–713.
79. Vega GL. Results of expert meetings: obesity and cardiovascular disease. Obesity, the metabolic syndrome and cardivascular disease. Am Heart J 2001;142:1108–1116.
80. Deen D. Metabolic syndrome: time for action. Am Fam Physician 2004;69:2875–2882.
81. Wilson PW, Grundy SM. The metabolic syndrome: practical guide to origins and treatment. Circulation 2003;108:1422–1424.
82. Knowler WC, Barnett-Conner E, Fowler SE. Diabetes Prevention Program Research Group. Reduction in the incidence of type 2 diabetes with lifestyle intervention or metformin. N Engl J Med 2002;346:393–403.

83. Zinman B, Ruderman N, Campaigne BN, Devlin JT, Schneider SH. American Diabetes Association. Physical activity, exercise and diabetes mellitus. Diabetes Care 2003;26 (Suppl. 1):S73–S77.
84. Rossouw JE, Anerson GL, Prentice RL. Risks and benefits of estrogen plus progestin in healthy postmenopausal women: principal results from the Women's Health Initiative randomized controlled trial. JAMA 2002;288:321–333.
85. Hulley S, Grady D, Bush T. Randomized controlled trial of estrogen plus progestin for secondary prevention of coronary heart disease in postmenopausal women. Heart and Estrogen/progestin Replacement Study (HERS) Research Group. JAMA 1998;280:605–613.
86. Manning P, Allum A, Jones S, Sutherland W, Williams S. The effect of hormone replacement therapy on cardiovascular risk factors in type 2 diabetes. Arch Intern Med 2001; 161:1134–1135.
87. Herrington DM, Vittinghoff E, Lin F. Statin therapy, cardiovascular events, and total mortality in the Heart and Estrogen/Progestin Replacement Study (HERS). Circulation 2002; 105:2962–2967.
88. Malmberg K. Prospective randomized study of intensive insulin treatment on long term survival after acute myocardial infarction in patients with diabetes mellitus. Diabetes Mellitus, Insulin Glucose Infusion in Acute Myocardial Infarction (DIGAMI) Study Group. BMJ 1997;314:1512–1514.
89. Kjekshus J, Gilpin E, Cali G, Blackey AR, Henning H, Ross J. Diabetic patients and beta-blockers after acute myocardial infarction. Eur Heart J 1990;27:1143–1150.
90. Chen J. Beta blockers in elderly diabetic patients post myocardial infarction. J Am Coll Cardiol 1999;34:1388–1394.
91. Bakris G, Bell D, Fonseca V. GEMINI Investigators. The rationale and design of the glycemic effects in diabetes mellitus. JAMA 2004;292(18):198.
92. Myers J, Prakash M, Froelicher V, Do D, Partington S, Atwood JE. Exercise mortality among men referred for exercise testing. N Engl J Med 2001;346:793–801.
93. Vinik A, Flemmer M. Diabetes and macrovascular disease. J Diab Complications 2002; 16:235–245.
94. Patterson JE, Andriole VT. Bacterial urinary tract infections in diabetes. Infect Dis Clin North Am 1995:9(1):25–51.
95. Patterson JE, Andriole V. Bacterial urinary tract infections in diabetes. Infect Dis Clin North Am 1997;11(3):735–750.
96. Lunt H. Women and diabetes. Diabet Med 1996;13(12):1009–1016.
97. Rayfield EJ, Ault MJ, Keusch GT. Infection and diabetes: the case for glucose control. Am J Med 1982;72(3):439–450.
98. Addison WA, Livingood CH, Hill GB. Recurrent necrotizing fasciitis of vulvar origin in diabetic patients. Obstet Gynecol 1984;63(4):473–479.
99. Bohannon NJ. Treatment of vulvovaginal candidiasis in patients with diabetes. Diabetes Care 1998;21(3):451–456.
100. Bell DS, Clements RS, Cutter GR, Whitey RJ. Condylomata acuminate in IDDM. Diabetes Care 1988;11(3):295–296.
101. Stenchever MA, Herbst AL, Mishell DR (eds). Comprehensive Gynecology. 4th ed.Mosby, St. Louis, MO; 2001.
102. Peer AK, Hoosen AA, Seedat MA. Vaginal yeast infections in diabetic women. S Afr Med J 1993;83(10):727–729.
103. Tobin MJ. Vulvovaginal candidiasis: topical versus oral therapy. Am Fam Phys 1995;51: 1715–1720.
104. Coats AJ. Angiotensin receptor blockers—finally the evidence is coming in: IDNT and RENAAL. Int J Cardiol 2001;79:99–102.

105. Heart Outcomes Prevention Evaluation Study Investigators. Effects of ramipril on cardiovascular and microvascular outcomes in people with diabetes mellitus: results of the HOPE study and MICRO-HOPE substudy. Lancet 2000;355:253–259.
106. Spanheimer RG. Reducing cardiovascular risk in diabetes. Which factors to modify first? Postgrad Med 2001;109:26–30, *see* also p. 33–36.
107. Adler AI, Stratton IM, Neil HA. Association of systolic blood pressure with macrovascular and microvascular complications of type 2 diabetes (UKPDS 36): prospective observational study. BMJ 2000;321:412–419.
108. Colwell JA. American Diabetes Association. Aspirin therapy in diabetes. Diabetes Care 2003;26(Suppl. 1):S87–S88.
109. Hansson L, Zanchetti A, Carruthers SG. Effects of intensive blood pressure lowering and low dose aspirin in patients with hypertension: principal results of the Hypertension Optimal Treatment (HOT) Randomized Trial (HOT) Study Group. Lancet 1998;351:1755–1762.
110. CAPRIE Steering Committee. Randomized, blinded trial of clopidogrel versus aspirin in patients at risk of ischemic events (CAPRIE). Lancet 1996;348:1329–1339.
111. Gaede P, Vedel P, Larsen N, Jensen GV, Parving HH, Pedersen O. Multifactorial intervention and cardiovascular disease in patients with type 2 diabetes. N Engl J Med 2003;348: 383–393.

10 Polycystic Ovary Syndrome

Katherine Sherif, MD

CONTENTS

INTRODUCTION

Polycystic Ovary Syndrome (PCOS) is the one of the common cause of menstrual irregularity in the United States and a leading cause of infertility. PCOS prevalence ranges from 6 to 10% in the United States. Because obesity may unmask PCOS, the incidence may increase as obesity rates increase. PCOS has been viewed as a collection of reproductive disorders, including polycystic ovaries, anovulation, infertility, and pregnancy loss, associated with hirsutism, acne, and obesity. More recently, PCOS has been linked with cardiovascular risk factors, such as elevated blood pressure, dyslipidemia, abnormal glucose metabolism, and coagulopathies. As many as one-third of PCOS women develop type 2 diabetes. Small observational studies have linked PCOS with early coronary artery disease.

From: *Current Clinical Practice: Women's Health in Clinical Practice*
Edited by: Clouse and Sherif © Humana Press Inc., Totowa, NJ

DEFINITION

PCOS presents with varied symptoms, which has created a lack of agreement in diagnostic criteria and has made studies difficult to compare. In 1990, the National Institutes of Health (NIH) convened a consensus conference regarding PCOS and published "probable" and "possible" criteria to define PCOS *(1)*. More recently, in 2003, the American Society of Reproductive Medicine and the European Society of Human Reproduction and Embryology developed a definition *(2)*. According to their criteria, PCOS is diagnosed in the presence of two out of three of the following factors: oligo-ovulation or anovulation, clinical or biochemical signs of hyperandrogenemia, and polycystic ovaries on ultrasound, in the absence of another etiology. Despite this widely accepted definition, there is still controversy because some experts think that PCOS cannot exist without oligo-ovulation or anovulation. The new definition does take into consideration the fact that not all women with PCOS exhibit polycystic ovaries, and as many as 20 to 30% of non-PCOS women have polycystic ovaries *(3)*. The failure to reach a universal definition arises from the heterogeneous nature of the syndrome, whose etiology is probably multifactorial.

Menstrual dysfunction may take any of several forms. Most commonly, menses are irregular since the onset of menarche, with varying intervals, but almost always longer than 35 days apart. Menses are often associated with significant menorrhagia and dysmenorrhea. In some women, menses may be regular after menarche for a year or two, and then become irregular. Other women may be somewhat regular, but frequently skip periods. Although irregular menses in adolescents are frequently ascribed to the "normal" variation in cycle length before the maturation of the hypothalamic–pituitary–ovarian axis, the most common cause of markedly irregular cycles (>90 d in length) is hyperandrogenemia. It is not unusual for some women to be amenorrheic for longer than a year.

Hyperandrogenemia refers to elevated serum concentrations of total testosterone and/or free testosterone. Hyperandrogenemia causes clinical hyperandrogenism, which presents as hirsutism, diffuse alopecia, and cystic acne. Dehydroepiandrosterone sulfate, often elevated in PCOS, is a weak androgen and probably does not contribute as much as testosterone does to clinical hyperandrogenism.

PATHOPHYSIOLOGY

The pathophysiology of PCOS is not completely understood; it is probably multifactorial. The most widely accepted hypothesis is that insulin resistance is a central feature, and that hyperinsulinemia stimulates ovarian production of androgens *(4)*. Although peripheral tissue is insulin resistant, ovarian theca cells are not and respond to hyperinsulinemia. Although insulin resistance is a common feature of obesity, studies comparing obese PCOS women with obese non-PCOS women reveal both a higher *prevalence* of insulin resistance and impaired glucose tolerance in PCOS women and a greater *degree* of insulin resistance *(5)*. Insulin is a potent growth hormone. Hyperinsulinemia not only leads to obesity (which worsens insulin resistance) but it has numerous other effects:

- Hyperinsulinemia is associated with endothelial dysfunction
- Hyperinsulinemia increases formation of free fatty acids and triglycerides
- Hyperinsulinemia is toxic to pancreatic β-cells, thereby decreasing insulin production and setting the stage for hyperglycemia

As many as 25% of women with PCOS are lean. The role of insulin resistance is less clear in non-obese PCOS women, although some studies have shown that thin women are also insulin resistant.

A second theory postulates that the primary pathophysiological process resides in the hypothalamic pituitary axis. In PCOS, the hypothalamus releases gonadatropin-releasing hormone (GnRH) in abnormally high-frequency and high-amplitude pulses, which causes abnormally elevated luteinizing hormone (LH). High LH concentrations favor the formation of androgens, which interfere with anovulation *(6)*. However, hyperinsulinemia has been demonstrated to increase GnRH pulse frequency and amplitude, resulting in elevated LH.

Although it is not clear whether hyperinsulinemia alone or abnormal GnRH pulsatility alone is responsible for hyperandrogenemia, there is no question that elevated serum testosterone, and/or increased receptor sensitivity to testosterone, results in clinical androgenization and anovulation. The most obvious manifestations of androgenization are hirsutism, cystic acne, and diffuse alopecia. In the ovaries, hyperandrogenemia prevents the formation of a dominant follicle, which, in turn, prevents atresia of nondominant follicles, resulting in the formation of multiple peripheral cysts. Androgens also affect metabolic parameters. For example, testosterone is associated with low high-density lipoprotein (HDL) cholesterol concentrations *(7)*.

DIAGNOSIS

The patient's history is the most important component of diagnosing PCOS.

The most common etiology of irregular periods is PCOS. However, if a woman has had regular menses for years and then develops irregular periods, she should first have a pregnancy test. If she is not pregnant, than the differential includes hypothyroidism, prolactin-producing pituitary adenoma, late-onset (non-classic) congenital hyperplasia (NCCAH), and androgen-secreting tumor. These diagnoses must be specifically excluded by laboratory testing before the diagnosis of PCOS can be made. There are historical clues that may lead to accurate diagnoses. Galactorrhea may signal a prolactin-producing pituitary adenoma or thyroid dysfunction. Hypothyroidism may be associated with typical symptoms of weight gain and constipation. The rarest of these, an androgen-secreting tumor, is signaled by the *sudden* onset of virilizing symptoms, such as hirsutism. A history of precocious puberty and Ashkenazi Jewish or Italian descent are suggestive of late-onset congenital hyperplasia.

PCOS can mimic and coexist with NCCAH, a variety of adrenal enzyme deficiencies that range from mild to moderate in the steps leading to glucocorticoid production. The most common enzyme deficiency is a 21-hydroxylase mutation, which interrupts cortisol production to varying degrees depending on the severity of enzyme impairment. Because adrenal enzyme deficiencies may result in elevated adrenal androgens, the symptoms often mimic those of PCOS *(8)*. Ethnic groups with a relatively high incidence of late-onset NCCAH include Ashkenazi Jews, Greeks, Italians, Latinas, and Slavs. Clues to NCCAH include precocious puberty (menses as early as 9 or 10 years of age) and menses that are not as irregular as observed in PCOS.

Conditions that are closely related to PCOS, but not included in any definition, include elevated blood pressure, hypothyroidism, diabetes, and dyslipidemia. PCOS is common enough in women with type 2 diabetes that some experts recommend screening for PCOS among all women with type 2 diabetes. Reproductive conditions include premature births, multiple miscarriages, a higher incidence of stillborn births, and endometrial cancer in middle age secondary to chronic anovulation.

HISTORY

The typical history reveals menarche at the average age of 12 to 13 years. Almost immediately, menses occur at irregular intervals. Often, teenagers are told that irregular menses are a normal part of development for a few years. Without establishing a diagnosis, physicians usually prescribe oral contraceptive pills (OCPs) to initiate regular menses. OCPs decrease ovarian androgen production and lower serum androgen levels by increasing hepatically synthesized sex hormone-binding globulin (SHBG). OCPs improve hirsutism and acne. Using an OCP for years delays the diagnosis and prevents the teen or woman in her 20s from understanding the reproductive and cardiovascular risks associated with PCOS. After discontinuing OCPs, many women are surprised to discover they have oligomenorrhea, are anovulatory, or are infertile. At this point, women may blame OCPs for their menstrual dysfunction or infertility. When the diagnosis of PCOS is finally confirmed, they may often be dismayed.

Women with PCOS generally do not discuss infertility with primary care providers. In fact, they may not have even tried to conceive. However, it is possible to elicit a history of infertility by asking patients whether they have ever had sexual intercourse without using contraception but did not become pregnant.

Although women will consult a gynecologist regarding the irregular menses, they may not mention other troublesome symptoms. These symptoms include rapid weight gain, extreme difficulty losing weight, hirsutism, acne, and alopecia. Patients may mention that they have central obesity, which is associated with type 2 diabetes. Some investigators hypothesize that eating disorders, especially bulimia, are more common in PCOS, but no clinical trials have addressed this issue.

Hair and skin changes are often noted. Women complain of hirsutism on the chin, cheeks/sideburns, neck, chest and between breasts, in the periareolar area, on the upper arms, and from the umbilicus to the pubic triangle. Patients should be questioned regarding hair removal using depilatories, shaving, waxing, bleaching, laser, or electrolysis; because body hair in women is culturally undesirable in many Western countries, women go to considerable efforts to hide it. One of the most distressing symptoms reported by patients is diffuse (or androgenic) alopecia, not to be confused with patchy alopecia. Acne can be mild to severe and may occur in areas more commonly associated with men, including the upper arms, upper back, and buttocks.

There is often a history of family members with irregular periods, severe acne, excess hair growth, infertility in a female relative, or few children. Type 2 diabetes is often present in parents, aunts, and uncles. PCOS is thought to be autosomal dominant in inheritance, but with variable manifestations. A family history of premature balding may be elicited in male family members.

PHYSICAL EXAMINATION

After the history, the next most important component in the diagnosis of PCOS is the physical examination. It is important to remember that not all women with PCOS have the typically described symptoms. Phenotypic presentations vary in several factors because the etiology is probably multifactorial. For example, some women may have few testosterone receptors in skin, preventing the expression of hirsutism (e.g., East Asians). Other women may have a normal body mass index (less than 25 mg/kg^2). Some women do not have acne or alopecia. A small number have regular menses, but have most of the other features of hyperandrogenism and polycystic ovaries. The absence of all classically described symptoms should not automatically exclude PCOS.

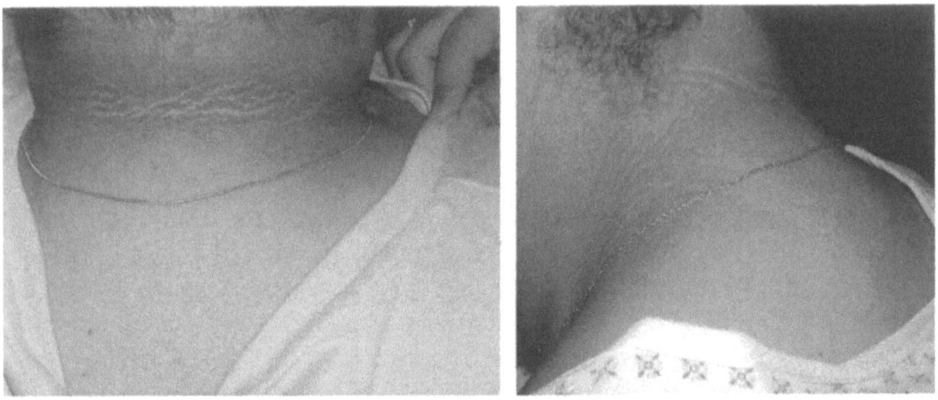

Fig. 1. Acanthosis nigricans on the neck.

Vital Signs

It is not unusual to find elevated blood pressures, with systolic pressures as high as 130 to 135 mmHg and diastolic pressures in the high 80 mmHg to low 90 mmHg range, even in young women. Most women with PCOS are obese, and, in particular, have central obesity consisting of fat deposition in the abdomen, upper arms, and upper back.

Hair and Skin

Hirsutism may or may not be present on the chin, neck, cheeks, chest, periareolar area, upper arms, back, or abdomen. Even if there are only a few terminal hairs on the chest, between the breasts, or on the lower abdomen; hair in these areas is indicative of elevated serum androgens. Hirsutism may also be relative to other family members. Women of some ethnic groups, for example, Asians, may not display any hirsutism in the presence of hyperandrogenemia. A history of *acute* onset of hirsutism accompanied by severe hirsutism on the trunk is suspicious for an androgen-secreting tumor. Acne may be non-existent, mild, or severe, and may be present on the face, neck, upper arms, upper chest, back, or buttocks. Diffuse alopecia, as opposed to patchy alopecia, is common and is usually mentioned by the patient. What may appear as a normal head of hair to the practitioner may not be normal to the patient and should be taken seriously.

Other signs of hyperandrogenemia include disproportionately small, underdeveloped breasts. Elevated androgens promote seborrhea production, which may increase cause seborrheic dermatitis, with flaking and erythema in the eyebrows, nasolabial folds, and below the lower lip.

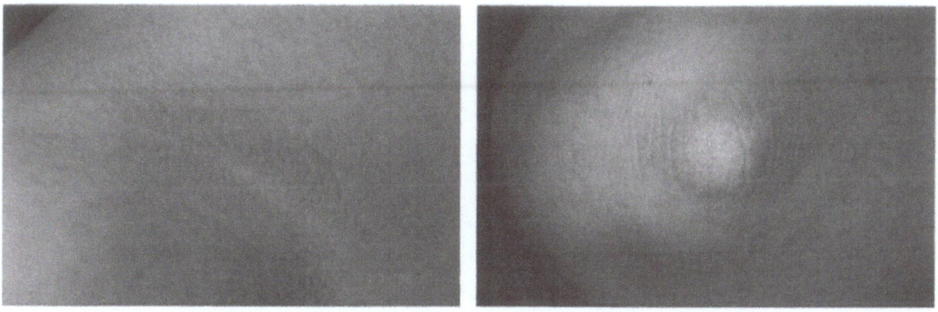

Fig. 2. Acanthosis nigricans of the axilla and elbow.

Signs of hyperinsulinemia include acanthosis nigricans and skin tags. Acanthosis nigricans is hypertrophied, hyperpigmented skin in skin folds, such as the posterior neck, axillae, elbows, under the breasts, between abdominal fat folds, or in the groin (Fig. 1). It is important to remember that hypertrophic skin caused by acanthosis nigricans is not necessarily dark; the degree of hyperpigmentation depends on skin color. Because textbooks typically show severe acanthosis nigricans in persons with dark skin, the more subtle findings of acanthosis nigricans in lightly pigmented patients may be missed. These include rough grey patches on the elbows and knees (Fig. 2). Skin tags are commonly found on the neck and axillae.

Extensive abdominal striations, a buffalo hump, facial plethora, and relatively thin limbs in contrast to abdominal obesity should prompt a work-up for Cushing's disease.

Pelvic Exam

Pelvic exam should be completed with specific attention to the clitoris, looking for signs of enlargement that would raise suspicion of an androgen-secreting tumor. Clitoromegaly and underdeveloped labia indicate early exposure to elevated androgens. Clitoromegaly, although multiple definitions exist, is defined as a clitoral diameter greater than 1 cm or a clitoral index (width times length of clitoris) greater than 35 mm^2.

LABORATORY TESTING

Laboratory testing in the evaluation of a patient with a clinical picture suspicious for PCOS involves obtaining tests to support the diagnosis, as well as those that exclude other serious causes of their symptoms.

It is important to note that hormone concentrations obtained while a patient is taking OCPs are not useful in diagnosing PCOS. Supraphysiological doses of estrogen in the OCP raise SHBG, which binds testoterone, decreasing the bioavailable testosterone. OCPs also elevate HDL cholesterol and triglycerides. OCPs suppress LH and follicle-stimulating hormone (FSH). To obtain accurate hormonal values, patients should discontinue OCPs for a minimum of 6 weeks. The desirability of such testing to confirm a diagnosis should be weighed against the significant contraceptive and noncontraceptive benefits of OCPs in managing PCOS.

Though LH and FSH levels are usually drawn on day 3 of the menstrual cycle for an infertility evaluation, it is not necessary to do so when evaluating for PCOS. The only exception to the need to assess timing FSH and LH values occurs when a level reveals an elevated LH, which is not only a hallmark of PCOS, but also normally present immediately before ovulation. This can be excluded by determining whether a menstrual period followed the day of phlebotomy by approx 14 days. LH and FSH usually show a greater than 2 or 3 to 1 ratio, and help confirm the diagnosis. However, the absence of the elevated ratio does not exclude PCOS.

Total testosterone greater than 50 ng/dL is considered elevated. Most laboratories in the United States list a reference range of somewhere between 14 and 70 ng/dL as "normal," but reference ranges refer to the mean plus or minus two standard deviations, not to values that are "normal" or optimal. It is unknown what an "optimal" range of serum testosterone is, but most women with a level greater than 50 ng/dL will have irregular menses and clinical hyperandrogenism. Free (unbound) testosterone is also usually elevated. There is no advantage in ordering total testosterone vs free testosterone, because both will be elevated in PCOS *(9)*.

Once a diagnosis of PCOS is made, testing should be performed to assess the patient for underlying insulin resistance and diabetes. There are many approaches to the evaluation and little evidence to support one over the other. Many investigators will diagnose impaired glucose tolerance resulting from insulin resistance using the 2-hour oral glucose tolerance test (GTT). Insulin is often tested but requires a frozen specimen for the assay to be performed correctly, and insulin values often return falsely low in the office setting. The reference range for insulin is usually designated as between 5 and 25 or 30 IU, however, most experts agree that an insulin greater than 10 IU is consistent with insulin resistance. Other investigators consider the clinical usefulness of measuring a fasting glucose and insulin ratio to be the desired screening test; a ratio of glucose to insulin less than 4.5 is considered abnormal, indicating developing insulin resistance. A normal fasting glucose can also be used to exclude diabetes. This is particularly helpful in young women, who are less likely to exhibit impaired glucose tolerance than are older women.

A fasting lipid profile is useful for assessing cardiovascular risk, and the typical pattern is elevated triglycerides and low HDL cholesterol. Other useful tests include SHBG, which is low in hyperandrogenemic and hyperinsulinemic states, as well as in obesity *(10)*.

Other tests to help exclude PCOS include:

- Thyroid-stimulating hormone. Hypothyroidism may cause oligomenorrhea. However, hypothyroidism is more common in women with PCOS than in women without PCOS.
- Prolactin. Elevated prolactin is seen with a pituitary adenoma.
- Dehydroepiandrosterone (DHEA) sulfate (S). DHEA-S is often elevated in the 200 to 300 ng/dL range in PCOS. However, levels greater than 700 ng/dL should prompt a search for an androgen-secreting tumor. Do not order DHEA, which is variable and unhelpful. DHEA-S measurement is useful if a patient presents with sudden onset of virilizing symptoms.
- 17-α-hydroxyprogesterone, if elevated in the morning (before 10 AM), may indicate NCCAH if levels are normal, but if there is a high suspicion of NCCAH, a corticotrophin stimulation test should be performed. After a baseline measurement of 17-α-hydroxyprogesterone, corticotrophin (250 μg) is administered intravenously or intramuscularly. Samples at 15, 30, and 60 minutes are drawn (although the author finds 60-min values most useful). If the 17-α-hydroxyprogesterone level increases fourfold, the test is diagnostic of 21-hydroxylase deficiency, and the patient should be referred to an endocrinologist.
- Cortisol should be measured in a patient with Cushingoid features. One method to measure cortisol is a 24-hour urine collection; if the cortisol is greater than 100, the patient should be referred to an endocrinologist. An alternative screening test is the overnight dexamethasone suppression test, 1 mg of dexamethasone is administered at 11 PM, and serum cortisol is measured at 8 AM.

TRANSVAGINAL SONOGRAPHY

Many clinicians, especially in Europe, consider transvaginal sonography (TVS) essential to diagnose PCOS. TVS may be necessary for infertility evaluation and management. However, if a patient does not wish to conceive, and if she has a classic history and signs of PCOS, a TVS without evidence of polycystic ovaries probably would not change management. The classic PCOS finding on TVS is a "string of pearls," which describes typical cysts that are peripheral, multiple, and less than 10 mm in diameter. There is a large body of literature in reproductive endocrinology that attempts to classify PCOS according to ovarian morphology.

Key Points in the Diagnosis of PCOS are:

- PCOS is a clinical diagnosis
- Presentation is highly variable and women do not typically have all of the common symptoms of PCOS

- Thyroid disease, prolactinoma, congenital adrenal hyperplasia, and testosterone-secreting tumors must be specifically excluded
- Laboratory testing for PCOS can be supportive of the diagnosis but not definitive
- Transvaginal ultrasound is not necessary to make the diagnosis of PCOS, and polycystic ovaries can be observed in normally cycling women without PCOS

TREATMENT

The most important strategy to address all symptoms of PCOS is to improve diet, increase physical activity, and lose weight. *The role of proper nutrition and adequate physical activity cannot be overemphasized.* Patients need to be encouraged to exercise, and it may help to prescribe specific activities. Patients may benefit from group support, such as in Weight Watchers. Referral to a nutritionist may be helpful.

Treatment beyond lifestyle changes must be guided by the patient's goals and desire for fertility. In addition, comorbidities, such hypertension, diabetes, dyslipidemia, and obesity must be addressed.

Combined Hormonal Contraception

Traditional treatment has focused on restoring regular menses with OCPs, which contain supraphysiological doses of estrogens. In addition to causing monthly menstrual cycles, OCPs increase SHBG production by the liver, which binds free (unbound) testosterone. Acne may improve dramatically, and hirsutism and alopecia often decrease. However, OCPs may not cause sufficient improvement in metabolic parameters and may increase insulin resistance in some cases *(11)*. One approach to treatment involves the use of OCPs for initial therapy coupled with lifestyle changes—weight loss and increased exercise. If insulin resistance persists or worsens with this approach, insulin sensitizers, such as metformin, may be added or substituted for OCPs.

Metformin

Although some patients do exercise and eat well, many still have such a high degree of insulin resistance that they are unable to lose weight or ovulate. At this point, the addition of metformin may help to surmount the obstacle created by hyperinsulinemia by decreasing insulin resistance. There are no guidelines on dosage and duration, but most clinicians prescribe 1000 mg metformin twice a day. This dose is similar to that of treatment of type 2 diabetes. There are few studies reporting the use or long-term effects of metformin in adolescents with PCOS, although they are currently being prescribed for this population based on the theoretical benefits of lowering long-term cardiovascular risk. Compliance is an issue in the use of metformin in adolescents, and careful ongoing discussions of potential side effects coupled with very gradual increases in dosage are required.

Metformin is a relatively safe medication that is available in several doses and formulations. Because metformin is commonly associated with gastrointestinal effects, such as nausea, bloating, and diarrhea, it is prudent to titrate up slowly. Metformin is contraindicated in renal insufficiency and the elderly, and should be used with caution in those with liver disease or significant alcohol use. Baseline creatinine should be obtained to exclude renal disease. Lactic acidosis is a severe but rare complication that is usually observed in those with renal failure. The starting dose of metformin is usually 500 to 1000 mg once a day after the evening meal.

- Immediate-release metformin (500 mg or 850 mg Glucophage®) is administered three times a day after meals
- Extended-release metformin (500 mg or 750 mg Glucophage XR®) is administered once or twice daily after meals
- Extended-release metformin (500 mg or 1000 mg Fortamet is administered once daily after dinner

The dose is usually titrated by doubling the starting dose after 1 to 2 weeks, if the patient does not have adverse effects that warrant discontinuation of the medication. The maximum dose is 2500 mg daily. In studies of patients with type 2 diabetes, 2000 mg has been established as the optimal dose *(12)*. As long as the baseline creatinine is normal, and the patient is not taking other medications that affect renal function, there is no need to recheck the serum creatinine.

Ovulation and spontaneous menses usually occur by 3 months, especially in combination with improved diet and exercise. There are hundreds of case reports of patients conceiving while taking metformin, and no fetal abnormalities have been reported. Some obstetricians advocate the use of metformin during the first trimester to prevent miscarriage, and a few are comfortable using metformin during the entire pregnancy. Metformin should not be used during breastfeeding. Caution should be used in prescribing metformin as sole therapy for PCOS in adolescents and young adults because of the increase in fertility. Metformin causes previously anovulatory women to ovulate, thus, leading to an increased risk of unintended pregnancy if alternative contraception is not used. Adolescents may find it difficult to divulge or admit their sexual activity to clinicians, and typically do not seek medical contraception until many months after first initiating intercourse.

A meta-analysis of the use of metformin in PCOS concludes that metformin is effective for inducing ovulation and increasing pregnancy rates *(13)*. Metformin was shown to decrease androgens, decrease blood pressure, and low-density lipoprotein cholesterol. There was no evidence supporting a weight loss effect, or improvement in hirsutism, alopecia, or acne.

Metformin frequently causes gastrointestinal side effects, such as bloating, loose stools/diarrhea, and nausea. Metformin should be started at the lowest dose (500 mg) and titrated up slowly. It should be taken after meals. There are no guidelines for dosage and duration, but, in general, 1000 mg metformin twice a day is used. Many patients report that if they eat refined carbohydrates with metformin, they develop diarrhea. The high risk of pregnancy must be emphasized in women starting metformin. Often, they are unconcerned about pregnancy because they have been infertile for so long that they may not think they could conceive. Sometimes conception occurs before the onset of the first spontaneous menses.

Hirsutism and Alopecia

In addition to OCPs, androgen receptor antagonists, such as spironolactone, may be effective in diminishing hirsutism and alopecia. In the past, spironolactone has been thought to be of little value, but the doses used then were 25 to 50 mg/d. More recently, doses as high as 100 mg once or twice a day have been effectively used. Higher-dose spironolactone diminishes hirsutism both in the frequency of new terminal hair growth, and in the return of hair that has been removed. A recent systematic review of the literature concluded that 6 month treatment with 100 mg spironolactone compared with placebo was associated with a statistically significant subjective improvement in hair growth *(14)*. Diffuse alopecia may respond dramatically to 100 mg spironolactone once or twice a day. Other antiandrogens include flutamide (250 mg twice a day) and finasteride (5 mg daily); both drugs require monitoring of liver function tests. All antiandrogens are contraindicated in pregnancy. Eflornithine is a topical hair growth retardant that is applied twice a day to hirsute areas. Response rates, indicating diminished but not absent growth, are approx 30%.

Acne

Acne improves with reduction of serum testosterone, and subsequent reduction of sebum production. Patients with cystic acne should be referred to dermatologists for possible Accutane® use. Otherwise, the combination of oral and topical antibiotics will improve acne, especially in conjunction with the reduction of serum androgens.

Ovulation and Infertility

Ovulation may be restored with the use of medications. With the discovery that insulin plays an important role in PCOS, and that the ovaries contain receptors that respond to insulin to upregulate production of androgens, clinicians began experimenting with insulin-sensitizing medications in the mid 1990s. A large body of data supports the use of metformin in restoring ovulation, presumably by decreasing testosterone production indirectly by lowering serum insulin. Other insulin sensitizers used include pioglitazone and rosiglitazone; troglitazone was used before it was removed from the market. A systematic review concludes that metformin is significantly more effective than placebo in restoring ovulation *(12)*. If a woman has not had spontaneous or induced menses for the last 3 months, a withdrawal bleed should be induced with either medroxyprogesterone acetate (5–10 mg daily for 5–10 d), or oral micronized progesterone (400 mg before bed for 10 d). If the patient does not have a withdrawal bleed, she may have endometrial atrophy, which could be treated by use of an OCP (containing at least 30 μg ethinyl estradiol) for 2 months.

The recent explosion of research on the association of PCOS and insulin resistance has added a welcome new dimension in the treatment of PCOS-associated infertility, allowing for more treatment options for patients. PCOS causes anovulation or oligo-ovulation by interfering with normal follicle growth. Anovulation undoubtedly reduces fertility by reducing the number of ovulatory cycles per year in women. Cycles that happen to be ovulatory are probably more likely to be suboptimal for fertility. It is now well-known that most women with PCOS, if not the vast majority, are insulin resistant, and many are obese. Thus, insulin-sensitizing agents and lifestyle modifications have been studied as treatment options for infertile patients with PCOS, and have yielded acceptable results.

In the past, treatment options for PCOS-associated infertility were limited to oral or injectable ovulation-inducing medications. Clomiphene, an oral agent, has been used as first-line therapy, and injectable gonadotropins (FSH plus LH or FSH alone) were used in failure to ovulate with clomiphene.

The treatment options for infertile women with PCOS can be customized to the patient's individual situation. Insulin sensitizers now seem to be gaining more favor as the first option or as adjunctive medication. Clomiphene, the first and most widely used ovulation-inducing medication, has been used in patients with PCOS for more than 3 decades with reasonable success. Ovulation rates of up to 90%, and average pregnancy rates of 50% have been reported. Clomiphene is an oral nonsteroidal compound with only a very weak estrogen effect. It exerts its effects on the hypothalamus and pituitary to induce ovulation by occupying their cellular estrogen receptors and simulating a hypoestrogenic environment. It also enhances FSH action on the ovarian follicle. It is typically administered for 5 days straight of a fixed dose, starting on day 5 of the menstrual cycle. Patients are monitored for evidence of ovulation by over-the-counter urinary LH testing or by basal body temperature charting. The dose is increased monthly if no ovulation is noted. Some clinicians will choose to monitor follicle growth by transvaginal ultrasound. Side effects may include hot flashes or central nervous system complaints, such as moodiness, headache, or visual symptoms. Cervical mucus, normally thin and watery in consistency at ovulation, may become thick and inhospitable to sperm from antiestrogen effect of clomiphene. Multiple births rates, primarily twins rather than higher-order multiple births, are approx 5 to 8%. Although clomiphene has long been the medication of first choice for PCOS ovulation induction, injectable gonadotropins are available in a combination of purified urinary FSH and LH, purified FSH only, and recombinant FSH. They are administered subcutaneously. Indications for ovulation induction with injectable gonadotropins in PCOS are essentially the lack of an ovulatory response to or occurrence of side effects from clomiphene. They are started on the second or third day of menses (or induced menses) and usually administered in a variable dose protocol, generally during an 8- to 10-day period. Serial ultrasound and blood hormonal monitoring are essential to reduce the risk of multiple births (~20% of pregnancies) and ovarian hyperstimulation. In addition to these risks, injectable fertility medications are much more costly to patients than clomiphene, and are much less likely to be covered by prescription plans. Ovulation rates for clomiphene-resistant patients are greater than 90% and pregnancy rates are greater than 50%.

Ovulation induction may be treated conservatively with the lifestyle alterations of diet modification and exercise. Realistically, this is successful in only a small number of patients, and can not be offered to patients with PCOS of normal weight. It requires strict adherence to a program that may be difficult to complete, and may take too long for patients interested in conception immediately. Insulin sensitizers have become an excellent option for the conservative treatment of PCOS-associated infertility. Those studied have included metformin, troglitazone (but has since been removed from the market) and d-chiro-inositol (a complex carbohydrate that has not cleared phase 2 trials). Of these, metformin has been the most thoroughly studied. Metformin may be used alone as monotherapy and has been shown to allow for regular ovulation to occur. One of its advantages is its induction of monofollicular ovulation, as opposed to exogenous fertility drugs that have side effects of multiple births and ovarian hyperstimulation. Monitoring costs (ultrasound, and serum hormonal assays) associated with these medications can also be avoided. It does not induce cervical mucus abnormalities. Some patients experience some weight loss with metformin, an advantage before their pregnancy. Diet and exercise plans may be used along with metformin to enhance the response and take advantage of its initial effect. Results have been very encouraging. Ovulation rates of 77 to 82% have been reported when doses ranging from 1500 to 1700 mg/d were administered during 3 to 4 months.

Pregnancy rates on metformin alone have not been reported in multiple studies. However, it may be reasonable to consider that these strong rates of ovulation may result in respectable pregnancy rates. Metformin monotherapy as a first-line treatment may be used in younger reproductive age patients, for those who prefer to reduce their costs or risk of multiple gestations with fertility medications, and for obese patients who prefer to lose weight before conceiving. If regular ovulation does not occur in 6 to 8 weeks, clomiphene treatment may be added. Preliminary studies have reported a lower risk of first trimester miscarriage and gestational diabetes with metformin use, but further research is needed to confirm these findings.

Patients taking clomiphene and metformin alone for ovulation induction may not ovulate while on their respective medications. Metformin, administered to clomiphene-resistant women as an adjunct in a multicenter study, seems to be useful as an adjunctive medication by increasing clomiphene's ovulation and pregnancy rates. There has been one report of metformin vs placebo pretreatment of clomiphene-resistant patients undergoing injectable FSH treatment *(15)*. A tendency to reduce the risk of ovarian hyperstimulation (and perhaps multiple gestations) was noted. Metformin may have promise as an adjunctive treatment for in vitro fertilization in women with PCOS. One study has reported that low-dose metformin treatment increases oocyte maturity and fertilization rates, and enhances embryo numbers.

SUMMARY

PCOS, a leading cause of menstrual irregularities and infertility, is also associated with obesity, hirsutism, and cardiovascular risk factors, such as elevated blood pressure, dyslipidemia, and diabetes. Insulin resistance seems to play a central role in the pathophysiology. Diagnosis is based on history of menstrual dysfunction and evidence of hyperandrogenemia. Physical examination usually shows hirsutism and central obesity. Laboratory tests that support the diagnosis of PCOS include a serum testosterone concentration greater than 50 ng/dL and LH to FSH ratio of greater than 2 or 3:1. Measurement of hormone levels is not useful when patients are taking OCPs. Treatment includes physical activity, proper nutrition, and weight loss. OCPs induce monthly menstrual cycles and improve acne and hirsutism. Insulin sensitizers, such as metformin, induce ovulation and improve some metabolic parameters. Insulin sensitizers play an important role in PCOS-associated infertility. Patients should be aggressively screened and treated for hypertension, diabetes, and hyperlipidemia. There are no long-term studies to evaluate the ability of insulin sensitizers to prevent cardiovascular disease.

REFERENCES

1. Zawedzki JK, Dunaif A. Diagnostic criteria for polycystic ovary syndrome: towards a rational approach. In: Polycystic Ovary Syndrome (Dunaif A, Givens JR, Haseltine FP, Merriam GR, eds.). Glasckwell Scientific, Boston, 1992; pp. 377–384.
2. Rotterdam ESHRE/ASRM-Sponsored PCOS Consensus Workshop Group. Revised 2003 consensus on diagnostic criteria and long-term health risks related to polycystic ovary syndrome. Fertil Steril 2004;81(1):19–25.
3. Balen A, Michelmore K. What is polycystic ovary syndrome? Hum Repro 2002;17(9): 2219–2227.
4. Dunaif A. Insulin resistance and the polycystic ovary syndrome: mechanism and implications for pathogenesis. Endocr Rev 1997;18:774–800.
5. Dunaif A, Segal KR, Futterweit W, Dobrjansky A. Profound peripheral insulin resistance, independent of obesity, in polycystic ovary syndrome. Diabetes 1989;38:1165–1174.
6. Rebar R, Judd HL, Yen SS, Rakoff J, Vandenberg G, Naftolin F. Characterization of the inappropriate gonadotropin secretion in polycystic ovarian syndrome. J Clin Invest 1976;57: 1320–1329.
7. Sherif K, Kushner H, Falkner BE. Sex hormone-binding globulin and insulin resistance in African-American women. Metab Clin Experim 1998;47(1):70–74.
8. Deaton MA, Glorioso JE, McLean DB. Congenital adrenal hyperplasia: not really a zebra. Amer Fam Physician 1999;59(5):1190–1196.
9. Luthold WW, Borges MF, Marcondes JA, Hakohyama M, Wajchenberg BL, Kirschner MA. Serum testosterone fractions in women: normal and abnormal clinical states. Metab Clin Exper 1993;42(5):638–643.
10. Sherif K. Benefits and risks of oral contraceptives. Amer J Obstet Gyn 1999;180(6): S343–S348.
11. Hull MGR. Epidemiology of infertility and polycystic ovarian disease: endocrinological and demographic studies. Gyn Endocrinol 1987;1:233–245.
12. Garber AJ, Duncan TJ, Goodman AM, Mills DJ, Rohlf JL. Efficacy of metformin in type 2 diabetes: results of a double-blind, placebo-controlled, dose-response trial. Amer J Med 1997;103(6):491–497.
13. Lord JM, Flight IHK, Norman RJ. Metformin in polycystic ovary syndrome: systematic review and meta-analysis. BMJ 2003;327:951.
14. Farquhar C, Lee O, Toomath R, Jepson R. Spironolactone versus placebo or in combination with steroids for hirsutism and/or acne. Cochrane Database of Systematic Reviews. 2001;(4):CD000194.
15. George SS, George K, Irwin C, et al. Sequential treatment of metformin and clomiphene citrate in clomiphene-resistant women with polycystic ovary syndrome: a randomized, controlled trial. Human Repro 2003;18(2):299–304.

11 Cervical Cancer Detection and Prevention

New Guidelines for Screening and Managing Abnormal Pap Tests

Amy L. Clouse, MD

Contents

INTRODUCTION

Since the introduction of the Papanicolaou (Pap) test in 1943, cervical cancer mortality has decreased by more than 70%. Once the number one cancer killer of women, cervical cancer now ranks 13th in cancer deaths for women in the United States *(1)*. In 2005, the American Cancer Society (ACS) estimates 10,370 new cases of invasive cervical cancer and 3710 cervical cancer deaths. Five-year survival rates for women with preinvasive lesions have reached nearly 100%, whereas the 5-year survival rate for cervical cancers detected at an early stage is close to 92% *(2)*.

Approximately 93 to 100% of squamous cell carcinomas of the cervix contain DNA from the human papillomavirus (HPV). This common sexually transmitted

From: *Current Clinical Practice: Women's Health in Clinical Practice*
Edited by: Clouse and Sherif © Humana Press Inc., Totowa, NJ

disease, with an estimated 5.5 million new infections in the United States each year, is now known to be the major cofactor in the development of cervical cancer *(1)*. Studies of the natural history of HPV suggest that most infections are from low-risk types and generally will resolve spontaneously or produce only low-grade lesions. The high-risk types of HPV are associated with high-grade intraepithelial lesions and can progress to cervical cancer if left untreated *(3–5)*. The role of the Pap test is to detect these high-grade abnormalities so they can be treated before the development of cervical cancer.

This new information regarding HPV as well as newer technologies both for obtaining cervical specimens and identifying high-risk HPV DNA have prompted a review of previously published cervical cancer guidelines. During the last few years, new recommendations for appropriate cervical cancer screening protocols and the management of abnormal Pap tests have been published.

NEW SCREENING GUIDELINES

The ACS and the American College of Obstetricians and Gynecologists (ACOG) have updated their cervical cancer screening guidelines with new recommendations for the initiation and frequency of screening. They also make recommendations regarding when to stop screening, screening in women after hysterectomy, and the role of liquid-based Pap tests and HPV testing *(1,6)*. The US Preventive Services Task Force (USPSTF) also reviewed newly available evidence and weighed in on these same topics in 2003 *(7)*.

Both the ACS and ACOG guidelines recommend the initiation of screening approx 3 years after the onset of intercourse but no later than age 21 years. According to the ACS, women younger than 30 years should have a yearly Pap test if the conventional smear is used and a test every other year if liquid-based sampling is used.

ACOG recommends yearly Pap testing for all women under age 30 years regardless of method. After age 30 years, both organizations agree that the frequency of screening can be reduced to every 2 to 3 years in those women who have had three consecutive normal results. These guidelines for initiation and frequency of screening have been supported by the Centers for Disease Control (CDC) and also given an "A" recommendation from the USPSTF. Screening that is more frequent, at least annually, is recommended in HIV-positive or immunocompromised women or in those who were exposed to diethylstilbestrol (DES) *in utero*.

The upper limit for screening for cervical cancer differs slightly among organizations. According to the ACS, women may decide to stop screening at age 70 years if they have had three consecutive normal cytology results and no history of abnormal results within the preceding 10 years. ACOG, on the other hand, does not offer an upper age limit for screening, and recommends that the decision to stop screening be made on an individual basis. The USPSTF recommends against routine screening of low-risk women older than age 65 years with a history of normal Pap tests in the past ("D" recommendation).

Both sets of guidelines and the USPSTF support discontinuing screening in women who have had a total hysterectomy for benign disease and no history of abnormal or cancerous lesions. The ACS specifically addresses the nonbenign nature of moderate-to-severe dysplasia or cervical intraepithelial neoplasia (CIN) grades 2 and 3 (CIN-2,3). With a history of CIN-2,3, the ACS recommends discontinuing screening after results from three consecutive tests have been normal and no abnormal results have occurred in the past 10 years. If the hysterectomy was because of CIN-2,3, then screening every 4 to 6 months is recommended by the ACS, with continuation until three consecutive normal results occur within 18 to 24 months.

NEW TECHNOLOGIES

Liquid-Based Pap Technology

Currently, the Food and Drug Administration (FDA) has approved using a liquid-based Pap collection system as an acceptable alternative to the conventional Pap smear. Compared with the conventional smear on the glass slide, the liquid-based samples are thought to have improved sample adequacy, improved cellular sampling, and decreased amount of obscuring background factors *(1)*. Most studies also suggest an increased sensitivity but a decreased specificity for high-grade lesions, leading to an increase in number of colposcopy referrals and potentially more samples lacking an endocervical component *(1)*.

This decreased specificity led the ACS to suggest the longer interval between testing, as reviewed above, for women under age 30 years, to avoid unnecessary procedures. Furthermore, the USPSTF gave an "I" recommendation to the use of liquid-based technologies in 2003. They concluded that there is not enough evidence to determine whether these were more effective than conventional smears in reducing cancer detection or mortality *(7)*.

HPV Typing

HPV DNA testing has been shown in multiple studies to have a higher sensitivity than cytology alone but a lower specificity for detecting high-grade lesions *(1)*. In 2003, the FDA approved the use of HPV typing through the Digene's Hybrid Capture II (HC2) High-Risk HPV DNA test to screen for cervical cancer. Whereas previously, HPV DNA typing was used solely as a triage method for abnormal Pap test results, this new indication allows the test to be used in conjunction with a Pap test in women older than age 30 years to screen for HPV infection. In women under age 30 years, the more transient nature of an HPV infection makes HPV typing unlikely to be useful as a screening strategy. A negative Pap test and no high-risk HPV confer a very low likelihood of developing cervical cancer. However, consensus guidelines for the management of women with normal cytology results and a positive test for high-risk HPV DNA still need to be developed.

The ACS guidelines, published before the FDA approval, preliminarily suggested that HPV typing could be used in conjunction with a Pap test every 3 years in women 30 years and older. The ACOG guidelines, released later, recommend the combination of HPV typing and cervical cytology every 3 years in women 30 years and older. ACOG further recognizes that annual testing with cytology alone continues to be an acceptable screening plan. HPV testing alone, however, is still not considered appropriate for cervical cancer screening. The USPSTF concluded that there was insufficient evidence to recommend for or against the use of HPV testing as a primary screening test for cervical cancer, giving it an "I" recommendation.

MANAGING ABNORMAL CERVICAL CYTOLOGY AND CIN

Seven percent of the nearly 60 million women who undergo Pap testing each year in the United States will be told they have abnormal results. In the past, deciding who gets a colposcopy, when to repeat the Pap test, and which patients should be treated has been both confusing and controversial. The publication of two sets of guidelines from the American Society for Colposcopy and Cervical Pathology (ASCCP) has greatly clarified these issues. These new evidence-supported, consensus-based guidelines provide algorithms for managing cervical cytological abnormalities and histologically confirmed CIN. They were developed out of a consensus workshop convened by ASCCP in 2001 and subsequently published in *JAMA* and the *American Journal of Obstetrics and Gynecology (8,9)*.

These new guidelines were preceded by revisions to the Bethesda System of nomenclature for cervical cytology *(10)*. This updated terminology as well as advances in the understanding of HPV as a cervical cancer precursor and the increased use of advanced technologies, such as liquid-based cervical cytology and HPV DNA typing, were key in developing these guidelines.

The 2001 Bethesda System

The National Cancer Institute (NCI) organized a workshop in 2001 to update the 1991 Bethesda System used by pathologists to report cervical cytology results *(10)*. There are three components of a Pap test result as reported under the new Bethesda System: specimen adequacy, a general categorization, and the interpretation or result.

Specimens are categorized as either "satisfactory" or "unsatisfactory." The once potentially confusing designation of "satisfactory but limited by…" has been eliminated. A specimen is considered adequate if it contains at least 8000 to 12,000 well-visualized squamous cells for conventional smears and at least 5000 cells with newer liquid-based technologies. The presence or absence of the endocervical/transformation zone component is noted here.

The general categorization section is considered an optional part of the interpretation, designed to offer rapid triage of abnormal results. Here a single category, "negative for intraepithelial lesion or malignancy" replaces the previous two designations "within normal limits" and "benign cellular changes." This was changed to more clearly indicate that reactive changes are considered negative. Any abnormal cellular findings will be categorized as an "epithelial cell abnormality." An additional category of "other" has also been added here to indicate findings that, although benign, may impart some increased risk to the patient, such as benign-appearing endometrial cells in a woman older than 40 years.

The third section to the revised Bethesda System is the actual interpretation or result section. This has been renamed from the diagnosis section to reflect the concept that a Pap test is a screening test and should be interpreted in its full clinical context. Specimens that are without any epithelial abnormalities are designated "negative for intraepithelial lesion or malignancy." Other findings, such as *Trichomonas vaginalis*, fungal organisms, or atrophy may also be reported under this heading.

Abnormal specimens are reported as "epithelial cell abnormalities" and are further categorized as either involving squamous cells or glandular cells. Of the squamous abnormalities, the old term "atypical squamous cells of undetermined significance" has undergone the most change. Atypical squamous cells (ACS) can now be reported as either "of undetermined significance" (ASC-US) or as "cannot exclude high-grade squamous intraepithelial lesions" (ASC-H). The previous term "atypical squamous cells favor reactive" has been eliminated.

The designations "low-grade intraepithelial lesion" (LSIL) and "high-grade squamous intraepithelial lesion" (HSIL) have remained unchanged in the new Bethesda System. LSIL continues to include HPV/mild dysplasia and CIN-1. Moderate and severe dysplasia, carcinoma *in situ*, CIN-2, and CIN-3 are clustered under the HSIL category.

The other type of epithelial cell abnormality that can be reported is glandular cell. These are now designated as "atypical glandular cells" (AGC) instead of the previous "atypical glandular cells of undetermined significance," which could have been confused with ASC-US. The category is further qualified as

AGC that are either endocervical, endometrial, or not otherwise specified; AGC favor neoplasia; and endocervical adenocarcinoma *in situ* (AIS).

Managing Women Who Have Cervical Cytological Abnormalities

Using this new terminology and incorporating information from the large, randomized ASC-US/LSIL Triage Study, the ASCCP published consensus-based guidelines for managing cervical cytological abnormalities *(8)*.

ACS

There is a 5% to 17% chance that a cytology result of ASC will turn out to be CIN-2,3 on biopsy. This risk increases to 24 to 94% in those with ASC-H. However, the risk for invasive cervical cancer after an ASC Pap test is as low as 0.1%. The guidelines recommend follow-up for these ASC results, but caution that unnecessary inconvenience, anxiety, cost, and potential patient discomfort should be avoided.

ASC-US

According to the guidelines, clinicians may choose one of three options for managing an initial Pap result of ASC-US: repeat cytology, immediate colposcopy, and HPV DNA testing for high-risk DNA types. The HPV DNA testing route is the preferred approach when both a liquid-based cytology system and reflex HPV DNA typing are available. This approach has the advantages of a higher sensitivity than a single repeat Pap test as well as the potential to avoid an unnecessary procedure.

If the HPV DNA testing is negative for high-risk types, those women can be followed with repeat Pap testing at 12 months. Those with high-risk types of HPV DNA should be triaged to colposcopy. Any CIN discovered after colposcopy should be managed according to the ASCCP guidelines as outlined below. However, if CIN is not identified during this colposcopy, either cytology testing at 6 and 12 months or HPV DNA testing at 12 months should be performed. If any Pap reveals ASC or greater, or if the HPV test is positive for high-risk types, repeating the colposcopy is recommended. Otherwise, a return to routine screening is appropriate.

If the clinician chooses to repeat the cervical cytology at 4- to 6-month intervals with an initial Pap result of ASC-US, another Pap result of ASC or greater warrants a colposcopy. When two consecutive "negative for intraepithelial lesion or malignancy" results are confirmed, the guidelines recommend resuming routine screening.

Immediate colposcopy is the third option for management of ASC-US. CIN found on colposcopic biopsies should be treated according to the ASCCP guidelines. Without evidence of CIN, women may have the Pap test repeated at 12 months. Management that is more aggressive of an ASC-US Pap with a diagnostic excisional procedure, such as loop electrosurgical excision procedure (LEEP) is not appropriate without evidence of biopsy-confirmed CIN.

ASC-US in Special Circumstances

Postmenopausal women are at lower risk for CIN-2,3 than their premenopausal counterparts, and immunosuppressed women are more likely to have both CIN-2,3 and high-risk HPV DNA types. Pregnant women with ASC-US should be managed the same way as nonpregnant women.

For postmenopausal women with ASC-US, the guidelines suggest a course of intravaginal estrogen followed by a repeat Pap test approx 1 week later. This is considered an acceptable alternative in those women with evidence of atrophy and no contraindication for estrogen therapy. If this test is negative and a follow-up Pap in 4 to 6 months is also negative, the patent can return to routine screening. A colposcopy is indicated if either repeat Pap test result shows ASC or greater.

Immunosuppressed women with ASC, including those with HIV, regardless of CD4 count or viral load, should be triaged to a colposcopy.

ASC-H

A colposcopy is the only recommended approach for managing women with ASC-H. Biopsy-confirmed CIN should be managed according to the ASCCP guideline for managing CIN. If a lesion is not identified at the time of colposcopy, then the cytology and histology results should be reviewed to determine whether there is a change in the interpretation. If this review changes the diagnosis to include identified CIN, this would be managed according to the CIN guidelines. If no change in the original interpretation can be confirmed. cytology should be repeated in 6 and 12 months, or HPV DNA testing can be performed at 12 months. Another colposcopy is suggested when results of ASC or greater is found during cytology follow-up or if high-risk HPV DNA is identified at the year mark.

LSIL

Of those women with LSIL on cervical cytology, approx 15 to 30% will subsequently have CIN-2,3 found on biopsy. This higher risk of more significant disease in addition to the risk of losing a patient to follow-up has prompted ASCCP to recommend immediate colposcopy for women with LSIL. Further management is dictated based on the adequacy of the colposcopic exam and whether or not a lesion is identified. Diagnostic excisional procedures and ablative procedures are unacceptable as the initial management of LSIL.

With a satisfactory colposcopy and an identified lesion, endocervical sampling is considered an accepted approach in nonpregnant women. Even when there is not a lesion identified or the colposcopy is not satisfactory, endocervical sampling is still preferred in the management of LSIL. Any biopsy-proven CIN should be treated according the ASCCP guidelines outlined below. If biopsy and/or endocervical sampling does not identify CIN, either cytology at 6 and 12 months or HPV DNA testing at 12 months is the appropriate next step. If both Pap test results are negative or no high-risk HPV types are found, it is safe to return to routing screening. Otherwise, a repeat colposcopy is recommended.

LSIL in Special Circumstances

Postmenopausal women with LSIL can be managed with conservative follow-up instead of an immediate colposcopy. Repeat cytologic testing at 6 and 12 months or HPV DNA typing at 12 months are both acceptable alternatives. A colposcopy should be recommended if either of the Pap tests reveal ASC or greater or if high-risk types of HPV DNA are identified. Similar to the approach to ASC-US in the postmenopausal woman, a course of vaginal estrogen may also be offered, provided there are no contraindications to estrogen therapy and there is atrophy present. Another Pap test should follow this, 1 week after the estrogen is completed. Colposcopy is recommended if this repeat shows ASC or greater. Otherwise, cytology should be repeated again in 4 to 6 months.

Adolescents with LSIL may also be followed with repeat Pap testing at 6 and 12 months or with HPV DNA testing at 12 months. Again, triage to colposcopy is appropriate if either the cytology tests show ASC or greater or if testing reveals high-risk types of HPV DNA.

For pregnant women with LSIL, see HSIL in special circumstances.

HSIL

Although relatively uncommon, women with HSIL cytology results have up to a 75% chance of having biopsy-confirmed CIN-2,3 and a 1 to 2% chance of invasive cervical cancer. The ASCCP continues to recommend colposcopy coupled with endocervical sampling for these women. Immediate treatment of the transformation zone with a LEEP is an acceptable option, especially in those who may be lost to follow-up or if fertility is not an issue.

With a satisfactory colposcopy, biopsy-confirmed CIN-2,3 should be treated according to the CIN management guidelines under the Subheading CIN-2,3. However, when no lesion or only CIN-1 is identified on a satisfactory colposcopy, there remains a considerable risk of missing disease that is more significant. In these cases, a thorough review of the material, including the cytology, colposcopic findings, and all biopsies, is recommended. If this review results in an upgrade of the diagnosis to CIN-2,3, the woman should be managed in accordance with the revised diagnosis. If still no lesion or only CIN-1 is identified after the review, a diagnostic excisional procedure is recommended to ensure there is no higher-grade dysplasia.

With an unsatisfactory colposcopy, review is again appropriate when no lesion is identified. If review is not possible or the original diagnosis is upheld, a diagnostic excisional procedure is recommended. Any biopsy-confirmed CIN should be managed according to the ASCCP guidelines.

HSIL in Special Circumstances

Pregnant women with HSIL (and also LSIL) on initial cytology should undergo a colposcopy performed by an experienced clinician. Lesions suspicious for high-grade disease can be biopsied, however, endocervical sampling is not recommended. If the colposcopy is unsatisfactory, it should be repeated in 6 to 12 weeks, because the transformation zone may become more easily visualized as pregnancy progresses. Neither treatment of the transformation zone nor a diagnostic excisional procedure is acceptable during pregnancy unless invasive disease is identified.

In adolescents with HSIL cytology results and no CIN-2,3 identified on colposcopy, observation with cytology and colposcopy at 4 to 6 month intervals for 1 year instead of a diagnostic excisional procedure is acceptable. This more conservative approach may only be followed if the initial colposcopy was satisfactory, endocervical sampling was negative, and the patient understands the risk of occult disease. The diagnostic excisional procedure should eventually be performed if there is any evidence of disease progression or if the HSIL cytology persists.

AGC and AIS

AGC abnormalities have a greater risk for cervical neoplasia than the ASC or LSIL categories. Studies have found that women with AGC have up to a 54% chance of having biopsy-confirmed CIN, an 8% chance of having AIS, and a 1 to 9% chance of invasive carcinoma.

The three methods used to evaluate AGC—repeat cytology, colposcopy, and endocervical sampling—have low sensitivity for detecting glandular abnormalities. Those women in whom cervical neoplasia is not found during the initial work-up may continue to be at risk for cancer and its precursors.

Women with all the subcategories of AGC or AIS, except atypical endometrial cells, should undergo colposcopy with endocervical sampling. The guidelines recommend endometrial sampling for those with atypical endometrial cells. Furthermore, endometrial sampling should accompany colposcopy in women aged 35 years and older with AGC and in those with unexplained vaginal bleeding. It is not acceptable to use repeat Pap testing for AGC or AIS results and there is not a role for HPV DNA typing in the management of these lesions.

If the initial Pap test showed AGC "favor neoplasia" or AIS, and invasive disease is not identified with the initial colposcopy and biopsies, further evaluation with a diagnostic excisional procedure is recommended, preferably with a cold knife conization. Invasive disease requires referral to an appropriate specialist. If the initial Pap showed AGC that are not otherwise specified, biopsy-confirmed CIN should be managed according to the ASCCP guidelines. If no CIN is identified in these women, they should be followed with repeat cytology at 4- to 6-month intervals until four consecutive "negative for intraepithelial lesion or malignancy" results are obtained. At this point, results of ASC or LSIL warrant another colposcopy and results of HSIL or AGC warrant a diagnostic excisional procedure.

Managing Women With CIN

The prevention of cervical cancer not only involves performing Pap tests and following up on abnormal cytology results but also in the destruction or removal of cervical cancer precursors. Using information from the same consensus conference referenced above, the ASCCP published further guidelines to help clarify management options for biopsy-confirmed intraepithelial neoplasia *(9)*.

CIN-1

Most untreated CIN-1 spontaneously regresses without treatment. Research indicates that CIN-1 lesions may regress in up to 57% of women but advance to CIN-2,3 or cancer in only 11% of women. Overall, there is a 0.3% chance of progression to invasive cancer and most of these cancers are in those lost to follow-up. The management guidelines, therefore, recommend a conservative follow-up strategy for CIN-1. However, when the colposcopy is not satisfactory, there is still the risk that higher-grade dysplasia could be missed, therefore, the guidelines suggest managing these women more aggressively.

With a satisfactory colposcopy, follow-up without treatment using either repeat cytology at 6 and 12 months or HPV DNA testing at 12 months is the preferred approach. After two consecutive negative Pap tests or no high-risk HPV at the year mark, a return to annual screening is appropriate. If either Pap reveals ASC or greater or if high-risk types of HPV are found, the colposcopy should be repeated. An acceptable alternative strategy is to perform both colposcopy and Pap testing at 12 months after the initial CIN-1 diagnosis. If colposcopic and cytologic regression is demonstrated, annual cytologic screening may be resumed. Otherwise, any CIN found should be treated according to these guidelines. Persistent CIN-1 can be treated depending on provider and patient preferences.

Treating biopsy-confirmed CIN-1 is also an acceptable management option if the colposcopy was satisfactory. Cryotherapy, electrofulguration, laser ablation, cold coagulation, and LEEP are all acceptable treatment modalities. Although the choice of method is based on provider experience and available resources, endocervical sampling should precede any ablative method. Excisional methods are preferred in the setting of recurrent CIN-1 after previous ablative therapy. Hysterectomy is not an appropriate treatment for CIN-1.

When the colposcopy is not satisfactory, a diagnostic excisional procedure is preferred to manage biopsy-confirmed CIN-1. However, one of the conservative follow-up protocols above may be used for immunosuppressed or pregnant women (*see* "CIN-2,3 in Special Circumstances"). Adolescents with CIN-1 and an unsatisfactory colposcopy may also be treated conservatively because higher-grade disease is unlikely in this population.

CIN-2,3

Unlike CIN-1, untreated moderate dysplasia, severe dysplasia, and carcinoma *in situ* are all more likely to persist or progress rather than regress. Forty-three percent of CIN-2 lesions will regress spontaneously, whereas 35% will persist, and 22% will progress to carcinoma *in situ* or cancer when left untreated. Likewise, 32% of untreated CIN-3 lesions will regress; 56% will persist and 14% will progress. The similarities in the behavior of these two lesions have led the ASCCP to combine their management in the 2001 consensus guidelines.

With a satisfactory colposcopy and biopsy-confirmed CIN-2,3, the guidelines recommend treatment with either excision or ablation of the transformation zone. Excisional methods are preferred in the case of recurrent CIN-2,3. When the colposcopy is unsatisfactory, a diagnostic excisional procedure is recommended as initial management of CIN-2,3. Following these lesions without treatment is generally unacceptable. This would only be appropriate in pregnancy or with adolescents (*see* "CIN-2,3 in Special Circumstances" below). Hysterectomy is also not acceptable as initial management for CIN-2,3 but could be considered for recurrent or persistent lesions.

Follow-up After Treatment for CIN-2,3

Recommendations for follow-up after the initial treatment for CIN-2,3 include either cervical cytology and colposcopy or cytology alone at 4 to 6 month intervals. Once three consecutive "negative for squamous intraepithelial lesion or malignancy" results are obtained, the woman may return to annual screening. However, if any of the Pap tests during this follow-up period reveals ASC or greater, another colposcopy is warranted.

Another option for follow-up after treatment of CIN-2,3 is HPV DNA testing at least 6 months after treatment. If high-risk types are identified at this point, another colposcopy should be performed. Annual cytologic screening can be resumed if this testing is negative for high-risk HPV DNA types.

If the margins of a diagnostic excisional procedure or a postprocedure endocervical sampling contain CIN, the 4- to 6-month follow-up visit should include colposcopy as well as another endocervical sampling. When CIN-2,3 is identified at the margins or in the endocervical sampling, it is also acceptable to repeat the diagnostic excisional procedure. If this is not possible, an acceptable alternative is a hysterectomy in this circumstance. A hysterectomy is also acceptable for treatment of recurrent or persistent biopsy-confirmed CIN-2,3.

CIN-2,3 in Special Circumstances

Because of the minimal risk of progression of CIN-2,3 to invasive cervical cancer during pregnancy and a reported 69% spontaneous regression rate after delivery, pregnant women with CIN-2,3 can be treated conservatively. The guidelines suggest shifting management goals to identifying invasive cervical cancers only and avoiding diagnostic excisional procedures unless invasive cancer cannot be excluded.

Likewise, some adolescents can also be treated more conservatively. Invasive cervical cancer is rare in adolescents and there is a relatively higher rate of spontaneous regression with CIN-2 compared with CIN-3. Follow-up with Pap tests and colposcopy at 4- to 6-month intervals for 1 year is an appropriate alternative in adolescents with CIN-2, assuming the following conditions are met: the initial colposcopy was satisfactory, endocervical sampling results were negative, and the patient understands the risk of occult disease. Treatment with either ablation or excision is the only acceptable option for biopsy-proven CIN-3 in this population.

In immunosuppressed women with HIV, there is a high rate of recurrence and persistence of CIN-2,3 even after appropriate treatment. Treatment does, however, seem to be effective in preventing the progression of CIN-2,3 to invasive cervical cancer.

FUTURE TRENDS

The most promising new development in cervical cancer prevention is the HPV vaccine. HPV types 16 and 18 are responsible for 60 to 70% of cervical cancers, whereas HPV types 6 and 11 account for 95% of external warts, as well as laryngeal, conjunctival, and esophageal papillomas *(11)*. Two recent randomized controlled trials of a monovalent HPV type 16 vaccine and a bivalent HPV types 16 and 18 vaccine both demonstrated 100% efficacy in preventing persistent HPV type 16 or HPV types 16 and 18-related infections, respectively *(12,13)*. An additional randomized controlled trial of a quadrivalent vaccine against HPV types 6, 11, 16, and 18 induced seroconversion in all recipients and was 100% efficacious in preventing disease attributable to these four HPV types *(14)*. The bivalent vaccine, Cervarix®, is projected to be FDA approved in late 2007. The quadrivalent vaccine, Gardasil®, was FDA approved in 2006 for women and girls aged 9 to 26 years as a three-shot series at zero, two and six mo. Although multiple studies confirmed this nearly 100% efficacy in preventing precancerous cervical lesions, HPV vaccines are not thought to be effective in preventing cervical abnormalities in those already infected with the HPV types against which the vaccine is directed. The widespread use of these vaccines, especially before sexual activity commences, could dramatically reduce the rate of cervical cancer deaths worldwide.

CONCLUSION

Cervical cancer is a preventable and curable disease. By following established guidelines for screening, early detection and treatment of precancerous lesions, cervical cancer morbidity and mortality will continue to decline. Future preventive efforts with both an effective vaccination against HPV and thorough education regarding the importance of screening will move us closer to eradicating cervical cancer entirely.

REFERENCES

1. Saslow D, Runowicz CD, Solomon D, et al. American Cancer Society Guideline for the early detection of cervical neoplasia and cancer. CA Cancer J Clin 2002;52:342–362.
2. American Cancer Society. Cancer Facts and Figures. 2005.
3. Hildesheim A, Schiffman MH, Gravitt PE, et al. Persistence of type-specific human papillomavirus infection among cytologically normal women. J Infect Dis 1994:169:235–240.
4. Moscicki AB, Shiboski S, Broering J, et al. The natural history of human papillomavirus infection as measured by repeated DNA testing in adolescent and young women. J Pediatr 1998;132:277–284.
5. Ho GY, Bierman R, Beardsle L, et al. Natural history of cervicovaginal papillomavirus infection in young women. N Engl J Med 1998;338:423–428.
6. ACOG Committee on Practice Bulletins. ACOG Practice Bulletin: Clinical management guidelines for obstetrician-gynecologists. Number 45, August 2003. Cervical cytology screening (replaces committee opinion 152, March 1995). Obstet Gynecol 2003;102:417–427.
7. US Preventive Services Task Force. Screening for cervical cancer (accessed August 7, 2005 at http://www.ahrq.gov/clinic/uspstf/uspscerv.htm.).
8. Wright TC, Cox JT, Massad LS, et al. 2001 Consensus Guidelines for the management of women with cervical cytological abnormalities. JAMA 2002;287:2120–2129.
9. Wright TC, Cox JT, Massad LS, et al. 2001 Consensus Guidelines for the management of women with cervical intraepithelial neoplasia. Am J Obstet 2003;189:295–304.
10. Solomon D, Davey D, Kurman R, et al. The 2001 Bethesda System. Terminology for reporting results of cervical cytology. JAMA 2002;287:2114–2119.
11. Harper DM. Are we closer to the prevention of HPV-related diseases? J Fam Pract 2005;54(7 Suppl):s10–s16.

12. Koutsky LA, Ault KA, Wheeler CM, et al. A controlled trial of a human papillomavirus type 16 vaccine. N Engl J Med 2002;347:1645–1651.
13. Harper DM, Franco EL, Wheeler C, et al. Efficacy of a bivalent L1 virus-like particle vaccine in prevention of infection with human papillomavirus types 16 and 18 in young women: a randomized controlled trial. Lancet 2004;364(9447):1757–1765.
14. Villa LL, Costa RL, Petta CA, et al. Prophylactic quadrivalent human papillomavirus (types 6, 11, 16, and 18) L-1 virus-like particle vaccine in young women: a randomized double-blind placebo-controlled multicentre phase II efficacy trial. Lancet Oncol 2005;6(5):271–278.

12 Breast Disorders

Lori Jardines, MD

CONTENTS

BREAST CANCER SCREENING

Women in their 20s and 30s should undergo a clinical breast examination every 2 to 3 years. At the age of 40 years, the examination should be performed annually. It is recommended that women age 40 years and older should undergo

From: *Current Clinical Practice: Women's Health in Clinical Practice*
Edited by: Clouse and Sherif © Humana Press Inc., Totowa, NJ

mammography annually. There is no upper age limit for mammography. It should be continued annually as long as the woman remains in good health. Breast self-examination is also an option for women and, if done, should be performed monthly beginning in the 20s *(1)*.

SCREENING MAMMOGRAPHY

Screening mammography is performed as two views of each breast (craniocaudal [CC] and mediolateral oblique) and is used in women who are asymptomatic. The purpose of screening mammography is to detect breast cancer before it can be appreciated clinically. For every 1000 women screened, approx 10 women will require biopsy and two to three breast cancers will be identified *(2)*.

To aid in the interpretation of the mammogram report, the radiologist must provide a clear, concise report and categorize the results into one of the six Breast Imaging Reporting Data System classifications (Table 1) *(3)*. The probability of malignancy with a class 1 or 2 mammogram is zero. A class 3 mammogram suggests that there is less than a 2% chance of the lesion being associated with an underlying malignancy *(4)*. A class 4 mammogram is associated with a 20% chance of malignancy. There is a 90% chance of identifying breast cancer when a mammogram has been categorized as class 5.

MAMMOGRAPHIC SIGNS OF MALIGNANCY

Microcalcifications observed on mammography should be evaluated for morphology and pattern of distribution *(5)*. Calcifications observed on a routine screening mammogram should be further evaluated by diagnostic mammography with magnification views in the 90° lateral and CC views. If the calcifications form a meniscus in the 90° lateral view and appear rounded on the CC view, they can be safely followed because they are associated with milk of calcium and microcystic disease. Microcalcifications that are punctate and scattered tend to be benign as well. However, calcifications that are pleomorphic, linear, or branching in shape are suspicious. In addition, patterns of distribution that are concerning are calcifications that are clustered, where at least 5 to 6 microcalcifications are observed in a small volume of breast tissue. Calcifications in a ductal distribution are suspicious for malignancy because they suggest that calcifications are contained within a ductal system within the breast. It is less common to see diffuse malignant-appearing microcalcifications.

Masses on mammography require further evaluation using compression views, which allow better definition of the margins. Low-density masses with smooth margins have a low probability of being malignant. Masses that are high density with spiculated or poorly defined margins have a much higher rate of being associated with an underlying breast cancer. Ultrasound is extremely

Table 1
Breast Imaging Reporting Data System Classification of Mammographic Abnormalities[a]

Category	*Assessment*	*Recommendation*
0	Abnormality observed	Needs additional imaging Diagnostic mammogram Possible breast ultrasound
1	Normal mammogram	Annual screening
2	Benign lesion	Annual screening
3	Probably benign lesion	Short-term follow-up
4	Suspicious	Recommend biopsy
5	Highly suggestive of malignancy	High probability of cancer, appropriate action should be taken
6	Biopsy-proven malignancy	Treatment

[a]From ref. *3*, with permission.

helpful in the evaluation of a mass observed on screening mammogram. If a mass on mammogram is consistent with a simple cyst, it requires no further intervention. Solid breast masses often require biopsy to provide histological confirmation and ensure that there is no evidence malignancy.

Architectural distortion occurs when the normal breast parenchymal pattern formed by Cooper's ligaments is pulled eccentrically away from the nipple. This mammographic finding must be very carefully evaluated to ensure that it is not associated with an underling malignancy. In the absence of previous surgery in that site within the breast, cancer is a major cause for this mammographic finding. Scar tissue associated with surgery should become less apparent with time. When the mammogram report suggests that a radial scar is present, the patient should undergo a surgical rather than a percutaneous biopsy. These lesions tend to pathologically complex and are often associated with a small focus of cancer.

An area of asymmetric density on mammography requires further evaluation to determine whether it is associated with normal breast tissue or an underlying breast cancer. This is usually accomplished with compression views of the breast and a targeted ultrasound.

BIOPSY OPTIONS FOR NONPALPABLE LESIONS IDENTIFIED BY BREAST IMAGING

As the use of screening mammography has increased, the recommendation for biopsy of image-detected breast abnormalities has increased. Nonpalpable breast abnormalities can be approached by percutaneous core needle biopsy or surgical needle localization breast biopsy. Patients who require chronic aspirin or nonsteroidal anti-inflammatory drug therapy or anticoagulation are best served by open surgical biopsy because of the risk of bleeding.

Ultrasound-Guided Core Needle Biopsy

Whenever possible, a percutaneous core needle biopsy is performed under ultrasound guidance for patient comfort because the patient can lie supine and the breast in not in compression. In most instances, an 11-gauge core needle is inserted through a small skin incision via a trocar. Vacuum assistance is applied to the needle when it is the correct location, which allows a greater volume of tissue to be excised. Multiple samples of the mass can be taken as the needle moves in and out through the trocar. Masses up to approx 2 cm can be removed with this technique and may no longer be visible radiographically. At the completion of the procedure, a clip is placed to mark the location of the biopsy site. Less frequently, a 14-gauge core needle without vacuum assistance is used to perform the biopsy. If this is the case, the lesion will be sampled and not completely removed. In addition, there may be a higher chance for a sampling error. At the completion of the biopsy procedure, hemostasis is achieved with pressure, and Steri-strips™ are applied to the incision site. The patient can apply ice to the area to reduce swelling.

Stereotactic Core Needle Biopsy

When a lesion cannot be visualized on ultrasound and the patient prefers a percutaneous biopsy, it is performed stereotactically. The woman lies prone on the table, where there is a hole cut out, though which the breast hangs down. The breast is then compressed in the location of the lesion, which is imaged via digital mammography, and the location of the lesion is determined by computer. The skin and deeper breast tissue is anesthetized with lidocaine. A small (3 mm) skin incision is made to allow passage of the needle through the skin into the breast tissue. The biopsy procedure is then performed with either an 8- or 11-gauge needle through a trocar, where vacuum assistance is applied. The opening of the needle can be rotated to allow for greater sampling of the target lesion. A clip is place at the completion of the procedure to mark the biopsy site. When the biopsy is performed for microcalcifications, a specimen radiogram is performed to document that the calcifications have been sampled. The likelihood of a false-negative biopsy performed with a large core needle biopsy and vacuum assistance is approx 1%. Hemostasis is achieved with pressure, the skin incision is closed with a Steri-strip™, and ice is often applied to reduce swelling.

Lesions close to the areola or chest wall may not be amenable to stereotactic biopsy for technical reasons. In addition, patients who are unable to lie prone for any length of time may not be candidates for this procedure. Women with small or thin breasts may also not be candidates for a minimally invasive mammographically guided biopsy. This is related to technical considerations and the size of the chamber within the needle for acquiring the specimen.

Interpretation of the Results

After a minimally invasive breast biopsy has been performed, the results of the biopsy must be compared with the imaging studies to determine whether they are concordant. If they are and the results are benign, the patients requires no further intervention and, in most cases, may return to annual screening mammography. If there is a discrepancy, a surgical biopsy is required. Further intervention is also warranted when malignancy is demonstrated.

When atypical ductal hyperplasia (ADH) is identified on core needle biopsy, a surgical biopsy is recommended because there is a 20% chance of identifying an associated breast cancer *(6)*. When atypical lobular hyperplasia (ALH) or lobular carcinoma *in situ* (LCIS) is identified after core biopsy with vacuum assistance, it is controversial whether the patient requires a surgical biopsy to obtain additional tissue for study *(7,8)*. When a diagnosis of ALH or LCIS is detected on core biopsy, it is important to determine whether the results of the pathology are concordant with the findings on the breast imaging studies. If they are not in concordance, surgical biopsy may be necessary to ensure that there is no evidence of an associated ductal carcinoma *in situ* (DCIS) or invasive carcinoma. Pleomorphic LCIS is an uncommon variant of LCIS and is often associated with pleomorphic invasive lobular carcinoma. When pleomorphic LCIS is identified on core biopsy, additional tissue sampling is recommended *(9)*. If additional tissue is needed after a minimally invasive breast biopsy, the procedure is performed under needle localization guidance because the initial lesion was nonpalpable.

Needle Localization Breast Biopsy

Needle localization breast biopsy is a surgical biopsy that is most often performed under local anesthesia with or without sedation. In some instances, general anesthesia may be recommended.

The target lesion is first localized with a needle, under either ultrasound or mammographic guidance. Once the needle is in the correct position, a thin wire is placed through it to mark the correct site. Most wires have a barb on the end to prevent movement of the wire within the breast. Mammogram films are taken and accompany the patient to the operating room to facilitate the procedure. The incision is planned so that there will be minimal dissection within the breast to identify the correct location along the wire and remove the target lesion with a small amount of surrounding normal breast tissue. The breast tissue and wire are removed and oriented for subsequent pathology examination. The specimen is first sent for a specimen radiogram to confirm that the lesion has been excised. The tissue is then sent to pathology for examination. If the lesion is not within the specimen, it is unlikely that removing more tissue will be beneficial. In most instances, it is best to close the incision, allow the patient to heal somewhat and repeat the process.

BREAST CLINICAL EVALUATION

The are many reasons why a woman will present for a breast evaluation. She may have a breast mass, nipple discharge or an abnormal mammogram. During the course of the evaluation, a large amount of information is gathered. Not only is the present problem evaluated, but all other relevant information concerning the patient's past breast history, family history, and medical history to allow an accurate assessment of the problem and the patient's risk for breast cancer.

History

A thorough breast history is the initial part of the evaluation, which includes specific questions concerning the problem. If she is presenting with a breast mass, the patient should be questioned regarding when she first noted the mass and whether it changes with her menstrual cycle, if she is premenopausal. It is helpful to ask where the mass is located in the breast and how large it is to facilitate the breast examination. The woman should also be questioned regarding whether she has any other breast complaints, such as focal breast pain, nipple discharge, or changes in the skin of breast or nipple, including erosion or retraction. In addition, she should be questioned regarding whether she has noted a mass or pain. Menstrual and reproductive histories, use of exogenous hormones, family history of breast and/or ovarian cancer, and social history, including the use of tobacco and alcohol, should also be elicited. The family history for breast and ovarian cancer should be detailed and cover two or three generations on the maternal and paternal side of the family to determine whether there could be a genetic predisposition to breast cancer. It is also helpful to know whether the patient has had previous breast surgery and, if so, what the pathology results showed. There are certain conditions (ADH and ALH, and LCIS) which increase a woman's risk for the development of a breast cancer. The purpose of the breast history is to provide the examiner information regarding the breast mass and the level of breast cancer risk for the patient (Table 2).

Clinical Breast Examination

The patient should be undressed from the waist up and the exam should be performed in a well-lit room. With the patient in a sitting position, the breasts

Table 2
Breast Cancer Risk Factors

Age
Sex
Family history of breast and/or ovarian cancer
Previous history of breast cancer
History of breast biopsy showing atypical hyperplasia or lobular carcinoma *in situ*
Age at menarche (younger than 12 years)
Age at menopause (older than 55 years)
Exogenous hormone use
Previous breast or mantle irradiation
Age at first full term pregnancy (older than 30 years)
Alcohol consumption
Tobacco abuse
Previous breast biopsy

should first be visually inspected for symmetry. If one breast is larger than the other, the patient should be questioned as to whether this is a new finding for her.

The cervical, supraclavicular infraclavicular and axillary nodes are then examined. The patient should then press her hands on her hips and raise her arms above her head. Cooper's ligaments, the suspensory ligaments of the breast insert onto the dermis of the skin and the pectoralis fascia. A breast cancer can grow into the suspensory ligaments of the breast and these maneuvers can produce skin and/or nipple retraction. If the patient is complaining of spontaneous nipple discharge or nonspontaneous bloody nipple discharge, the nipple and breast are compressed with the patient in the upright position to determine whether the fluid is emanating from a single duct or multiple ducts. Pressure is applied to each quadrant of the breast and areola to determine the origin of the discharge. The nipple fluid should be tested for occult blood. With the patient still sitting upright, a bimanual exam is performed of each breast. The patient is then asked to lie back in a semi-recumbant position, with the head of the exam table raised to approx 15°. When breast palpation is performed, the patient is asked to bring her ipsilateral arm up and place it behind her head. The flat portion of the fingertips are used. At each site, three concentric circles are made using varying amounts of pressure to appreciate superficial, intermediate depth, and deep masses. There are several different techniques for breast palpation (radial, horizontal strip, vertical strip, and circular) (Figs. 1–4). If a mass is identified, it should be measured and its location within the breast and the distance from the nipple should be determined and documented. The margins of the mass should also be evaluated to determine whether they are circumscribed as opposed to

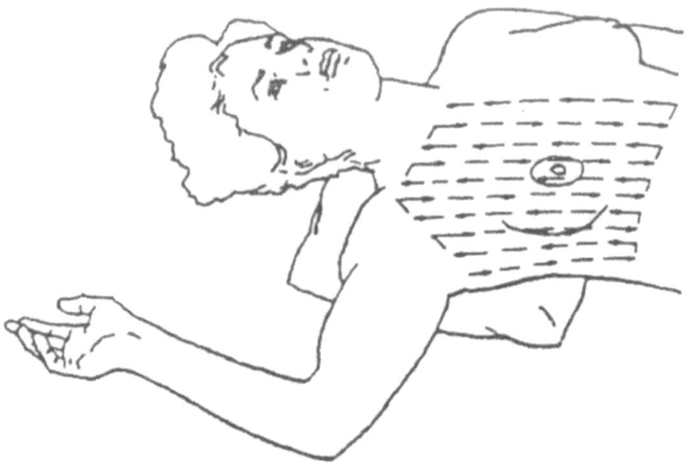

Fig. 1. Clinical Breast Exam: Circular method.

indistinct. If a mass is present, it should be noted whether there is retraction of or fixation to the skin, or fixation to the underlying chest wall.

The skin of the breast should be evaluated for edema (*peau d'orange*) which may be associated with an underlying inflammatory breast cancer. The skin should also be evaluated for erythema, nodules, and ulceration.

The nipples should be examined to determine whether there is retraction or erosions. If there are any suspicious findings on breast examination, the woman should be referred for a breast imaging evaluation. If no abnormality is identified on exam but the patient thinks that there has been a change in her exam, she should also be referred for breast imaging evaluation.

Breast Ultrasound

Breast ultrasound is beneficial for problem solving and is used in the evaluation of palpable masses and mammographically detected masses or asymmetric densities. Ultrasound will determine whether a mass is solid, complex with solid and cystic components, or a cyst. At this point, ultrasound is not used as a screening tool. It is also important to note that the quality of breast ultrasound is operator dependent. Therefore, it is best to have a skilled breast ultrasonographer perform the evaluation.

A breast cyst appears as a well-circumscribed anechoic mass, with thin walls and well-defined borders. A complex mass can be filled with debris or have both solid and cystic components. Ultrasound can help to determine whether a mass is likely to be benign or malignant. Benign solid masses tend to be ovoid

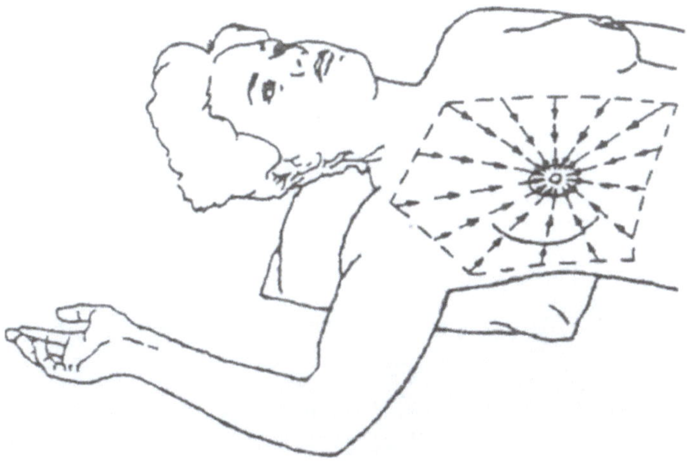

Fig. 2. Clinical Breast Exam: Radical method.

and homogeneous and have smooth margins or macrolobulations. Malignant solid masses tend to be taller than wide, with heterogeneous echotexture and have irregular margins or microlobulations. Ultrasound can also be used to determine whether a palpable finding is associated with a solid mass or a ridge of prominent breast tissue.

Mammography

When mammography is performed for a breast problem, a diagnostic mammogram is performed as opposed to a screening study.

Management of a Palpable Breast Mass

The patient should undergo a thorough breast history and examination. Women younger than 35 years of age who have an average risk for breast cancer and an examination that is not suspicious should undergo breast ultrasound to determine whether the mass is solid or a cyst. Women older than 35 years and young high-risk women should be evaluated by mammography and breast ultrasound.

If the mass is a cyst, it can be aspirated. If the mass resolves completely after aspiration and the fluid is not bloody, the patient should be reexamined in approx 6 weeks to ensure the cyst has not recurred. When a cyst recurs, despite repeated aspirations, it should be excised. If the mass does not resolve completely or the fluid is bloody and there is no evidence of a traumatic aspiration, the mass should be excised.

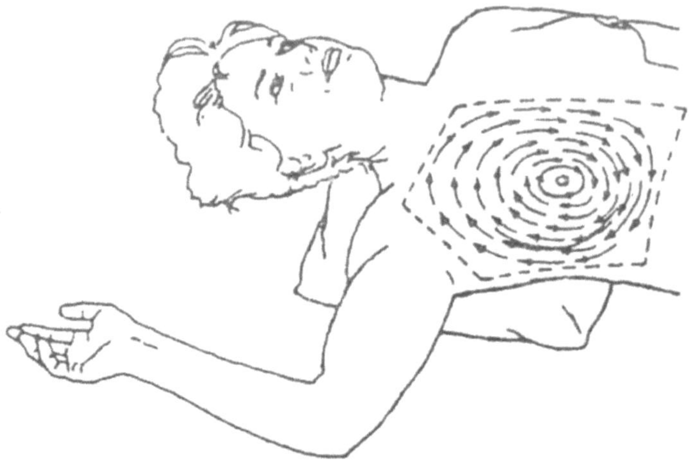

Fig. 3. Clinical Breast Exam: Vertical strip.

When a woman younger than 35 years is found to have a solid mass with benign features on breast examination and ultrasound, she can opt for needle biopsy *(10)*. If the results of the needle biopsy, ultrasound, and clinical examination are concordant and benign, she can be followed clinically. If, at any time, the mass increases in size, it should be excised. If the mass is solid and the ultrasound is suspicious, a biopsy should be performed. If a percutaneous biopsy is performed and the results of the breast examination, biopsy, and ultrasound are not concordant, excisional biopsy of the mass is recommended.

After breast imaging studies, a woman older than 40 years with a solid palpable mass should undergo biopsy. If the biopsy was performed percutaneously and all of the data point to a benign process, the mass can be followed *(11)*. If the examination, imaging studies, or percutaneous biopsy is not concordant or any reveal suspicious findings, excision is recommended.

BREAST PAIN

Breast pain is a common complaint and, for the most part, resolves without any intervention. At the time of evaluation, the pain can be categorized into cyclical, noncyclical, or chest wall. Part of the history should include whether the pain is cyclical, intermittent vs constant, and diffuse vs focal. The patient should also be questioned regarding how long she has had the pain, and should be asked about the severity of the pain.

A complete breast examination should be performed, with careful attention to the areas of pain to determine whether the discomfort can be demonstrated and to ensure that there is no palpable abnormality associated with the pain. When there is a suspicion that the pain is associated with the chest wall, the patient can be examined in the decubitus position, which allows the breast tissue to fall away from the chest wall and direct pressure can be applied to the chest wall.

When the discomfort is related to the chest wall or the costochondral junctions, the patient can be reassured. When the breast examination is unremarkable and the pain is diffuse and intermittent, the patient can also be reassured. If the patient has focal pain or the pain is constant, breast imaging appropriate for age should be performed.

In most patients, simple reassurance results in the resolution of the pain. For patients whose pain does not resolve, has been present for more than 4 months and is significant, treatment can be considered. The most effective agents are endocrine agents and include danazol *(12)*, bromocriptine *(13)*, and tamoxifen *(14)*. There are significant toxicities of the medications and many women stop because of the side effects. Nonhormonal means for treating breast pain include the use of a sports bra, low-fat diet, evening primrose oil, and caffeine reduction.

NIPPLE DISCHARGE

Nipple discharge is a common complaint and can be divided into three categories *(15)*:

1. Galactorrhea.
2. Physiological.
3. Pathological.

Galactorrhea is defined by bilateral, milky fluid being produced from multiple ducts not associated with pregnancy or lactation. The most common causes of galactorrhea are idiopathic with normal menses, pituitary tumors, idiopathic with abnormal menses, and certain medications, including oral contraceptives, tricyclic antidepressants, some antihypertensive medications, and phenothyazines. It has also been associated with hypothyroidism.

The first piece of the evaluation entails a thorough history to include the menstrual history and a review of the medications the woman is taking. Physical examination should include a breast examination and evaluation of visual fields, which may be impaired when a large pituitary adenoma is present. Prolactin and thyroid-stimulating hormone levels are sent to ensure that there is no endocrine abnormality. If the prolactin level is elevated, a MRI study of the sella turcica should be performed.

Physiological discharge most often occurs when the breast or nipple is stimulated. It may also be related to exogenous hormone use. The discharge is not spontaneous and is usually from multiple ducts. The color of the fluid varies and may be milky, yellow, green, or brown. If there is no evidence of blood in the discharge, there is no need for intervention, and the patient can be reassured. If the fluid is bloody, further evaluation is warranted.

Pathological nipple discharge is spontaneous, unilateral, from a single duct, and is persistent. Patients with this complaint should have a thorough breast history and examination. When the patient is sitting, the areola should be compressed in specific locations to determine the site of the lesion producing the fluid. If the fluid is not bloody, it can be tested for occult blood using a guaiac card. Whether the fluid is bloody or not, this type of discharge warrants evaluation and most often, surgical intervention. Preoperatively, the patient should be evaluated by mammogram and breast ultrasound directed to the retroareolar region of the breast. A ductogram may be helpful in identifying an intraductal lesion deep within the breast, particularly in women with large breasts. This is a procedure in which the secreting duct is cannulated, a radio-opaque dye is injected, and a mammogram is obtained. A negative ductogram should not be used as reason to not recommend surgery because of the possibility of a false-negative study. Cytology of nipple fluid is also not helpful in guiding the need for surgery, because there is a high incidence of false-negative and false-positive readings.

Patients who have a pathological nipple discharge should undergo a duct excision to determine the cause of the discharge. If an abnormality is identified on the preoperative imaging studies, it should be localized preoperatively and excised at the time of the duct excision. Young women who are interested in maintaining the ability to lactate can be offered a selective duct excision in which only the secreting duct is removed. The secreting duct can be identified preoperatively by ductography or intraoperatively, where it can be cannulated with a lacrimal duct probe to aid in the selective excision. Ductoscopy is a relatively new technology in which a fiberoptic scope is inserted into the secreting duct to identify other areas of intraductal abnormalities.

The causes of pathological nipple discharge are intraductal papilloma (50%), mammary duct ectasia (25%), fibrocystic changes (20%), and breast cancer (5%). When breast cancer is associated with only pathological nipple discharge, it is often noninvasive.

BENIGN BREAST MASSES

Fibrocystic Changes

Fibrocystic changes of the breast are extremely common and affect many women. It is associated with the hormonal effects of estrogen and progesterone on the ducts, lobules, and stroma of the breast. Cysts are fluid filled spaces that develop from the terminal ductal lobular unit or from an obstructed duct. Benign simple cysts are extremely common and occur most frequently in the fifth decade of life. Epithelial hyperplasia without atypia can be observed in the ducts and/or lobules. When the hyperplasia is mild, there is no increased risk for breast cancer. When the hyperplasia is moderate to florid, there is a small increase in the relative risk for breast cancer (1.5–2 times). Sclerosing adenosis is a form of proliferative fibrocystic changes that is most often found incidentally after biopsy. It may present as a palpable mass (adenosis tumor) or as microcalcifications on mammogram. It is important to note that sclerosing adenosis can sometimes be confused with an infiltrating carcinoma and special stains may sometimes be required to differentiate one from the other. Fibrosis of the breast is associated with a decrease in the numbers of lobules in the breast and an increase in the stroma. Focal fibrosis may present as a palpable mass of as a density on mammogram. In woman with long-standing insulin-dependent diabetes mellitus, this is known as diabetic fibrous mastopathy.

Fibroadenoma

Fibroadenoma is the most common solid benign breast mass observed in women younger than 35 years. There are no race-associated differences associated with their development or age at presentation. They are usually single, although in 10 to 15% of women, they are multiple. When palpable, they are most often well-circumscribed and mobile. Fibroadenomas are thought to arise from hyperplasia of the terminal duct lobular unit and contain both an epithelial and stromal component. Because there is an epithelial component, atypical hyperplasia *(16)* and carcinomas *(17)* have been identified in fibroadenomas; however, this is extremely rare.

Most fibroadenomas are approx 2 to 3 cm in size. Giant fibroadenomas are 5 cm in size or greater. Juvenile fibroadenomas are observed around the time of puberty and can increase in size rapidly. Excision is recommended because of the size and concern regarding possible malignancy.

Adenoma

Adenomas of the breast are divided into tubular adenomas and lactating adenomas. Both are well-circumscribed on breast examination. Microscopically, tubular adenomas appear as a proliferation of uniform small tubular structures with minimal stroma. Lactating adenomas are observed during pregnancy and in the postpartum period. They may undergo infarction postpartum secondary to loss of their vascular supply.

Hamartoma

Breast hamartomas are uncommon lesions, which, on physical examination, are well-circumscribed. They are composed of fat, glandular breast tissue, and stroma. Most occur in women older than 35 years. On mammography, one sees a mass composed of fat and fibroglandular tissue surrounded by a capsule of connective tissue.

Phyllodes Tumor

Phyllodes tumors are uncommon and account for less than 1% of breast tumors in women. They can present as a new mass or as a long-standing breast mass that is increasing in size *(18)*. The average age at presentation is in the 40s, but they have been observed in girls younger than 10 years and in women older than 70 years. Phyllodes tumors are divided into benign, intermediate, and malignant categories. They have an epithelial and stromal component. Tumors are stratified based on the degree of stromal cellular atypia, the mitotic activity of the stromal cells, the presence of stromal overgrowth, and the tumor margins.Most phyllodes tumors are benign. It can be difficult to distinguish a benign fibroadenoma from a phyllodes tumor based on fine needle aspiration biopsy or core biopsy. When there is a question of a phyllodes tumor, an excisional biopsy is often necessary to establish a diagnosis. Phyllodes tumors are most often treated with wide excision *(19)*. In some instances, the patient may require a mastectomy, particularly if the lesion is large and the breast is small and cannot accommodate a wide excision. If the patient has a benign phyllodes tumor, it may be reasonable to follow the patient carefully because the risk of recurrence is less than 10%.

Granular Cell Tumor

Granular cell tumors can occur anywhere in the body, and approx 6% of them are observed in the breast. They can be difficult to distinguish from a breast carcinoma because they are hard and may be fixed to the overlying skin or to the underlying pectoralis muscle. In addition, they often have suspicious features on mammogram. The mean age at diagnosis is 40 years and they occur more commonly in blacks. Most granular cell tumors are benign and are treated by wide excision.

Intraductal Papilloma

An intraductal papilloma usually presents as pathological discharge but can sometimes present as a palpable mass, generally, in the central portion of the breast. They are most frequently single and confined to the major lactiferous ducts of the breast. Solitary intraductal papillomas are most often observed in women between the ages of 30 and 50 years and are generally less than 1 cm in size.

Papillomas may contain areas of atypical hyperplasia, DCIS, and or invasive carcinoma. Patients with multiple peripheral papillomas tend to be younger and are at higher risk for developing carcinoma. Papillomatosis is diagnosed when there are microscopic foci of intraducal hyperplasia in which papillary architecture is observed. This lesion falls under the category of proliferative breast disorders without atypia and carries a small increased risk for breast cancer.

HIGH-RISK BREAST LESIONS

ADH and ALH

ADH and ALH are proliferative breast disorders with some but not all features of carcinomas *in situ*. There is a continuum of the disease process and it can sometimes be difficult to distinguish ADH from a low-grade DCIS. The presence of one or both of these obtained on breast biopsy increase a woman's risk for developing breast cancer in the future. In the past, when biopsies were performed primarily for palpable masses, the incidence of finding either ADH or ALH was approx 5%. With the increased use of minimally invasive breast biopsy techniques, the incidence increases to approx 12 to 17% when the biopsy is being performed for microcalcifications *(20)*.

ADH increases a woman's relative risk for breast cancer by approximately five times that of the general population. The increase in breast cancer risk associated with ALH is slightly higher. In the face of atypical hyperplasia and a family history of breast cancer, the risk for developing breast cancer is further increased, to approximately nine times that of the general population *(21)*.

LCIS is not considered a true breast cancer but is considered a high-risk breast lesion. ALH and LCIS represent a continuum of disease and are sometimes referred to as lobular neoplasia *(22)*. Most often, it is identified as an incidental finding when a breast biopsy is performed for other reasons. Because there are no characteristic signs for LCIS on mammography or physical examination, the true incidence of this entity is unknown. The peak age for the diagnosis of LCIS is in the fifth decade of life. LCIS tends to be multifocal and bilateral.

The risk for developing an invasive breast cancer is approx 1% per year. The time from diagnosis of LCIS to the development of a true breast cancer can be as long as 30 years, although most patients who develop breast cancer will do so within the first 15 to 20 years after diagnosis *(23)*. If the patient develops breast cancer, it is more likely to be ductal in origin, although the incidence of invasive lobular carcinoma is greater in women with a history of LCIS than in the general population. Each breast is at risk; however, if a breast cancer develops, it is three times more likely to occur in the breast in which the LCIS was identified *(24)*.

INHERITED RISK FOR BREAST CANCER

Approximately 5 to 10% of breast cancers are associated with an inherited susceptibility for breast cancer. Patients with inherited breast cancer tend to be younger at the time of diagnosis when compared with patients with sporadic breast cancer. In addition, there is a higher risk for the development of bilateral disease.

BRCA1 is a tumor suppressor gene that is inherited in an autosomaldominant fashion. Therefore, when evaluating a patient, it is important to ascertain the entire family history, including the maternal and paternal sides of the family. There is incomplete penetrance and not all affected individuals will manifest the disease. Patients with a mutated *BRCA1* gene has up to an 85% chance of developing breast cancer in her lifetime and, if she develops breast cancer, she has a 65% chance of developing contralateral disease. In addition, she will have up to a 50% chance of developing ovarian cancer. There is also an increased risk for colorectal cancer. There are two specific mutations in *BRCA1* that are observed with high frequency in women of Ashkenazi Jewish descent. Twenty percent of breast cancer cases in Ashkenazi Jewish women younger than 40 years of age at diagnosis are associated with one of these mutations.

BRCA2 is another tumor suppressor gene that is also inherited in an autosomal dominant fashion. Up to 80% of patients with a mutation in *BRCA2* develop breast cancer. There is a smaller risk for ovarian cancer (up to 20%). In addition, there is an increased risk for melanoma, pancreatic cancer, and male breast cancer. There is one mutation in *BRCA2* that is observed in high frequency in patients of Ashkenazi Jewish descent.

Li-Fraumeni syndrome, Cowden disease, Peutz-Jehger syndrome, and ataxia-telangiectasia are all associated with a specific gene mutation and are associated with an increased risk for breast cancer. They are also uncommon diseases.

MANAGEMENT OF WOMEN AT HIGH RISK FOR BREAST CANCER

Women may be at a high risk for developing breast cancer because of the pathology results from a breast biopsy and/or from their family history.

When evaluating a woman who seems to have a high risk secondary to family history, careful medical and family histories, including ethnic background, are necessary. Patients who have a 10% chance of having a mutation in either *BRCA1* or *BRCA2* should consider genetic counseling and genetic testing. When a patient presents with a family history of ovarian cancer, multiple cases of early onset beast cancer, breast cancer and ovarian cancer in the same relative, bilateral breast cancer, or male breast cancer, there is an increased incidence of finding a mutation in either *BRCA1* or *BRCA2*. She should consider genetic counseling and genetic testing.

If she tests positive for a mutation, she can discuss her options for management. Patients with mutations in either of these genes are at high risk for developing ovarian cancer and should discuss prophylactic oophorectomy to reduce their risk for this disease. Because there is a higher incidence of fallopian tube cancers in mutation carriers, the fallopian tubes should be removed at the time of oophorectomy *(25,26)*. There is no truly effective screening for ovarian cancer. Patients at high risk for the disease who do not wish to proceed with oophorectomy may opt for clinical exam, pelvic ultrasound, and testing for CA-125 levels, although these measures are not always reliable. Women who are mutation carriers who undergo prophylactic oophorectomy before the age of 50 years have a significant reduction in their risk for breast cancer *(25, 26)*. Women may also opt for bilateral prophylactic mastectomy with or without breast reconstruction. Studies have shown that high-risk women can reduce their risk for developing breast cancer by 90% after prophylactic mastectomy *(27)*. Patients must be aware that this procedure is not 100% effective and must seek prompt attention if they develop a chest wall nodule or mass because this could represent breast cancer. Women who are mutation positive and do not desire prophylactic breast surgery can be observed two to three times per year for clinical breast examination and undergo annual mammography. Breast MRI may be helpful in women who are mutation carriers.

Another result of genetic testing may be that a gene variant of unknown significance is identified. In this case, testing of other members of the family may be helpful in determining whether the mutation is associated with elevated breast cancer risk.

A patient is considered a true negative when she tests negative for known deleterious mutations observed in other members of her family. If this is the case, this individual is not at increased risk for breast cancer and can be followed accordingly.

If a woman is the first person to be tested in her family and is negative for a known mutation, it is possible that a mutation is present but not detectable by the methodology available today, there is a mutation in another gene associated with increased breast cancer risk or that she has developed a sporadic cancer. These possibilities should be discussed with the patient to guide her in the decision-making process.

The Gail model is a statistical method to evaluate a woman's risk for breast cancer. It takes into consideration the patient's age, race, age at menarche, age at first live birth, the number of breast biopsies and whether the biopsies revealed atypical hyperplasia or LCIS *(28)*. A woman whose 5-year risk for breast cancer based on her individual risk factors is equal or greater than 1.66% is thought to be at significant risk for breast cancer and should consider tamoxifen as a chemopreventive agent. The National Surgical Adjuvant Breast and Bowel Project (NSABP) completed a clinical trial in which 13,388 high-risk women were randomized to receive tamoxifen vs placebo for 5 years *(29)*. There was a significant reduction in the incidence of breast cancer in women who received tamoxifen, particularly in women with LCIS and atypical hyperplasia. The Gail model for breast cancer risk assessment may underestimate the risk for women with a family history of the disease because it does not allow the consideration of breast cancer in second-degree family members.

BREAST INFECTIONS

Lactational Infections

Mastitis and breast abscesses associated with lactation are relatively uncommon in developed countries. They most often occur in the first 3 to 6 weeks of breast feeding. The infection is related to a crack in the skin of the nipple allowing bacteria to enter the breast. Initially, mastitis develops in which the entire breast can become erythematous, hard, and painful. The common organism is *staphylococcus aureus (30)*. Antibiotic therapy should be directed to cover these bacteria, keeping in mind the increasing presence of community-acquired methcillin-resistent *s. aureus*. In some instances, the mastitis progresses to a breast abscess. The abscess can be treated with aspiration and antibiotic therapy providing that the skin overlying the abscess is not too thinned. The patient may require multiple aspirations to control the infection. If aspiration fails to resolve the problem or if the skin is overly thin, the patient may require operative incision and drainage in which the abscess is opened and explored in the operating room to ensure there are no deep loculations. The wound is then packed and heals by secondary intention. It is important to consider the diagnosis of inflammatory breast cancer in a woman who presents with what seems to be a mastitis or breast abscess.

Nonlactational Infections

Most nonlactational breast infections are centrally located and are more likely to occur in premenopausal women. Most are related to periductal mastitis and mammary duct ectasia. There is a relationship between cigarette smoking and the development of nonlactational beast abscesses *(31)*. These infections are generally polymicrobial and involve both gram-positive and gram-negative organisms *(32)*. Therefore, antibiotic coverage should be broad spectrum. If the patient presents with a central mastitis, the infection can generally be controlled with oral antibiotics. In some instances, the patient has repeated retroareolar infections with or without abscess formation. Those patients should undergo a mammary duct excision in an attempt to control the infection. Rarely, patients will require excision of the nipple and central breast tissue to eliminate the source of infection, the central ductal system. Patients who present with an apparent breast infection who are unresponsive to antibiotics should undergo biopsy to ensure there is not an underlying breast cancer.

BREAST CANCER STAGING

Staging for breast cancer is based on the size of the primary tumor, the presence of disease in the regional notes, and whether there is distant metastatic disease *(33)*. The clinical stage is based on the information available by clinical evaluation before definitive treatment. This includes a careful physical examination, imaging studies, and pathological examination of tissues used to establish the diagnosis of breast cancer. Pathological staging includes the information obtained from the clinical staging as well as the data obtained from the resection of the primary tumor, regional nodes, and any sites of distant disease, if present. When ductal carcinoma is present along with an invasive breast cancer, the tumor size is measured as the size of the invasive component.

DCIS

DCIS or noninvasive breast cancer is a heterogeneous disease with variability with respect to its potential to progress to invasive cancer. DCIS has been diagnosed more frequently with the increased use of screening mammography. In some institutions, where there are active screening programs, 25 to 50% of all breast cancers diagnosed are DCIS. The average age at diagnosis is between 54 and 56 years of age.

DCIS is most commonly diagnosed after biopsy of microcalcifications observed on mammography *(34)*. Less commonly, it may present as a palpable mass on breast examination, an asymmetric density or mass on mammography, or pathological nipple discharge. The likelihood that pathological nipple discharge is associated with an underlying breast malignancy increases with the age of the patient and if there is an associated breast mass on examination or a suspicious abnormality on mammogram. Paget's disease of the nipple is associated with an erosion of the nipple–areolar complex and is an uncommon presentation of breast cancer. In rare instances, changes of the skin may involve only the areola because there may be ducts that connect directly with the areola. Most often, Paget's disease is associated with DCIS alone, generally involving the terminal ducts of the breast. Approximately 20% will have an associated invasive breast cancer. It is commonly mistaken for eczema or chronic dermatitis of the skin. When there is an erosion of the nipple and/or areola that is not resolving, biopsy is necessary to exclude the presence of Paget's disease.

Not all DCIS will proceed to invasive breast cancer. However, at this point, there is no reliable way to know which DCIS will remain indolent and confined to the breast and which will progress to invasive disease with the potential to metastasize. Retrospective studies have been performed that have evaluated the natural history of untreated DCIS. Approximately 25% of women in these studies developed invasive carcinoma in the breast and the quadrant in which the DCIS was diagnosed *(35)*. The time between the diagnosis of the DCIS and the development of the invasive cancer ranged from approx 3 to 10 years.

DCIS has been classified into different subtypes based on the architectural features, including micropapillary, papillary, solid, cribiform, and comedo. Subsequently, a classification system was developed in which the DCIS was graded based on the nuclear grade, the presence of necrosis within the ductal lumen, and architectural features as a means to predict risk for local recurrence and risk of invasive disease *(36)*. Low-grade lesions have less cytological and nuclear atypia, and central necrosis within the lumen of the involved ducts is absent. Intermediate-grade lesions have a low-to-intermediate nuclear grade and central necrosis. High-grade DCIS is characterized by a high nuclear grade with or without central necrosis. High-grade DCIS is also called comedo DCIS.

Low-grade DCIS is more likely to grow in a discontinuous fashion and "skip" along the ducts. If there is discontinuous growth, the gaps between the disease are often less than 5 mm. The growth of high-grade DCIS is more likely to be continuous along the duct.

Treatment of DCIS has evolved over the years. Before the widespread use of mammography, DCIS often presented as a large palpable mass and the disease was treated with mastectomy. As the size of most DCIS decreased and there was widespread use of breast-sparing treatment for invasive breast cancer, the role of breast preservation has also increased.

The most important prognostic factor with respect to local control of this disease within the breast is margin status *(34)*. At this point, the optimal size of the surgical margin remains unknown. The risk for local recurrence with a margin width of 10 mm is quite low but this may be impractical because of the volume of breast tissue required to obtain that margin width. When considering a patient for surgery alone, there should be wide surgical margins, the size of the tumor should be relatively small, and the tumor should be low grade. When surgery is combined with breast irradiation, less extensive margin widths are acceptable.

Table 3

Category	*Assessment*
Primary Tumor	
TX	Primary tumor cannot be assessed
T0	No evidence of primary tumor
Tis	Carcinoma *in situ* Ductal carcinoma *in situ* (DCIS) Lobular carcinoma *in situ* (LCIS)
T1	Tumor 2 cm or less
T1mic	Microinvasion 0.1 cm or less
T1a	Tumor 0.1–0.5 cm in maximal dimension
T1b	Tumor 0.5–1 cm in maximal dimension
T1c	Tumor 1–2 cm in maximal dimension
T2	Tumor 2–5 cm in greatest dimension
T3	Tumor >5 cm in greatest dimension
T4	Tumor of any size with direct extension to chest wall or skin
T4a	Extension to chest wall, not including pectoralis minor muscle
T4b	Edema (including *peau d'orange*) or ulceration of the skin of the breast, or satellite nodules confined to the same breast
T4c	T4a and T4b
T4d	Inflammatory breast cancer
Regional nodes The regional lymph nodes are evaluated by clinical and pathological examinations	
Clinical	
NX	Regional nodes cannot be assessed (previously removed)
N0	No regional nodal metastasis
N1	Metastasis to moveable ipsilateral axillary nodes
N2	Metastasis to ipsilateral axillary nodes fixed or matted, or clinically apparent internal mammary nodes without clinically positive axillary nodes
N3	Metastasis in: 1. Ipsilateral infraclavicular lymph nodes with or without axillary nodal involvement 2. In clinically apparent ipsilateral internal mammary nodes and in the presence of clinically evident axillary nodal metastasis 3. Metastasis to ipsilateral supraclavicular nodes with or without axillary or internal mammary node involvement
Pathologic Staging	
pNX	Regional nodes cannot be assessed (previously removed or not removed for pathologic study)

(*Continued*)

Table 3 (*Continued*)

Category	*Assessment*
pN0	No regional nodal metastasis histologically, no additional examination for isolated tumor cells. Isolated tumor cells are defined as single tumor cells or small clusters of tumor cells <0.2 mm. These are usually identified by IHC or molecular examination, such as PCR studies of the nodes and may be confirmed by routine hematoxylin and eosin staining
pN0(i–)	No regional nodal metastasis histologically, negative IHC
pN0(i+)	No regional nodal metastasis histologically, positive IHC, no IHC cluster >0.2 mm
pN0(mol–)	No regional lymph node metastasis histologically, negative molecular findings (RT-PCR)
pN1	Metastasis in 1–3 axillary nodes and/or in internal mammary nodes detected by sentinel node biopsy but not clinically apparent
pN2	Metastasis in 4–9 axillary nodes or in clinically apparent internal mammary lymph nodes in the absence of axillary lymph node metastasis
pN3	Metastasis in 10 or more axillary nodes
Distant Metastasis	
MX	Distant metastasis cannot be assessed
M0	No distant metastasis
M1	Distant metastasis

IHC, immunohistochemical.

NSABP B-17 evaluated the benefit of adjuvant breast irradiation in the treatment of women with DCIS that had been completely excised with negative surgical margins *(37)*. Patients were enrolled and randomized to receive whole breast irradiation vs observation. After 12 years of follow-up, the incidence of ipsilateral breast tumor recurrence (IBTR) in patients treated with breast radiotherapy was 15.7%. Patients treated with surgery alone had a local failure rate of 31.7%. In each arm of the study, approximately half of the failures were related to recurrent DCIS and half of the failure were related the development of an invasive breast cancer within the treated breast. There was no difference in overall survival between the two groups. Traditionally, adjuvant breast irradiation has been delivered to the entire breast with or without a boost to the primary tumor site. A prospective clinical trial is underway to evaluate the role of partial breast irradiation in which the primary tumor site, along with a 1-cm margin of normal tissue, is radiated for the treatment of DCIS.

Table 4
Stage Grouping

Stage 0	Tis	N0	M0
Stage I	T1	N0	M0
Stage IIA	T0	N1	M0
	T1	N1	M0
	T2	N0	M0
Stage IIB	T2	N1	M0
	T3	N0	M0
Stage IIIA	T0	N2	M0
	T1	N2	M0
	T2	N2	M0
	T3	N1	M0
	T3	N2	M0
Stage IIIB	T4	N0	M0
	T4	N1	M0
	T4	N2	M0
Stage IIIC	Any T	N3	M0
Stage IV	Any T	Any N	M1

The NSABP also evaluated the role of adjuvant tamoxifen in the treatment of DCIS in NSABP B-24 *(38)*. Approximately 1800 women with DCIS were enrolled and were treated with wide excision and breast irradiation. The women were then randomized to receive tamoxifen vs placebo for 5 years. Surgical margins could be involved in this study. After 7 years of follow-up, 11% of the women who received surgery and radiotherapy developed local recurrences. Half of these were invasive breast cancer and half were associated with DCIS. In the group that received adjuvant tamoxifen, 7.7% developed recurrences, and there were twice as many of the recurrences with DCIS as opposed to invasive breast cancer. The group of women who had positive surgical margins was small. Those women in this group who were treated with tamoxifen were found to have an 11% rate of IBTR and those treated with placebo had a local recurrence rate of 18%. Only patients whose tumors were hormone receptor positive had a reduction in IBTR with the addition of tamoxifen. There were no differences in overall survival.

There are studies that have evaluated wide excision alone for the treatment of DCIS. Because these studies have not been prospective, randomized studies, there is inherent selection bias. Patients treated by wide excision alone have tended to be smaller with low-grade histology and wide negative surgical margins. There may be patients who can be treated by wide excision alone, but this should be evaluated on an individual basis.

Some women with DCIS are best served by mastectomy. Women with DCIS who have persistently positive surgical margins after attempts to clear the margins have been unsuccessful are not candidates for breast conservation. In addition, women with extensive residual malignant-appearing microcalcifications after wide excision should undergo mastectomy. Lastly, women with multicentric disease (disease in more than one quadrant of the breast) are not candidates for conservative treatment.

The likelihood for metastatic disease to the axillary nodes in women with DCIS is uncommon. In older surgical series, in which mastectomy was routinely performed, the incidence of positive axillary nodes was 1 to 2%. Therefore, routine axillary node dissection for women with DCIS is not recommended. There are some instances in which evaluation of the axilla should be considered because sentinel node biopsy, a minimally invasive technique to evaluation the axilla in breast cancer, is available. Women who require mastectomy for DCIS should undergo sentinel node biopsy. This will provide evaluation of the axilla should invasive breast cancer be identified on the final pathology evaluation of the breast specimen or if there were occult invasive cancer not identified on the original specimen.

INVASIVE BREAST CANCER

Approximately 211,240 new cases of invasive breast cancer will be diagnosed in 2005 and approx 40,000 will die of this disease in the same time interval. Overall, breast cancer is being diagnosed in earlier stages when compared with the recent and remote past. In addition, options for adjuvant treatments have expanded and now include a wide range of chemotherapy, hormonal therapy, and biological therapy options.

The surgical treatment of invasive breast cancer has evolved slowly during the last 100 years, during which radical mastectomy has been replaced by breast conservation. The surgical therapy has changed as women presented with earlier stage disease and as it became evident that larger and more radical surgery was not associated with an improved survival. Breast cancer becomes invasive when the cancer cells break through the wall of the duct or lobule and invade the stroma of the breast. It is at this point that the cancer has the ability to metastasize via either the lymphatic system or hematogenously.

Most invasive cancers of the breast are ductal cancer in origin. Invasive lobular carcinomas are the second most frequent invasive cancer observed. A small proportion of breast cancers are mixed with both ductal and lobular features. There are certain breast cancer histologies, such as tubular carcinomas and mucinous carcinomas, that are associated with outcomes that are more favorable *(39)*.

The most important prognostic factor with respect to disease-free and overall survival in patients with invasive breast cancer is the status of the axillary nodes.

Treatment as well as prognosis are determined through accurate evaluation of the axillary nodal basin. The 5-year survival changes dramatically when lymph nodes contain metastatic disease and diminishes as the number of positive nodes increase. The disease-free survival for all patients with negative nodes is approx 70%. When patients have 4 to 10 positive nodes, the 10-year disease-free survival drops to approx 40% *(40)*.

Tumor size is also an important prognostic factor and, as the tumor size increases, the risk of axillary nodal metastases increases. However, even in the face of negative axillary nodes, as the tumor increases in size, the 5-year survival rate decreases *(40)*. The 5-year survival in a woman with a tumor less than 1 cm and negative nodes is greater than 98%. When the tumor is greater than 5 cm and the axillary nodes are free of disease, the 5-year survival rate diminishes to 82%. Pathological tumor size is more accurate than clinical staging.

Histological grade of the tumor and nuclear grade are also used to determine the patients risk for recurrence *(41)*. The evaluation of histological grade is somewhat subjective and there is variation between pathologists interpretations of the slides. The grading system looks at the degree of differentiation and pleomorphism of tumor cells, as well as the mitotic index.

There are certain histological subtypes of breast cancer that are considered favorable prognosis lesions. Most breast cancers are invasive ductal carcinoma and are of no specific type. Pure papillary, tubular, and mucinous carcinomas are subtypes of invasive ductal cancer and tend to be associated with improved outcomes *(39)*. Patients with these subtypes who have tumors that are up to 3 cm in diameter and have negative axillary nodes have an extremely good prognosis. They may not require adjuvant systemic chemotherapy because their risk for recurrence is so low.

Age at diagnosis remains an important prognostic factor; young women (younger than 35 years) are at greater risk for local breast recurrence after breast conservation therapy and for the development of systemic disease when compared with older women *(42)*. The numbers of young women with breast cancer is small and only 6.5% of women diagnosed with breast cancer are younger than 40 years. However, younger women have a greater likelihood of having high-grade tumors, lymphatic and vascular invasion, hormone negative tumors, large primary tumors, and positive axillary nodes. Younger premenopausal women have worse outcomes when compared with older premenopausal women.

Minority patients, particularly black and Hispanic women, have worse outcomes when compared with white women. This may be related, in part, to minority women having larger numbers, positive nodes, or tumors that are hormone insensitive. However, even when these other factors are adjusted, black women tend to have a diminished over-all survival stage for stage when compared with white women *(43)*.

The presence of estrogen receptors (ER) and progesterone receptors in a given tumor will predict response to hormonal therapy. ER positivity is associated with an improved disease-free survival in short-term follow-up. However, as time progresses, that benefit is lost and the risk of relapse and death gradually increases and the initial benefit is lost *(40)*. Most ER-positive tumors will respond to hormonal therapy. A certain fraction will not and, in some instances, patients who initially responded to endocrine manipulation will become resistant.

HER2/neu or c-erb-B2 is a member of the Erb-B (HER) growth factor receptor family that includes three other tyrosine kinase growth factor receptors. Overexpression of *HER2/neu* is observed in 10 to 35% of invasive breast cancers and is extremely common in high-grade DCIS *(44)*. No ligand has been identified for HER2/neu and the receptor is activated by dimerizing with other activated receptors in the HER2 family, resulting in signal transduction.

Overexpression of *HER2/neu* has been associated with aggressive disease and poor-prognosis breast cancer *(45)*. In addition, patients whose tumors overexpress *HER2/neu* tend to be hormone receptor negative. Recently, treatments for breast cancer are targeting specific molecular changes in the breast cancer cell. Traztuzamab (Herceptin®) is a humanized monoclonal antibody directed against the HER2/neu receptor. This new medication was tested in women with metastatic breast cancer whose tumors overexpressed *HER2/neu*. The traztuzamab was combined with chemotherapy and was compared with chemotherapy alone. The combination therapy resulted in a significantly higher response rate when compared with chemotherapy alone *(46)*. The use of traztuzamab in the adjuvant setting in high-risk women was recently reported, with dramatic improvements in survival *(47,48)*.

Most patients with invasive breast cancer will present with Stage I to II disease and are, therefore, potential candidates for breast-conserving therapy. Numerous prospective randomized clinical trials have demonstrated that survival from early stage breast cancer treated with breast conservation vs mastectomy have similar overall survival rates. The addition of breast radiotherapy to conservation surgery improves disease-free survival rates *(49)*.

Local recurrence or IBTR within the breast after conservative treatment tends to be the most frequent within the first 7 to 8 years after completion of therapy and most of those recurrences are in the region of the primary tumor site *(50)*. Breast recurrences are divided into true recurrences, marginal misses, and elsewhere cancers. True recurrences occur at the primary tumor site. Marginal miss recurrences are located just outside of the radiotherapy boost site. Elsewhere recurrences occur at other locations within the breast and are most likely new a new primary tumor within the breast. The annual rate of true or marginal miss recurrences between years 2 through 7 after completion of therapy is approx 1.5% per year. The rate of true or marginal miss recurrences then diminish significantly. Recurrences can occur outside the primary tumor site and are called "elsewhere" cancers. The rate of developing an elsewhere cancer is approx 0.7% per year *(50)*.

Patient Selection for Breast Conservation Therapy

There are many considerations when discussing options for the treatment of breast cancer and include estimating risk for IBTR as well as cosmetic appearance of the breast after surgery and radiotherapy.

Considerations for Breast Conservation Therapy

The size of the tumor relative to the patient's breast size is important with respect to the ultimate cosmetic appearance of the breast after treatment has been completed. A woman may desire breast conservation but has a breast size that may not accommodate a wide excision of the primary tumor and result in an acceptable cosmetic outcome. She may consider neoadjuvant chemotherapy or hormonal therapy (if the tumor is hormone sensitive) to reduce the size of the tumor and increase the likelihood the tumor will be excised with clear surgical margins.

To proceed with breast conservation therapy, patients must also be reliable. They must come for appointments, undergo the prescribed course of radiation and must agree to return for routine follow-up appointments after the treatment has been completed. Patients must understand that a small number of women who undergo breast conservation will develop an IBTR and most can undergo salvage mastectomy without an effect on overall survival. This can best be accomplished by early detection of the recurrence.

Young age is not a contraindication for breast conservation. However, young women (younger than 35–40 years) have a higher risk for IBTR than older women who are treated conservatively *(51)*. This may be related to the higher frequency of poor-risk breast cancer in young women. Young age is also associated with a higher risk for systemic relapse and recurrence after mastectomy.

Patients with alterations in *BRCA1* or *BRCA2* can be treated with breast conservation and there does not seem to be an increased short-term risk for local recurrence within the treated breast *(52)*. There may be an increased risk for recurrence with long-term follow-up, although there is not a significant experience with this specific patient population. Women who harbor mutations in either *BRCA1* or *BRCA2* have up to a 65% lifetime risk for developing a contralateral breast cancer. It is reasonable to consider bilateral mastectomy with or without immediate reconstruction to reduce the risk of a second breast cancer in the future.

The most important risk factor for local control in breast preservation is the margin status after wide excision *(49)*. At the time of a wide excision for breast cancer, the tumor is excised with approx 1 cm of surrounding normal breast tissue. When the breast specimen is removed, it should be oriented for the pathologist. Each specimen has six margins and each is inked with a different color. The pathologist can then evaluate the specimen and determine the adequacy of the surgical margins. If a re-excision is required, only the tissue at the involved margin(s) is removed, to ensure that the smallest amount of tissue is removed to provide a surgical margin where no tumor is observed at the inked surface. In cases in which the cancer presented with microcalcifications on mammography, it is prudent to obtain a postsurgical mammogram to ensure that all the malignant-appearing microcalcifications have been excised. If there are residual calcifications, they should be excised under needle localization guidance.

Patients treated by wide excision with a negative surgical margin and adjuvant breast irradiation have a low risk for local recurrence, which ranges from 2 to 7% with 10 years of follow-up *(53,54)*. "Close" margins are defined in a variety of ways and can vary between 1 and 3 mm of normal tissue between the tumor and the cut surface of the breast specimen. When the surgical margin is "close," the rate of recurrence between 2 and 14% with 8 to 10 years of follow-up *(54,55)*. Patients who have a positive surgical margin have up to a 25% risk of local failure within the breast, despite addition of breast radiotherapy *(56)*. Therefore, patients with positive margins require additional surgery to improve the rate of local control. Patients who have a focally positive margin have a relatively low rate of recurrence; however, the numbers of patients in this category is small.

It is common to see DCIS in association with invasive ductal carcinoma. When the DCIS comprises more than 25% of the total tumor volume and DCIS is present in the surrounding normal tissue, the tumor is classified as having an extensive intraductal component (EIC) and is EIC+. In early studies in which surgical margins were not routinely evaluated by inking the specimen, women with EIC+ tumors who underwent breast conservation treatment were found to have extremely high rates of local failure within the breast. The most likely reason for the high rate of local failure is the presence of additional disease within the breast. To reduce the risk of local failure within the breast, patients who are EIC+ should be treated with wide excision and have negative surgical margins. Postoperative radiation should not be added to less than adequate surgery to control the disease within the breast.

Multicentric breast cancer is defined by the presence of two or more foci of breast cancer in two or more quadrants of the breast, on either physical examination or mammogram. This is a contraindication for breast conservation because there is likely to be significant residual disease within the breast that cannot be controlled with wide excision and radiotherapy. Patients with diffuse malignant-appearing microcalcifications on mammogram are not candidates for breast conservation. Multicentric breast cancer is best treated with mastectomy.

Multifocal breast cancer is defined as more than a single tumor in the same quadrant of the breast. A distinction is made between microscopic multifocal and gross multifocal disease. Patients with microscopic multifocal disease can be safely treated with breast conservation, provided that negative surgical margins can be obtained *(57)*. Patients with multiple gross tumors within the same quadrant must be carefully evaluated before offering conservative treatment because there may be a residual large tumor burden within the remainder of the breast and a higher risk for local failure.

Tumor location is not a contraindication for breast conservation. Patients whose tumors are centrally located may sometimes require excision of the nipple–areolar complex to attain negative surgical margins. Tumors located in the upper inner quadrant can also offer a challenge in breast conservation because there is the least amount of breast tissue in this area. Oncoplastic surgical techniques can be used to optimize cosmetic appearance of the breast if a wide excision is performed in this location.

Histology of the tumor is not a contraindication to breast conservation. Patients with invasive lobular cancer can be offered breast-sparing surgery; although it may be more difficult to obtain negative surgical margins in this situation. Preoperatively, the patient should be carefully screened to ensure that the disease is unifocal.

There are contraindications for the use of adjuvant breast irradiation and they should be kept in mind when making recommendations for care. Patients who have had previous chest wall radiation, such as mantle irradiation for the treatment of Hodgkin's disease, are not candidates to receive additional radiation to the chest area. Patients with certain forms of collagen vascular disease, specifically lupus and scleroderma, tolerate radiation poorly and should not be treated with radiation. Patients with rheumatoid arthritis can be considered potential candidates; however, they should be evaluated before treatment by the radiotherapist. Women with pregnancy-associated breast cancer can be treated with breast conservation therapy, although the experience is somewhat limited. It is suggested that breast irradiation be held until the patient is postpartum.

The decision-making process in determining which local treatment option is best for any given patient can be complex and may involve several discussions with the patient to determine which surgical therapy is best for her. Patients should understand that when there is no contraindication to breast conservation, the overall survival is equal to mastectomy.

Evaluation of the Axilla

Until very recently, axillary node dissection was the standard of care for evaluating whether there was spread of the cancer to the regional nodal basin. Most women with Stage I and II breast cancer have no metastatic disease identified in their nodes after routine node dissection. Therefore, they receive the morbidity of the procedure and no true benefit other than the staging information. Common complications of axillary nodes dissection include seroma formation, infection, paresthesias, shoulder immobility and lymphedema, and chronic pain. Less frequently, the long thoracic or thoracodorsal nerves or the axillary vein can be injured.

Sentinel node biopsy was developed initially as a minimally invasive way to evaluate the regional nodes in the treatment of melanoma. When the sentinel node is negative for metastatic disease, the patient required no additional axillary surgical and the morbidity is minimized. Because this procedure involves the removal of fewer nodes when compared with a routine node dissection, the morbidity is diminished. If the patient has metastatic disease to the axillary nodes, a completion node dissection is standard treatment.

In 1991, pilot studies were performed in women with breast cancer to determine whether lymphatic mapping and sentinel node biopsy was applicable in the surgical staging of breast cancer. Two methods for identifying the sentinel node were used, vital dye and radioguided surgery with or without lymphoscintigraphy. Both methods have proven to be accurate with respect to localizing the sentinel node. In a small number of patients, the sentinel node is extra-axillary and will not be identified using the vital dye technique.

As experience with this technique has increased, the identification rate of the sentinel node has increased and the false-negative rate has decreased *(58)*. For most surgeons, there was a steep learning curve as the technique was refined. At this point, the identification rate for most experienced surgeons is 90% or greater. The false-negative rate is approx 5%.

The sentinel node is most often evaluated intraoperatively, using either frozen section or touch preparation for cytology analysis. If the sentinel node is positive, a completion node dissection is performed. If the sentinel node is negative, no further axillary surgery is performed at that time. The patient should be advised that the frozen section may not reveal the presence of metastatic disease, but all decisions are based on the final and more thorough pathology examination. The lymph node(s) are fixed and then sections are taken though the node every 2 to 3 mm. The nodal tissue is then stained using hematoxylin and eosin staining. In some institutions, the sections are studied further with immunohistochemistry. If disease detected in the lymph node is isolated tumor cells or clusters of cells measuring less than 0.2 mm, the node is considered negative. When the disease is between 0.2 and 2 mm, it is considered a micrometastasis. When the metastatic focus is greater than 0.2 mm, consideration should be given for additional axillary treatment with either a completion node dissection or axillary irradiation. The likelihood for additional positive nodes being identified at the time of completion node dissection increases with the size of the primary tumor and the size of the metastatic deposit in the sentinel node *(59,60)*. In addition, the presence of lymphovascular invasion associated with the primary tumor increases the chance of identifying metastatic disease in nonsentinel nodes. The likelihood of an axillary recurrence after a negative sentinel node biopsy is 1% or less in most series *(61)*.

There are many considerations when offering lymphatic mapping and sentinel node biopsy to a patient. Failure to identify a sentinel node has been associated increasing patient age and high body mass index. When intramammary lymphatic channels are plugged with tumor, the sentinel node may not be identified because the vital dye and or the radioisotope may track to another node. Therefore, digital examination of the operative site is an essential piece of the procedure. Previous breast or axillary surgery is not a contraindication to sentinel node biopsy and the success for identifying the sentinel node is related to the length of time between the surgical procedures. Patients with multicentric and multifocal breast cancer are candidates for sentinel node biopsy, although the experience with this group of patients is not extensive. Patients with palpable axillary nodes may be candidates for lymphatic mapping and sentinel node biopsy. Many patients may have enlarged nodes that are negative for metastatic disease. Enlarged nodes can be evaluated preoperatively be fine needle aspiration for cytology. If positive, a node dissection should be performed. If the cytology is negative, sentinel node biopsy can be performed and, at the same time, the enlarged nodes can be excised during the course of the procedure.

The role of sentinel node biopsy after neoadjuvant chemotherapy is controversial. The major concern is that there may be occult disease in the axilla that is not reflected by the status of the sentinel node. The false-negative rate can be as high as 11 to 12% in experienced hands *(62)*.

Neoadjuvant or Preoperative Therapy

Patients who are marginal candidates for breast preservation because of the tumor size to breast size ratio can consider neoadjuvant chemotherapy or hormonal therapy, if the tumor is hormone sensitive. The NSABP performed two large clinical trials comparing the results of chemotherapy followed by surgery and surgery followed by chemotherapy *(63,64)*. More women who were treated with neoadjuvant chemotherapy were able to undergo breast conservation. There was no difference in overall survival between the two groups *(63)*. The studies using neoadjuvant hormonal therapy are small but there is a similar reduction in size of the primary tumor, facilitating breast conservation.

Inflammatory Breast Cancer

Inflammatory breast cancer accounts for approx 1 to 5% of all patients at initial presentation. It may be initially misdiagnosed because it can be confused with mastitis. The breast symptoms are rapidly progressive and evolve over weeks. The patient presents with unilateral breast enlargement. The skin of the breast is erythemetous, edematous (*peau d'orange*), and may be warm to touch. On breast palpation, the breast tissue is generally thickened, and a defined breast mass may not be appreciated. In addition, the patient often has clinically positive axillary nodes. Mammography often reveals thickening of the breast tissue and skin. Breast ultrasound may be helpful in distinguishing inflammatory breast cancer from other conditions. This condition requires prompt diagnosis and treatment because this form of breast cancer is aggressive and rapidly progressive. Therefore, one must have a high level of suspicion and refer the patient for biopsy and definitive treatment.

Patients with inflammatory breast cancer are best treated with multimodality therapy including neoadjuvant chemotherapy, modified radical mastectomy, and chest wall irradiation. Adjuvant hormonal therapy should be administered if the tumor is hormone receptor positive. If the *HER2/neu* gene is amplified, adjuvant Herceptin® is recommended. With aggressive multimodality therapy, the 5-year survival rate is approx 50%.

Mastectomy

Patients who are candidates for breast conservation may opt for mastectomy. Alternatively, some may be advised to undergo mastectomy because they are not candidates for breast preservation. Women who are undergoing immediate reconstruction at the time of mastectomy, can be offered skin-sparing mastectomy. The surgical incision is made to encompass the nipple and areolar complex as well as the scars from the previous biopsy. This technique has been shown to be safe oncologically and enhances the cosmetic outcome. Patients undergoing mastectomy are candidates for sentinel node biopsy. In some instances, the lymphatic mapping and sentinel node biopsy is performed before the definitive breast surgery and reconstruction so the final pathology is available and decision for a node dissection will be not be based on frozen section results of the sentinel node.

Breast Reconstruction

Breast reconstruction can be performed immediately at the time of mastectomy or in a delayed setting after all the treatments have been delivered.

Each type of reconstruction has its own risks and benefits. Therefore, each patient must be evaluated in a team setting to determine what is best in her individual situation.

Tissue Expander and Permanent Implant

A tissue expander is a small sac that is placed below the pectoralis major muscle. There is a port within the expander that can be accessed with a needle, and the expander is filled with fluid over time to allow expansion of the skin over time. When the expansion is complete, the expander is removed and exchanged for a permanent implant. Most reconstructions performed in the United States are of this type. The advantage is that it provides an adequate reconstruction for most women and is a smaller surgical procedure. It is best suited for women with small-to-moderate size breasts because it is not possible to obtain ptosis with this type of reconstruction. Because the implant is a foreign material, the body may form a capsule around the implant, resulting in capsular contracture. This may lead to distortion of the shape of the reconstructed breast or pain. Patients who have had previous radiotherapy to the chest may not be good candidates for this type of reconstruction because the skin may not be pliable enough.

Latissimus Dorsi Myocutaneous Flap Reconstruction

In most instances, this flap does not have enough volume to be used alone for breast reconstruction and is often used with a tissue expander and permanent implant. The flap is hardy and the incidence of flap loss is less than 1%. There is minimal donor site morbidity. In instances in which no skin is required to close the mastectomy defect, the muscle can be harvested with endoscopic techniques to minimize scarring on the back. Patient satisfaction with this type of reconstruction is high.

Transverse Rectus Abdominus Myocutaneous Flap

The transverse rectus abdominus myocutaneous flap is a more complex surgical procedure, although it offers the most natural cosmetic outcome. The skin and fat from the lower abdomen is used to create a breast mound. The rotation flap is based on the superior epigastric artery through a portion of the rectus abdominus muscle and can be either unipedicle or bipedicle. The flap is then tunneled through the upper abdomen to the chest. The transverse rectus abdominus myocutaneous can also be performed as a free flap and the blood supply is based on the deep inferior epigastric vessals. This type of reconstruction is not recommended for patients who smoke cigarettes, are obese, or who have many other comorbidities.

OTHER CANCERS OF THE BREAST

Primary Breast Sarcomas

Sarcomas are rare tumors that arise from the soft tissues in the body. Less than 1% of all tumors of the breast are sarcomas. They will often present as a painless mass in the breast and occur most frequently in older women, although they have been observed in the second decade of life.

Primary Breast Lymphoma

Primary breast lymphoma is also an uncommon malignancy and accounts for 0.5% of breast malignancies. This disease most often presents as a painless breast mass or as an abnormal mammogram.

REFERENCES

1. Smith RA, Cokkinides V, Eyre HJ. American Caner Society Guidelines for the early detection of cancer. CA Cancer J Clin 2006;56:11–25.
2. U.S. Department of Health and Human Services. Quality determinants of mammography. Clinical practice guideline no. 13. U.S. Government Printing Office, Washington DC, 1994.
3. American College of Radiology. Breast imaging reporting and data system, 3rd ed. American College of Radiology, Reston, VA, 1998.
4. Sickles EA. Periodic mammographic follow-up of probably benign lesions, results of 3,184 consecutive cases. Radiology 1991;179:439–442.
5. Kopans DB. Breast Imaging. J.B. Lippencott Co., Philadelphia, pp 137–155.
6. Liberman L, Cohen MA, Dershaw DD, et al. Atypical ductal hyperplasia diagnosed at stereotactic core biopsy. AJR Am J Roentgenol 1995;164(5):1111–1113.
7. Foster MC, Helvis MA, Gregory NE, et al. Lobular carcinoma in situ or atypical lobular neoplasia at core-needle biopsy: is excisional biopsy necessary? Radiology 2004;231: 813–819.
8. Berg WA, Mrose HE, Ioffe OB. Atypical lobular hyperplasia or lobular carcinoma in situ at core-needle breast biopsy. Radiology 2001;218:503–509.
9. Georgian-Smith D, Lawton TJ. Calcifications of lobular carcinoma in situ of the breast: radiologic-pathologic correlation. Am J Roentgenol 2001;176:1255–1259.
10. Morris KT, Vetto JT, Petty JK. A new score for the evaluation of palpable breast masses in women under 40. Am J Surg 2002;184:346–347.
11. Vetto J, Pommier R, Schidt W, et al. Use of the triple test for palpable breast lesions yields high diagnostic accuracy and cost savings. Am J Surg 1995;169:519–522.
12. Mansel RE, Wisby JR, Hughes LE. Controlles trial of the antigonadotropin danazol in painful nodular benign breast disease. Lancet 1982;1:928–933.
13. Mansel RE, Dogliotti L. European multicentre trial of bromocriptine in cyclical mastalgia. Lancet 1990;335:190–195.
14. Kontosolis E, Stefanidis K, Navrozoglou I, et al. Comparison of tamoxifen with danazol in the treatment of cyclical mastalgia. Gynecol Endocrol 1997;11:393–398.
15. Jardines L. Management of nipple discharge. The American Surgeon 1996;62:119–122.
16. Carter BA, Page DL, Schuyler, et al. No elevation in the long term breast carcinoma risk for women with fibroadenomas that contain atypical hyperplasic. Cancer 2001;92:30–36.
17. Diaz NM, Palmer JO, McDivitt RW. Carcinoma arising within fibroadenomas of the breast: a clinicopathologic study of 105 patients. Am J Pathol 1991;95:614–620.

18. Reinfrus M, Mitus J, Duda K, et al. The treatment and prognosis of patients with phyllodes tumor of the breast: an analysis of 170 cases. Cancer 1996;77:910–916.
19. Zurrida S, Bartoli C, Galimberti V, et al. which therapy for unexpected phyllodes tumour of the breast? Eur J Cancer 1992;28:673–675.
20. Rubin E, Visscher DW, Alexander RW, et al. Proliferative disease and atypia in biopsies performed for non-palpable lesions detected mammographically. Cancer 1988;61:2077–2082.
21. Dupont WD, Page DL. Risk factors for breast cancer in women with proliferative breast disease. N Engl J Med 1985;312:146–151.
22. Haagensen CD, Lane N, Lattes R, et al. Lobular neoplasia (so-called lobular carcinoma in situ) of the breast. Cancer 1978;43:737–769.
23. Page DL, Kidd TJ, Dupont WD, et al. Lobular neoplasia of the breast: higher risk for subsequent invasive cancer predicted by more extensive disease. Hum Pathol 1991;22:1232–1239.
24. Page DL, Dupont WD, Rogers LW, et al. Atypical hyperplastic lesions of the female breast: a long-term follow-up study. Cancer 1985;55:2698–2708.
25. Rebbeck TR, Lynch HT, Neuhausen SL, et al. Prophylactic oophorectomy in carriers of BRCA1 And BRCA2 mutations. N Engl J Med 2002;346:1616–1622.
26. Kauff ND, Satagopan JM, Robson ME, et al. Risk reducing salping-oophorectomy in women with a BRCA1 or BRCA2 mutation. N Engl J Med 2002;346:1609–1615.
27. Hartmann LC, Schaid DJ, Woods JE, et al. Efficacy of bilateral prophylactic mastectomy in women with a family history of breast cancer. N Engl J Med 1999;340:77–84.
28. Gail MH, Brinton LA, Byar DP, et al. Projecting individualized probabilities of developing breast cancer for white females who are being examined annually. J Natl Cancer Inst 1989;81:1879–1886.
29. Fisher B, Constatino JP, Wickerham DL, et al. Tamoxifen for the prevention of breast cancer: report of the National Surgical Adjuvant Breast and Bowel Project. P-1 study. J Natl Cancer Institute 1998;90:1371–1388.
30. Benson EA. Management of breast abscesses. World J Surg 1989;13:753–760.
31. Schafer P, Furrer C, Mermillod B. An association of cigarette smoking with recurrent subareolar abscess. Int J Epidemiol 1988;17:810–817.
32. Walker AP. A prospective study of the microflora of nonpuerperal breast abscesses. Arch Surg 1988;123:908–915.
33. Singletary SE, Connolly JL. Breast cancer staging: working with the sixth edition of the AJCC cancer staging manual. CA Cancer J Clin 2006;56:37–47.
34. Burstein HJ, Polyak K, Wong JS, et al. Ductal carcinoma in situ of the breast. N Engl J Med 2004;350:1430–1441.
35. Page D, Dupont W, Rogers L, et al. Intraductal carcinoma of the breast; follow-up after biopsy only. Cancer 1982;49:751–760.
36. Silverstein MJ. The Van Nuys prognostic index for ductal carcinoma in situ. Breast J 1996; 2:38–48.
37. Fisher B, Dignam J, Wolmark N, et al. Lumpectomy and radiation therapy for the treatment of intraductal breast cancer: findings from National Surgical Adjuvant Breast and Bowel Project B-17. J Clin Oncol 1998;16:441–452.
38. Fisher B, Dignam J, Wolmark N, et al. Tamoxifen in treatment of intraductal breast cancer: National Surgical Adjuvant Breast and Bowel Project B-24 randomised controlled trial. Lancet 1999;353:1993–2000.
39. Fisher ER, Anderson S, Redmond C, et al. Pathologic findings from the National Surgical Adjuvant Breast and Bowel Project protocol B-06: 10-year pathologic and clinical prognostic discriminants. Cancer 1993;71:2507–2514.

40. Hilsenbeck SG, Ravdin PM, de Moor CA, et al. Time-dependence of hazard ratios for prognostic factors in primary breast cancer. Breast Cancer Res Treat 1998;52:227–237.
41. Contessa G, Mourisse H, Friedman S, et al. The importance of histologic grade in long-term prognosis of breast cancer: a study of 1,010 patients, uniformly treated at the Institut Gustav-Roussy. J Clin Oncol 1987;5:1378–1386.
42. Nixon AJ, Neuberg D, Hayes DF, et al. Relationship of patient age to pathologic features of the tumor and prognosis for patients with Stage I or II breast cancer. J Clin Oncol 1994; 12:888–894.
43. Chlebowski RT, Chen Z, Anderson GL, et al. Ethnicity and breast cancer: factors influencing differences in incidence and outcome. J Natl Cancer Inst 2005;97:439–448.
44. Van de Vijar MJ, Peterse JL, Mooi WJ, et al. Neu-protein overexpression in breast cancer. Association with comedo-type ductal carcinoma in situ and limited prognostic value in Stage II breast cancer. N Engl J Med 1988;319:1239–1245.
45. Wistansley J, Cooke T, Murray GD, et al. The long term prognostic significance of c-erb-2 in primary breast cancer. Br J Cancer 1991;63:447–450.
46. Slamon D, Leyland-Jones B, Shak S, et al. Use of chemotherapy plus a monoclonal antibody against HER2 for metastatic breast cancer that overexpresses HER2. N Engl J Med 2001;344:783–792.
47. Romond EH, Perez EA, Bryant J, et al. Trastuzumab plus adjuvant chemotherapy for operable HER2-positive breast cancer. N Engl J Med 2005;353:1673–1684.
48. Piccart-Gebhart MJ, Procter M, Leyland-Jones B, et al. Trastuzumab after adjuvant chemotherapy in HER2-positive breast cancer. N Engl J Med 2005;353:1659–1672.
49. Fisher B, Anderson S, Bryant J, et al. Twenty-year follow-up of a randomized trial comparing total mastectomy, lumpectomy, and lumpectomy plus irradiation for the treatment of breast cancer. N Engl J Med 2002;347:1233–1243.
50. Gage I, Recht A, Gelman R, et al. Long-term outcome following breast conserving surgery and radiation therapy. Int J Radiati Oncol Biol Phys 1995;33:245–254.
51. Nixon AJ, Neuberg D, Hayes EF, et al. Relationship of patient age to pathologic features of the tumor and prognosis for patients with Stage I or II breast cancer. J Clin Oncol 1994;12: 888–895.
52. Pierce LJ, Strawderman M, Narod SA. Effect of radiotherapy after breast-conserving treatment in women with breast cancer and germline BRCA1/2 mutations. J Clin Oncol 2000;18:3360–3369.
53. Smitt MC, Nowels JW, Zdeblich MJ, et al. The importance of the lumpectomy surgical margin status in long-term results of breast conservation. Cancer 1995;76:259–269.
54. Freedman G, Fowble B, Hanlon A, et al. Patients with early stage invasive cancer with close or positive surgical margins treated with conservative surgery and radiation have an increased risk of breast recurrence that is delayed by adjuvant systemic therapy. Int J Radiati Oncol Biol Phys 1999;44:1005–1114.
55. Obedian E, Haffty BG. Negative margin status improves local control in conservatively managed breast cancer patients. Cancer J 1999;6:28–37.
56. Pittinger TP, Maronian NC, Poulter CA, et al. Importance of margin status in outcome of breast-conserving surgery for carcinoma. Surgery 1994;11:605–612.
57. Singletary SE, McNesse M. Segmental mastectomy and irradiation in the treatment of breast cancer. Am J Clin Oncol 1988;11:679–689.
58. Shivers S, Cox C, Leight G, et al. Final results of the Department of Defense multicenter breast lymphatic mapping trial. Ann Surg Oncol 2002;9:248–255.
59. Rahusen FD, Torrenga H, van Diest PJ, et al. Predictive factors for metastatic involvement of nonsentinel nodes in breast cancer. Arch Surg 2001;136:1059–1063.

60. Kamath VJ, Giuliano R, Dauway EL, et al. Characteristics of the sentinel lymph node in breast cancer predict further involvement of higher-echelon nodes in the axilla. Arch Surg 2001;136:688–693.
61. Loza J, Colo F, Nadal J, et al. Axillary recurrence after sentinel node biopsy for operable breast cancer. Eur J Surg Oncol 2002;28:897–898.
62. Mamounas E, Brown A, Smith R, et al. Accuracy of sentinel node biopsy after neoadjuvant chemotherapy in breast cancer: updated results form NSABP B-27. Proc Soc Clin Oncol 2002;21:36a.
63. Wolmark N, Wang J, Mamounas E, et al. Preoperative chemotherapy in patients with operable breast cancer: nine-year results from the National Surgical Adjuvant Breast and Bowel Project B-18. J Natl Cancer Inst Monograph 2001; p. 96.
64. Bear HD, Anderson S, Brown A, et al. The effect on tumor response of adding sequential preoperative docetaxel (taxotere) to preoperative doxorubicin and cyclophosphamide (AC): Preliminary results from the National Surgical Adjuvant Breast and Bowel Project (NSABP) Protocol B-27. J Clin Oncol 2003;21:4165–4174.

13 Thyroid Disorders

M. Hamed Farooqi, MD, FACE
and Serge A. Jabbour, MD, FACP, FACE

CONTENTS

Thyroid disorders in women can be divided into two broad categories, disorders of thyroid function, such as hyperthyroidism or hypothyroidism; and disorders related to structural or morphological abnormalities. The major areas of concern here are thyroid nodules and thyroid cancer.

HYPERTHYROIDISM

Introduction

Hyperthyroidism refers to the increase in production and secretion of thyroid hormones (free thyroxine [T4], free triiodothyronine [T3], or both); This, in turn, causes thyrotoxicosis, which is the clinical syndrome of hypermetabolism that results from this excess of thyroid hormones.

Causes

The common causes of thyrotoxicosis include Graves' disease, which is the result of abnormal production of thyroid-stimulating antibodies. Other causes include a single or multiple toxic adenomas. Inflammatory or infectious diseases

From: *Current Clinical Practice: Women's Health in Clinical Practice*
Edited by: Clouse and Sherif © Humana Press Inc., Totowa, NJ

of the thyroid (thyroiditis) can present with thyrotoxicosis by releasing the stored thyroid hormones. Ingestion of excess thyroid hormone can also lead to thyrotoxicosis.

Uncommon causes include excess thyroid-stimulating hormone (TSH) production by the pituitary gland in cases of pituitary adenomas. Human chorionic gonadotropin, which has molecular similarity with TSH, can act on the thyroid gland and, therefore, thyrotoxicosis can be observed in hyperemesis gravidarum as well as by trophoblastic tissues, such as hydatidiform moles and choriocarcinomas *(1)*.

Clinical Manifestations

Symptoms include nervousness, fatigue, weakness, increased perspiration, heat intolerance, tremors, hyperactivity, palpitations, changes in weight and appetite, as well as menstrual disturbances. These can include scanty menses and decreased frequency of the menstrual periods.

Signs include irregular heart rate, such as atrial arrhythmia and tachycardia; systolic hypertension; warm, moist smooth skin; retraction of eyelid and a stare; tremors; hyperreflexia; and muscular weakness.

The clinical manifestations of thyrotoxicosis are summarized in Table 1.

Evaluation

Third-generation TSH remains the ideal test for initial screening for any functional thyroid abnormality. If the clinical suspicion is high, a free T4 level may be performed at the same time. In cases of hyperthyroidism, TSH will be below normal or suppressed. However, there are certain instances in which TSH levels might be below normal without associated hyperthyroidism. This can occur in hypopituitarism, profound illness, or Cushing's syndrome. In the event that TSH levels are low but the patient has low thyroid hormone levels and clinical features of hypothyroidism, endocrine referral should be considered.

The next test is measurement of T4 and T3 levels, which are the two major thyroid hormones. These are present both as free (or active) and protein bound (or inactive) forms. A total T3 or T4 level is an estimate of both the free and bound forms. Measurement of free T3 and free T4 levels is available from all major laboratories and is a more accurate measurement of the actual active hormone levels. In comparison, total T4 and T3 levels are affected by many conditions that can increase or decrease the levels of these binding proteins. The conditions that increase these proteins and are important to remember include any condition associated with excess estrogen (estrogen in oral contraceptives, pregnancy, and so on), hepatitis, HIV, and drugs such as clofibrate. Conditions that decrease these proteins include nephrotic syndrome and drugs such as androgens and corticosteroids. The ideal way of measuring free T4 is by equilibrium dialysis.

Table 1
Major Symptoms and Signs of Thyrotoxicosis

Symptoms	
Nervousness	Hyperactivity
Fatigue	Palpitations
Weakness	Increased appetite
Increased perspiration	Weight loss
Heat intolerance	Menstrual disturbances
Tremor	Neck pain (De Quervain's thyroiditis)
Signs	
Tachycardia or atrial arrhythmia	Muscle weakness
Systolic hypertension	Ophthalmopathy (Graves')
Stare, lid lag, and eyelid retraction	Diffuse goiter (Graves'), solitary nodule, or multinodular goiter
Tremor and hyperreflexia (De Quervain's thyroiditis)	Thyroid tenderness.

In the event that a person does have a low TSH along with an elevated free T4/free T3 level and clinical manifestations of hyperthyroidism, this needs to be pursued further.

The next step toward the diagnosis is obtaining a radioactive iodine uptake and scan. This helps in further determining the underlying pathology. In case of Graves' disease, there would be a diffuse uptake by the entire gland. In case of toxic adenomas, depending on the number, those areas will show an increased uptake, whereas the rest of the thyroid does not take up as much. In the event that this is caused by inflammation of the thyroid gland (thyroiditis), there would be no or very minimal uptake by the thyroid. That is because thyroiditis causes release of the stored thyroid hormone and there is no excess hormone production.

Graves' Disease

Graves' disease is caused by an antibody to the TSH receptor of the thyroid gland. This results in the excess stimulation of the thyroid gland causing hyperthyroidism. This autoimmune activity generates the production of cytokines that lead to other manifestations of this disease, such as ophthalmopathy and dermopathy.

This disease, similar to many other autoimmune diseases, is more common in women. Genetic susceptibility and certain precipitating factors, such as infection and stress, can also play a role.

Clinical Presentation. In addition to the usual presentation of hyperthyroidism, ophthalmopathy is a widely recognized complication. This may be observed in up to 45% of patients, if a technique such as orbital CT is used *(2)*. However, this finding is quite evident in most people and no specialized testing is usually required. The usual presentation includes proptosis, which is the appearance of a stare. There may be retraction of the eyelid and that may result in damage to the cornea. Other findings include periorbital edema, blurry vision, and diplopia. These findings may be unilateral.

This ophthalmopathy gradually worsens during an initial period of 3 to 6 months. After a period of relative stability, remission may occur. The issue of whether radioactive iodine treatment worsens this ophthalmopathy remains controversial *(3)*. Smoking does seem to affect this condition adversely. There are some recommendations regarding the use of steroids, before treatment with radioactive iodine *(4)*.

Our recommendation for any patients with Graves' disease who exhibits moderate-to-severe ophthalmopathy is referral to not only an endocrinologist but also to an experienced neuro-ophthalmologist for further management.

Diagnosis Of Graves' Disease. Measurement of TSH along with levels of thyroid hormones is recommended. TSH level is usually very low or suppressed; T4 and T3 levels are above normal. These levels usually correlate well with the severity of the symptoms.

Thyroid-stimulating immunoglobulins levels are also found to be elevated. These antibodies can also help predict whether the patient is likely to relapse if the levels remain high after antithyroid drugs are stopped. Similarly, these can predict the occurrence of neonatal hyperthyroidism in pregnant patients.

A radioiodine uptake and scan usually reveals significantly high diffuse uptake.

Treatment. Three major modes of treatment are available. These include oral agents called thionamides, radioiodine therapy, and surgery. In the United States, the most commonly used modality in adults is radioiodine treatment. For pregnant females and children, oral agents are preferred. Surgery is usually the last resort in most cases and only 1% of patients are treated with surgery *(5)*.

1. For radioiodine treatment, referral to a nuclear medicine facility is recommended. The important issues to remember regarding radioiodine treatment include the following:
   a. Patients with profound hyperthyroidism or those in thyroid storm are not candidates for radioiodine treatment. They present with thyrotoxicosis, altered sensorium, and hyperthermia. These cases should be immediately referred to the emergency room and transferred to the ICU for appropriate management. They are usually in shock and need specialized care.

b. Patients in whom thyroid hormone levels are very high are not candidates for immediate radioiodine therapy because it can cause significant elevation of the hormone levels immediately after the treatment. These patients usually need to be pretreated with oral agents for 6 to 12 weeks before the radioiodine therapy. We would recommend referral to an endocrinologist in this case.
c. In cases of patients who smoke and have concomitant ophthalmopathy, there is a significant chance that the condition might worsen after this treatment. Use of steroids is an option that needs to be considered, as mentioned above.
d. In addition, all females who are fertile should have a pregnancy test before this treatment. It is recommended that they refrain from pregnancy for at least 6 months after receiving the treatment.
e. Treatment with radioiodine in the majority of cases will lead to hypothyroidism. This requires the replacement of thyroid hormone. Levothyroxine replacement in adequate doses is recommended. It is extremely important to note that TSH levels remain low or suppressed for an extended period of time even though the actual T4 and T3 levels may be below normal. Therefore, TSH levels should NOT be followed to measure the success of treatment or the thyroid status of the patient. Rather the free T4 level would be a good indicator to follow. As soon as it reaches the lower limit of the normal range, thyroid hormone therapy with levothyroxine should be commenced. Similarly, free T4 levels should be used to titrate the dosage of levothyroxine replacement until TSH levels return back to normal and then can be used to assess the thyroid status.

2. The second treatment modality is that of oral agents. There is only one class of agents that is available in the United States called thionamides. The two available products are propylthioracil (PTU) and methimazole (Tapazole®). They act inside the thyroid gland by inhibiting mechanisms such as the organification of iodine by the thyroid gland. Outside the thyroid gland, PTU blocks the conversion of T3 to T4, whereas some actions on the immune system have also been postulated.

The choice of either of these medications is mostly on a personal preference. However, in cases of pregnancy, lactation, and thyroid storm, PTU is recommended. The usual dose to start is 100 mg three times daily for PTU and 20 to 30 mg in single or divided doses for methimazole. The side effect profile includes rash, urticaria, arthritis, fever, hepatitis, jaundice, and bone marrow suppression. Agranulocytosis, thrombocytopenia, and aplastic anemia have all been reported. Currently, there are no recommendations regarding mandatory monitoring of either the liver enzymes or blood counts. Clinical judgment should be used. For example, patients should be instructed to be vigilant for any signs of infection, such as a sore throat or fever; in this case, they should discontinue the medication, and a blood count should be obtained to ensure the absence of agranulocytosis. Similarly, they should be aware of the symptoms of hepatitis or jaundice, and so on.

Finally, the issue of how long should oral agents be administered is also controversial. However, most authorities agree on a duration of 1 to 2 years, based on the observation that in most cases in which there has been a remission, it tends to occur within 1 to 2 years. For patients who have not gone into remission after 2 years of treatment (70% of patients), another definitive treatment modality should be considered.

Single or Multiple Toxic Adenomas

This is the next common cause of hyperthyroidism. The clinical presentation is that of hyperthyroidism, as outlined on page 250. These nodules are essentially autonomous areas of excess thyroid hormone production. The decision to intervene therapeutically is based on the severity of symptoms. If needed, oral agents or radioiodine therapy may be considered. Radioiodine is preferred because remission is not observed with antithyroid agents (as opposed to Graves' disease, in which remission can be observed after 1 to 2 years of treatment). Usually a larger dose of radioiodine is required in these cases as compared with Graves' disease.

Single toxic adenomas can also be removed surgically and mostly, in such cases, the remaining normal thyroid tissue starts to function normally.

Thyroiditis

Thyroiditis refers to the inflammation of the thyroid gland *(6)*. This usually results in the release of stored thyroid hormone causing excess levels, which leads to a hyperthyroid state. There is more than one type of thyroiditis:

1. De Quervain's thyroiditis is a self-limiting painful inflammation of the thyroid. Usually observed in women between the ages of 20 and 50 years. The exact cause is unknown. A viral etiology has been hypothesized. There is usually a viral prodrome that precedes this condition. Patients present with a pain in their neck. There can be a difficulty in terms of swallowing. Hoarseness and sore throat can be observed. Systemic symptoms can precede the actual symptoms of hyperthyroidism, which occur once the stored hormones are released. Once they subside, there can be a transient phase of hypothyroidism, which persists until the thyroid heals completely. Each of these phases can last 4 to 8 weeks. Diagnosis is made based on clinical symptoms. A thyroid profile will show elevated T3 and T4 levels along with a low TSH level. Sedimentation rate is always high. A radioiodine uptake and scan will show a very low uptake. If a biopsy is performed based on the firmness, which raises the suspicion of malignancy, giant cells, which are histiocytes, are observed. Treatment is usually symptomatic because the condition resolves on its own. For the neck pain, anti-inflammatory agents can be used. Severe cases require steroids. Antithyroid agents, such as PTU and Tapazole® are ineffective.

2. Silent thyroiditis (except the postpartum variant) is now very rare. This condition is similar to De Quevain's thyroiditis except for the absence of pain. Radioiodine uptake and scan does show the characteristic decreased uptake, but Erythrocyte Sedimentation Rate (ESR) is usually normal. Again, the condition resolves on its own.
3. Postpartum thyroiditis is the most common type of thyroiditis and is observed in 5 to 10% of all deliveries. It is a form of silent thyroiditis occurring after pregnancy. The likely mechanism is thought to be the resolution of the immune suppression that is observed during pregnancy. This condition occurs most commonly in the first 6 months after delivery. The usual phases of hyperthyroidism and hypothyroidism follow. Treatment remains the same as for other types of thyroiditis *(7)*.
4. Suppurative thyroiditis. Infection of the thyroid by various bacteria, fungi, and other infectious agents leads to this condition. The clinical picture again is that of pain and swelling in front of the neck, along with fever. Blood tests show an elevated white count. If the stored thyroid hormones are also released, symptoms of hyperthyroidism do occur. Treatment is based on the extent of the abscess. Options extend from drainage with the help of a needle to surgical removal. Involvement of a specialist (surgeon) is recommended.
5. Amiodarone-induced thyrotoxicosis occurs after the use of this antiarrythmic agent. The increased thyroid hormone levels result from one of two different mechanisms. In type 1, there is excess hormone production by the thyroid caused by the iodine load, whereas, in type 2, there is release of the stored hormones as a result of the damage done to the thyroid by this drug (destructive thyroiditis). Because there is excess hormone production in type 1, oral agents, such as methimazole or PTU, are effective. Type 2 is treated with glucocorticoids.
6. Riedel's thyroiditis refers to the progressive fibrosis of the thyroid gland. It is a part of a systemic process. It occurs rarely and the etiology is unknown. These patients present with a thyroid gland that is hard, fixed, and painless. Obstructive symptoms, such as esophageal or tracheal compression, may occur. If the fibrosis extends to the parathyroid glands, hypoparathyroidism may result. Depending on the level of fibrosis, function of thyroid gland is affected. If this involves all or most of the gland, hypothyroidism does occur. Treatment is surgical followed by thyroid hormone replacement. Other modalities have been tried in the early stages of this disease *(8)*.

SUBCLINICAL HYPERTHYROIDISM

Subclinical hyperthyroidism is defined as a condition in which there is a low TSH level associated with normal levels of both free T3 as well as free T4. This condition has become more common with the advent of third-generation TSH assays, which are very accurate.

Most patients with this presentation are asymptomatic. This condition has been divided into two categories based on whether the cause is endogenous, such as a primary thyroid disorder, or exogenous, secondary to thyroid hormone therapy. Exogenous cause is the more common of the two.

Data regarding the prevalence of this disorder is very variable. In the United States, a study from Colorado *(9)*, showed a 2.1% prevalence. More than half of these individuals were on thyroid hormone therapy, whereas the rest had endogenous causes. The prevalence increased with age. US National Health and Nutrition Examination Survey (NHANES) III data suggests a 1.3% prevalence. It is important to note that the cutoff was at most 0.3 μU/mL for the Colorado study and less than 0.1 μU/mL for the NHANES data.

Diagnosis is based on the patient's history and physical exam. If the TSH level is below normal, free T3 and free T4 levels are obtained. In case of a suspected endogenous cause, radioactive iodine uptake and scan is obtained to determine the possible underlying cause. These include Graves' disease, toxic single or multinodular goiter, or thyroiditis.

Half of the individuals usually revert to normal if the decrease in TSH is minimal. If the level of TSH is less than 0.01 μU/mL, the condition usually leads to clinical hyperthyroidism. The clinical effects on various organ systems have been documented. These include the cardiovascular system as well as bone mineral density. There might be an increased rate of fractures. This condition has also been associated with increased mortality *(10)*. Some experts recommend treating subclinical hyperthyroidism in the elderly (older than 60 years) and in patients with underlying atrial fibrillation and severe osteoporosis.

Because it is quite prevalent and is most likely secondary to exogenous administration of thyroid hormone, steps should be taken to avoid overreplacement, if possible. This is important particularly in the elderly population.

HYPOTHYROIDISM

Introduction

Hypothyroidism results from the decreased levels of thyroid hormones in the majority of cases. Rarely, it may occur when there is resistance in the body to the effects of the thyroid hormones.

Causes

Hypothyroidism is broadly categorized into two categories, primary and secondary. Primary hypothyroidism occurs when the cause lies within the thyroid gland itself; the most common cause in the United States being Hashimoto's thyroiditis. Other examples include damage or destruction of the thyroid by radiation or surgery. In such cases, there is a low level of thyroid hormones but the TSH level is significantly high.

Secondary hypothyroidism occurs because of inadequate stimulation of the thyroid gland by low or absent TSH in pituitary or hypothalamic disease. Here, both the TSH as well as thyroid hormone levels are low.

Clinical Manifestations

Symptoms of hypothyroidism include lethargy, cold intolerance, constipation, dry skin and coarse hair, menstrual disturbances, weight gain, depression, and so on.

Signs include delayed reflexes, dry skin, bradycardia, nonpitting edema (myxedema), and pericardial effusion (in profound hypothyroidism). There may also be an enlargement of the thyroid gland.

Infants with congenital hypothyroidism exhibit inactivity, hypotonia, feeding problems, umbilical hernia, enlarged tongue, mottled skin, and edematous facies.

The clinical manifestations of hypothyroidism are summarized in Table 2.

Evaluation

The best screening test for primary hypothyroidism is TSH. If the TSH level is normal, primary hypothyroidism is excluded; the only exception is secondary hypothyroidism, in which TSH levels could be normal or low; in this case, free T4 is used to make the diagnosis. The combination of low free T4 level and low/normal TSH level is diagnostic of secondary hypothyroidism.

Hashimoto's Thyroiditis

This is the most common cause of hypothyroidism and goiter in the United States. It is autoimmune in nature. There are various theories to explain the mechanism that leads to this disease, which involves the activation of T lymphocytes, which then induce the production of antibodies by the B lymphocytes. More than 90% of patients with this disease have high serum thyroid peroxidase antibodies and 20 to 50% have high serum thyroglobulin antibodies.

It is interesting to note that 10% of the general population and 25% of women older than 60 years in the United States have these antibodies. Detailed data in other subsets is also available *(9)*. The majority of these people do have a normal thyroid function.

Diagnosis of this disease is based on the elevated TSH and low thyroid hormone levels. Presence of the antibodies confirms the diagnosis. Twenty-four-hour radioactive iodine uptake is NOT helpful in the diagnosis. It is also important to remember that monitoring of these antibody levels once the diagnosis is made serves no useful purpose because they do not decrease once treatment starts.

Treatment essentially consists of replacement with levothyroxine and titrating the dose to achieve normal TSH levels. The recommendation is to start with a dose of 1.6 μg/kg/d except in the elderly and in patients with underlying

Table 2
Major Symptoms and Signs of Hypothyroidism

Symptoms	
Fatigue and lethargy	Decreased perspiration
Depression	Weight gain
Sleepiness	Decreased appetite
Mental impairment	Constipation
Dry skin	Menstrual disturbances
Cold intolerance	Arthralgias
Hoarseness	Paresthesias
Signs	
Slow movements	Hyporeflexia and delayed relaxation of reflexes
Slow speech	Ascites
Hoarseness	Pleural effusions
Bradycardia	Nonpitting edema (Myxedema)
Diastolic hypertension	Puffy face
Dry, coarse skin	Loss of lateral third of eyebrows
Carotenemia	Diffuse or nodular goiter

heart disease, in whom a low dose (12.5–25 μg) is given initially and then gradually increased *(10)*. TSH levels should be drawn every 4 to 6 weeks to adjust the dosage.

OTHER CAUSES OF HYPOTHYROIDISM

Other causes of hypothyroidism include central causes, such as pituitary disease or surgery, and diseases of the hypothalamus. Once the diagnosis is made, thyroid hormone replacement should be instituted. With these central causes of hypothyroidism, TSH levels should not be followed for dosage adjustment. Instead, free T4 levels should be measured and kept within a normal range.

SUBCLINICAL HYPOTHYROIDISM

Subclinical or mild hypothyroidism is frequently observed in clinical practice *(11,12)*. As is with subclinical hyperthyroidism, with the advent of sensitive third-generation TSH assays as well as increased emphasis on routine monitoring of thyroid activity, more and more cases are observed. TSH levels are in the 5 to 10 μU/mL range in the majority of cases, with the actual free T4 levels being normal. Prevalence ranges from 1 to 10% worldwide, with the highest rate is in women older than 60 years of age *(9)*. These patients have a higher incidence of goiter as well as having thyroid peroxidase antibodies.

Underlying causes include history of exposure to radiation and postpartum thyroiditis. Use of drugs such as amiodarone and lithium has been identified as a cause in some patients. Patients with type 1 diabetes also have a higher incidence.

Screening of the entire population remains somewhat controversial because of the lack of prospective trials. However, screening should be considered in women and men older than 35 years (American Thyroid Association), especially if the index of suspicion is high. If untreated, this commonly progresses to overt hypothyroidism *(13)*.

The signs and symptoms are similar to those of clinical hypothyroidism as noted above. However, these may be subtler.

There is data to indicate that patients with mild thyroid failure need to be treated. A Dutch study *(14)* showed that women with subclinical hypothyroidism were twice as likely to have atherosclerosis as well as myocardial infarction as compared with healthy controls, even after adjustment for other factors. Similarly, there is a higher incidence of depression and this condition may also contribute to infertility. The effects on lipids remain controversial.

A summary of the recommendations made by different groups is based on an initial TSH level. If it is elevated and free T4 levels are normal, thyroid peroxidase antibodies should be obtained. Therapy with levothyroxine should be considered if these antibodies are positive and the patient has mild symptoms, elevated lipids, or has an enlarged thyroid. If the TSH level is greater than 10 μU/mL (regardless of symptoms or antibodies), levothyroxine therapy should be initiated. In the event of a negative antibody result, no symptoms and a TSH level below 10 μU/mL, annual follow-up is recommended. The aim is to correct the TSH levels with the free T4 level remaining normal *(15)*. Requirements will increase if overt hypothyroidism occurs. In the event of no significant benefit, therapy can be discontinued in mild cases.

THYROID NODULES

Introduction

Thyroid nodules are commonly found in clinical practice *(16)*. Nodules may be detected by the patient, by a physician on routine physical examination, and are frequently found incidentally on radiological imaging. Prevalence rates range from 5 to 50%, depending on the population studied as well as the sensitivity of detection methods. In the United States, clinically apparent solitary nodules are present in 4 to 7% of the adult population. Ultrasonographic studies have found unsuspected thyroid nodules in 20 to 45% of healthy women and 17 to 25% of healthy men.

The discovery of a nodule may be quite concerning to patients because of the fear of thyroid carcinoma, although the risk of cancer in a thyroid nodule is only approx 5%. Nevertheless, any thyroid nodule should be considered clinically relevant and worked up in an appropriate manner.

Differential Diagnosis

The differential diagnosis of a thyroid nodule includes benign lesions (colloid or hemorrhagic cysts, Hashimoto's thyroiditis, adenomas, and colloid goiter) and malignant lesions (papillary, follicular, Hurthle cell, medullary and anaplastic carcinomas, and lymphoma and metastatic lesions). Discovery of a thyroid nodule creates anxiety in patients because of the fear of thyroid cancer. As mentioned, the risk of thyroid cancer in any nodule is only 5%, and even so, the majority of thyroid cancers (papillary and follicular carcinomas) are slow growing and easily treated. Clinically unapparent thyroid cancer is much more common than clinically perceptible thyroid cancer. Occult microcarcinomas (<1 cm) may be found in as many as 13% of thyroid glands studied at autopsy; these microcarcinomas almost never become clinically relevant and pose no threat to life *(17)*.

Thyroid incidentalomas are increasingly common in recent years; patients are sent for nonthyroid neck imaging, and clinically inapparent thyroid nodules are discovered. These nodules are termed thyroid incidentalomas and are extremely prevalent, from 19 to 46%, depending on imaging techniques *(18)*.

Patients with thyroid nodules, whether they are clinically apparent or incidentally discovered, should be sent for appropriate evaluation, including assessment of thyroid function, possible referral for imaging or biopsy, and consultation with an endocrinologist.

History and Physical

Any physician evaluating a nodule should be aware of three basic concerns with nodules: the possibility of thyroid cancer, thyroid dysfunction, and compressive symptoms. Primary physicians should become comfortable with an initial evaluation, which should include history, physical examination, and laboratory testing.

Some patients with nodules may be at increased risk for cancer. Historical features that may indicate increased risk of cancer are age (<20 years or >70 years), sex (men are twice as likely to have a malignancy than women), history of radiation exposure (primarily exposure during childhood), personal history of thyroid cancer, and family history of thyroid cancer (as in the Multiple Endocrine Neoplasia [MEN] syndromes). Other appropriate historical questions should include pain or tenderness associated with the nodule, signs or symptoms associated with hyperthyroidism or hypothyroidism, and family history of autoimmune or benign nodular disease. Although these features do not exclude the possibility of thyroid cancer, their presence favors benign disease.

Patients should be asked for the presence of compressive symptoms that may be associated with a larger nodule (hoarseness, dyspnea, and dysphagia).

Features on neck examination for the physician to be alerted to are firmness or fixed position, tenderness on palpation, irregularity of nodule borders, and the presence of cervical or regional lymph nodes. Small nodules or nodules occurring deep in the gland observed on previous imaging may not be palpable on physical exam.

Work-Up

Laboratory Testing

Serum TSH levels should be tested to assess thyroid function in all patients with thyroid nodules. TSH is the single best screening test to determine hypothyroidism or hyperthyroidism. The assessment of thyroid hormone levels (free T4 and T3) should be performed secondarily if the TSH is elevated or suppressed; free T4 and T3 are preferred over total T4 and T3 because they are not affected by thyroxine binding globulin changes.

When hypothyroidism is diagnosed, it may indicate the presence of autoimmune Hashimoto's thyroiditis, in which the gland often contains nodules. Positive thyroid peroxidase antibodies may help to confirm a diagnosis of autoimmune thyroid disease. Conversely, hyperthyroidism might indicate a toxic nodule, a toxic multinodular goiter, or a cold nodule in association with Graves' disease. In this case, a thyroid scan would help differentiate these three hyperthyroid conditions (*see* Imaging Studies). The presence of hypothyroidism or hyperthyroidism lowers the suspicion for, but does not exclude the possibility of, malignancy.

Calcitonin, which is a marker for medullary thyroid cancer (MTC), should certainly be drawn in anyone with a family history of medullary carcinoma or MEN syndrome. However, routine screening with calcitonin produces false positives and is not a cost-effective screen in patients without risk factors *(19)*.

Imaging Studies

Ultrasound is the best radiological test to evaluate thyroid nodules. Ultrasound is noninvasive, relatively inexpensive, and can accurately determine nodule size and distinguish cystic vs solid content. Although ultrasound cannot determine whether a nodule is benign or malignant, characteristics such as solid hypoechoic features (less echogenic), irregular margins, and calcifications may be more concerning for malignancy *(20)*. Ultrasound also gives the best quantification of nodule size, and it is the best objective measure to determine growth or change over time during follow-up.

Not all patients require ultrasound examination. If a nodule is found on exam, the patient should be referred to an endocrinologist for biopsy (if indicated); if the biopsy is benign, subsequent follow-up could be performed by palpation. However, if a nodule is not felt on exam but is found on imaging studies and decision is made to biopsy the nodule (*see* Thyroid Biopsy), then an ultrasound-guided biopsy is performed; if the biopsy is benign, subsequent follow-up is performed by repeating the ultrasound at periodic intervals.

We do not routinely perform radionuclide uptake and scans for thyroid nodules. This study cannot determine the presence or absence of nodules (unless large), but only can assess regions of uptake and functionality. Some authors suggest that uptake and scan be performed to assess whether a thyroid nodule is warm, cold, or hot, because the incidence of cancer is, in fact, lower in hot nodules. However, this is only true if the TSH level is suppressed with a hot nodule on scan and suppression of uptake by the rest of the gland; in this case, we are dealing with a toxic nodule, which has a risk of cancer of less than 1%. To clear the confusion regarding these terms, all toxic nodules are hot (with suppressed TSH), but not all hot nodules are toxic (you can have a hot nodule on a scan with a normal TSH level; this hot nodule will still carry a risk of cancer of almost 3–5%). In summary, an uptake and scan should be performed only if the TSH level is suppressed enough to indicate hyperthyroidism (toxic nodule); otherwise, you do not need to perform this test.

Patients who present with large or multiple nodules may complain of dysphagia, hoarseness, or choking. The physician should ask historical features related to gastroesophageal reflux or postnasal drip, which are common causes of similar symptomatology. Such patients may need to be referred for radiological testing (e.g., barium swallow, CT of neck) or to an otolaryngologist to determine whether the nodules are the cause of such complaints. Of note, when CT is used, iodinated contrast should not be administered, because it will not improve the sensitivity of the CT and there is a risk of inducing hyperthyroidism in autonomous nodules. If the nodule is found to be contributing to symptoms, then the patient should be referred to a surgeon for consultation and possible thyroidectomy. The decision on surgical resection (subtotal vs total thyroidectomy) is dependent on the presence of malignancy and, therefore, would be determined after a biopsy is performed as indicated.

Thyroid Biopsy

Any patient with a thyroid nodule greater than 1 cm or any thyroid nodule that appears suspicious for malignancy on thyroid ultrasound should be referred for fine-needle aspiration biopsy (FNAB).

FNAB is the most reliable test to diagnose malignant nodules. This is an outpatient procedure, which is simple and safe when performed by an experienced physician. A thin gauge needle is guided into the nodule at several different locations and cells are aspirated and sent for analysis. Thyroid nodules should be biopsied in several different sites to obtain an adequate yield of cells and to allow for sampling of cells from different areas of the nodule. FNAB has an overall accuracy of 95% if performed by an experienced physician and interpreted by an experienced cytopathologist.

Although the false-negative rate is low for FNAB, a high clinical suspicion for carcinoma should always overrule cytology in the decision to pursue surgery *(21)*. Another limitation to fine-needle aspiration includes insufficient or nondiagnostic yield of cells (insufficient cell material was obtained for the pathologist to formulate a diagnosis), which occurs in 10 to 15% of thyroid biopsies. Patients should be informed of these statistics before biopsy in the event that the biopsy may need to be repeated.

The use of ultrasound to guide FNAB has been shown to reduce the number of inadequate samples. Furthermore, ultrasound guidance enables FNAB of nonpalpable nodules. Ultrasound-guided FNAB should be performed if the initial biopsy attempt by palpation has produced nondiagnostic results, or if the nodule is not palpable (an incidentaloma).

Cytology may be interpreted as benign (80%, colloid nodules, chronic thyroiditis), malignant (5%), indeterminate, or suspicious (15%, follicular neoplasm).

Patients with malignant findings on FNAB should be referred to an experienced thyroid surgeon for total thyroidectomy and follow-up with an endocrinologist for postoperative management.

Follow-up for benign FNAB results should include periodic neck examination paired with ultrasound imaging (if nodule not palpable) every 6 to 12 months (depending on clinical judgment) to assess for change or growth in the nodule. If the nodule has enlarged or appears suspicious on repeat ultrasound, then repeat FNAB is recommended. If a nodule has grown in size and thought to be the etiology of compressive symptoms, then referral to an experienced thyroid surgeon is recommended.

Indeterminate or suspicious FNAB results include follicular or Hurthle cell neoplasms. Follicular and Hurthle cell cancer cannot be distinguished from benign adenomas on cytology. The only way to determine malignancy is by finding capsular or vascular invasion at surgery. Therefore, patients with an indeterminate or suspicious FNAB should have surgery. Many surgeons perform lobectomy on the side of the suspicious findings. If the surgical pathology is benign, then the patient is finished with surgery. If the surgical pathology does reveal capsular or vascular invasion, then the patient is brought back to remove the contralateral lobe (completion thyroidectomy), and should follow-up with an endocrinologist for postoperative thyroid cancer management.

For patients with insufficient or nondiagnostic specimens on initial FNAB, repeat FNAB is recommended, usually under ultrasound guidance.

Incidentally found nodules that are less than 1 cm do not need to be biopsied, unless there are major risk factors for cancer (history of radiation in childhood or family history of medullary carcinoma); nodules less than 6 mm may not be amenable to biopsy even by an experienced ultrasonographer. If biopsy is not indicated, these subcentimeter nodules can be followed with periodic neck examination and thyroid ultrasound (if not palpable). FNAB should be obtained for any nodule that increases in size with time.

Cystic Nodules

Cystic nodules may present with pain or tenderness, indicating hemorrhage or hemorrhagic infarction into the cyst. Many nodules may contain both a solid and cystic component *(22)*. Indications for an initial evaluation with FNAB for cystic nodules are the same as for solid nodules. Between 25 and 50% of predominantly cystic nodules may disappear after initial aspiration. However, cystic fluid will often reaccumulate, necessitating another FNAB. If the cyst recurs after two biopsies, then surgery is recommended. The use of sclerosing agents (tetracycline or ethanol) to shrink nodules is typically painful, and is not routinely used in the United States.

Natural History

Nodules may enlarge, shrink, or remain unchanged with time. Many benign nodules may increase in size slowly with time. One study suggests that there does not seem to be an increased risk of cancer in these slow-growing nodules based on repeat FNAB at 5 years *(23)*, however, current recommendations are to rebiopsy a nodule if it enlarges or seems clinically suspicious, even nodules with benign initial FNAB results. Most benign stable nodules can be managed conservatively. Indications for surgical referral in such nodules include patient anxiety regarding the nodule, cosmetic concern, and neck discomfort.

Thyroxine Suppressive Therapy

There is still controversy regarding the use of thyroxine (thyroid hormone) in euthyroid patients to suppress thyroid nodule growth. A meta-analysis *(24)* in 1998 reviewing the effect of thyroxine suppressive therapy in patients with thyroid nodules suggests that thyroxine therapy fails to shrink most nodules, and may not prevent the emergence of new nodules or the recurrence of nodules postoperatively. A double-blinded clinical trial revealed that thyroxine therapy may cause a mild decrease in nodule size, however, the results were not statistically significant compared with placebo patients *(25)*. Some patients even experienced an increase in nodule size even while taking thyroxine. Furthermore, suppressive therapy may cause osteoporosis and increase the risk for atrial fibrillation in certain patients. In our opinion, thyroxine therapy does not offer any benefit, and may pose more risk as far as cardiovascular and bone metabolic effects, therefore, we do not recommend the routine use of thyroxine to shrink thyroid nodules.

Toxic Nodules

Patients with nodules and a suppressed TSH (<0.1) should be sent for radionuclide uptake and scan. Toxic nodules are hyperfunctioning nodules, which display increased uptake on nuclear scanning (hot nodules), whereas the remainder of the gland usually has suppressed uptake. Patients may have overt hyperthyroidism (suppressed TSH level and elevated levels of T4 and/or T3) or subclinical hyperthyroidism (suppressed TSH level and normal T4 and T3 levels). The most appropriate definitive treatment for a toxic nodule with overt hyperthyroidism is radioiodine, because hyperthyroidism caused by a toxic nodule usually does not remit with time, like Graves' disease. In toxic nodules with subclinical hyperthyroidism, treatment is warranted in older patients or those with underlying atrial fibrillation or reduced bone mineral density. Other treatment options include antithyroid medication and surgery. Patients with toxic nodules and overt or subclinical hyperthyroidism should be referred to an endocrinologist for appropriate management.

THYROID CANCER

Introduction

Thyroid carcinomas are relatively rare, given the preponderance of thyroid nodules in the general population. Still, it is the most common endocrine malignancy.

Causes

Thyroid cancers basically fall into two categories. First are the follicular cell-derived cancers (FCDC) and second are MTC derived from the parafollicular or C cells, which produce calcitonin.

There are four subtypes of FCDCs: papillary, follicular, oxyphilic or Hurthle cell, and anaplastic. The majority of these cancers are papillary, which accounts for 80% of the total cases *(26)*, followed by follicular cancer with 10 to 15%.

MTC accounts for approx 10% of all thyroid cancers. Seventy-five percent of MTC cases are sporadic whereas 25% are hereditary or familial *(27)*. Familial MTC is a component of the MEN syndromes IIA and IIB.

Clinical Presentation and Diagnosis

These cancers are usually diagnosed with the discovery of a palpable mass on clinical exam. In some cases, it starts with the incidental finding on an imaging study performed for some other reason, such as a carotid ultrasound. In the next step, this is evaluated further as outlined above, in the section on thyroid nodules. FNAB is very helpful in the diagnosis of the papillary carcinoma. Diagnosis of follicular carcinoma is difficult on a FNAB. To make that diagnosis, invasion through the capsule of the nodule or into a blood vessel has to be demonstrated (on a pathology specimen).

Anaplastic carcinoma is also diagnosed by FNAB, but sometimes it is difficult to differentiate it from a metastatic carcinoma. Presence of thyroglobulin and cytokeratin is helpful in such instances.

Thyroid lymphoma is rare and difficult to diagnose on a biopsy. Most patients show a rapid increase in the size of a preexisting goiter. Presence of an underlying autoimmune thyroid disease is quite common. Most of these lymphomas are B cell in origin. Techniques such as flow cytometry can be helpful in the diagnosis.

MTCs are also diagnosed on a FNAB with special staining for calcitonin. Serum calcitonin levels are usually elevated. Calcitonin secretagogues can be used to detect this condition in the hyperplasia stage, even before the development of the carcinoma. Pentagastrin and calcium gluconate have been used for this purpose.

Preoperative ultrasound can help with the planning of surgery, particularly in reference to enlarged lymph nodes. Radioactive iodine scans usually show the nodules to be cold (underactive). It is rare to find a hot (overactive) nodule to be malignant. In the event that the TSH level is normal, a radioactive iodine scan is usually not helpful and is, therefore, not recommended.

Treatment

Primary treatment remains surgery. Some controversy exists regarding the extent of this surgery. Most experts recommend total or nearly total thyroidectomy in the setting of bilateral thyroid nodules. However, in case of a single thyroid nodule, unilateral thyroid lobectomy is performed pending outcome of final pathology. The extent of the surgery should be determined, keeping in view multiple factors such as age, metastasis, and extent of primary cancer. Multiple classification systems exist in this regard. Our recommendation is that these cases be handled by a team of specialists experienced in the management of thyroid cancer; the team would consist of endocrinologists, radiologists, pathologists, experienced thyroid surgeons, and nuclear medicine physicians.

Postoperatively, the "TNM" system is the most recommended means of classification at this time, as established by the American Joint Committee on Cancer. "T" refers to the size and extent of the lesion. T1 is 1 cm or less, T2 is between 1 and 4 cm, and T3 is larger than 4 cm. T4 refers to extrathyroidal extension or

Table 3
Staging System for Thyroid Carcinoma Established by the American Joint Committee on Cancer

	Papillary or Follicular		*Medullary*	*Anaplastic*
Stage	*Age < 45 yr*	*Age > 45 yr*	*(any age)*	*(any age)*
I	M0	T1	T1	—
II	M1	T2–3	T2–4	—
III	—	T4 or N1	N1	—
IV	—	M1	M1	Any

invasion through the thyroid capsule. "N" is involvement of the regional lymph nodes, and "M" indicates the absence or presence of metastasis.

These have been condensed into the four stages as shown in Table 3. Stage I refers to a FCDC with no metastasis in anyone younger than 45 years and older than 45 years if the tumor is less than 1 cm with no nodal involvement. Stage II is observed in patients with metastasis if younger than 45 years and between 1 and 4 cm with no nodes or metastasis older than 45 years. Stage III is determined by the presence of nodal involvement or tumors larger than 4 cm in patients older than 45 years. Stage IV refers to the presence of metastasis. For MTC there is no age limit. Stage I is size up to 1 cm tumor size, stage II is up to 4 cm in size, stage III is nodal involvement, whereas stage IV is defined by metastasis. All anaplastic tumors are stage IV.

Radioiodine Remnant Ablation

Radioiodine remnant ablation refers to the destruction of any remnant thyroid tissue after surgery with the use of radioactive iodine. This is performed once the primary tumor has been resected. This helps in detection of any recurrent disease later on a subsequent scan. In addition, there is an increased sensitivity in the measurement of thyroglobulin levels, as detailed under Tumor Markers. The use of this modality in low-risk cases is still undecided. Therefore, decisions regarding the use remains individualized according to each presentation. Nuclear medicine specialists, again on an individual basis, usually determine dosage.

Radioactive iodine remnant ablation is not needed in MTC because these cells do not take up iodine.

Thyroid Hormone Suppression

In patients with FCDC, after surgical resection, supraphysiological doses of levothyroxine are administered. The idea is to minimize the growth of any remnant cells by endogenous TSH. A level of TSH less than 0.01 μU/mL is aimed for in high-risk cases. In low-risk individuals, the range that is aimed for is between 0.1 and 0.4 μU/mL. However, there is a lack of prospective data in this regard. Given the risks of prolonged supraphysiological doses of thyroid hormone especially on the bones and heart, clinical judgment should be used.

TSH suppression is not required for MTC because these cells are not responsive to TSH. However, given the fact that there is a total removal of the thyroid gland, adequate levothyroxine replacement is necessary.

Tumor Markers

Thyroglobulin

Thyroglobulin is a glycoprotein produced by the thyroid as a prohormone. Thyroglobulin is used a tumor marker once the patient undergoes total thyroidectomy followed by radioactive iodine ablation. This takes away the body's ability to produce thyroglobulin and then thyroglobulin becomes a useful tumor marker for follow-up purposes.

A word of caution regarding the presence of antithyroglobulin antibodies: these antibodies are also found commonly in healthy individuals *(28)*. Presence of these antibodies can lead to both overestimation as well as underestimation and, therefore, should be measured together with the serum thyroglobulin levels. If present, the results should be interpreted with caution. In the absence of these antibodies, the thyroglobulin levels are very helpful and increasing levels point to a recurrence of the disease.

Calcitonin

As mentioned above, this is a product of the parafollicular C cells and is usually elevated in MTC. Calcitonin secretagogues, such as pentagastrin, are used in addition to basal calcitonin levels, to monitor persistent or recurrent MTC. In addition, it can also be used to screen first-degree relatives of patients with familial MTC.

Carcinoembryonic Antigen

This is a tumor marker for a number of malignancies and, with time, has proven to be quite effective in monitoring MTC *(29)*.

It is now used in combination with calcitonin for the monitoring of MTC.

Long-Term Follow-Up

The issue of long-term follow-up is again based on each individual's total clinical picture. Risk stratification is extremely important to determine what this would comprise.

Conventionally, whole body scanning is performed with radioactive iodine after increasing the serum TSH level. This level is usually greater than 25 to 30 μU/mL.

At this level, the uptake by any remnant tissue is much better. To achieve this level of TSH, traditionally the levothyroxine is held for a period of approx 6 weeks. This can be replaced by T3 (tri-iodothyronine) for the first 4 weeks followed by no replacement for the last 2 weeks. Serum thyroglobulin levels are also measured. Two to 5 mCi of radioactive iodine are administered and a whole body scan is obtained 2 days later. Results are then used to determine further course of action. If any remnants are observed, ablative doses of radioactive iodine are administered. In these situations, a posttreatment scan is also obtained to determine any additional sites. Levothyroxine therapy is resumed once this is all done.

Recombinant human TSH is now available and is being used to elevate the TSH levels to prepare for the whole body scan. A protocol is available for the administration of recombinant human TSH. However, the determination of the appropriate patient for this purpose should be deferred to specialized centers.

Similarly, the use of other imaging modalities, such as neck ultrasounds or PET scans, can also be best determined by such centers.

REFERENCES

1. Hershman JM. Hyperthyroidism caused by chorionic gonadotropin. In Werner and Ingbar's The Thyroid, 8th Ed (Braverman LE, Utiger RD, eds.). Lippincott-Raven Publishers, Philadelphia, 1996; p. 573–576.
2. Forbes G, Gorman CA, Brennan MD, et al. Ophthalmopathy of Graves' disease: computerized volume measurements of the orbital fat and muscle. Neuroradiol 1986;7:651–656.
3. Sridama V, DeGroot LJ. Treatment of Graves' disease and the course of opthalmopathy. Am J Med 1989;87:70–73.
4. Bartalena L, Marcocci C, Bogazzi F, Panicucci M, Lepri A, Pinchera A. Use of corticosteroids to prevent progression of Graves' ophthalmopathy after radioiodine therapy for hyperthyroidism. N Engl J Med 1989;321:1349–1352.
5. Wartofsky L, Glinoer D, Solomon B, et al. Differences and similarities in the diagnosis and treatment of Graves' disease in Europe, Japan and the United States. Thyroid 1991;1: 129–135.
6. Pearce EN, Farwell A, Braverman LE. Thyroiditis. N Engl J Med 2003;348:2646–2655.
7. Stagnaro-Green A. Recognizing, understanding, and treating postpartum thyroiditis. Endocrinol Metab Clin North Am 2000;29(2):417–430.
8. Vaida B, Harris PE, Barrett P, Kendall-Taylor P. Corticosteroid therapy in Riedel's thyroiditis. Postgrad Med J 1997;73:817–819.
9. Ross DS, Daniels GH, Gouveia D. The Colorado thyroid disease prevalence study. Arch Intern Med 2000;160:526–534.
10. Parle JV, Maisonneuve P, Sheppard MC, et al. Prediction of all cause and cardiovascular mortality in elderly people from one low serum thyrotropin result: a 10-year cohort study. Lancet 2001;358:861–865.
11. Hollowell GJ, Staehling NW, Falnders ED, et al. Serum TSH, T (4), and thyroid antibodies in US population (1988 to 1994): NHANES III. J Clin Endocrinol Metab 2002;87:489–499.
12. Burman KD. Hypothyroidism, Syllabus of Review of Endocrinology. Foundation for Advanced Education in the Sciences (FAES) at the National Institutes of Health, Oct. 2003; p. 594.

13. Vanderpump MP, Turnbridge WM, French JM, et al. The incidence of thyroid disorders in the community: a twenty-year follow-up of the Whickham survey. Clin Endocrinol (Oxf) 1995;43:55–68.
14. Hak AE, Pols HAP, Visser TJ, et al. Subclinical hypothyroidism is an independent risk factor for atherosclerosis and myocardial infarction in elderly women: the Rotterdam study. Ann Intern Med 2000;132:270–280.
15. Cooper DS, Subclinical hypothyroidism. N Engl J Med 2001;345:260–265.
16. McCaffrey TV. Evaluation of the thyroid nodule, cancer control 2000;7:223–228.
17. Pearce EN, Braverman LE. Papillary thyroid microcarcinoma outcomes and implications for treatment. JCEM 2004;89:3710–3712.
18. Burguera B, Gharib H. Thyroid incidentalomas, prevalence, diagnosis, significance, and management. Endocrinol Metab Clin North Am 2000;29:187–203.
19. Hodack SP, Burman KD. The calcitonin conundrum—is it time for routine measurements of serum calcitonin in patients with thyroid nodules? J Clin Endocrinol Metab 2004;89: 511–514.
20. Leenhardt L, Hejblum G, Franc B, et al. Indications and limits of ultrasound-guided cytology in the management of nonpalpable thyroid nodules. J Clin Endocrinol Metab 1999;84: 24–28.
21. Yeh MW, Demircan O, Ituarte P, et al. False-negative fine-needle aspiration cytology results delay treatment and adversely affect outcome in patients with thyroid carcinoma. Thyroid 2004;14:207–215.
22. de los Santos ET, Keyhani-Rofagha S, Cunningham JJ, et al. Cystic thyroid nodules. The dilemma of malignant lesions. Arch Intern Med 1990;150:1422–1427.
23. Alexander EK, Hurwitz S, Heering JP, et al. Natural history of benign solid and cystic thyroid nodules. Ann Intern Med 2003;138:315–318.
24. Gharib H, Mazzaferri EL. Thyroxine suppressive therapy in patients with nodular thyroid disease. Ann Intern Med 1998;128:386–394.
25. Zelmanovitz F, Genro S, Gross JL. Suppressive therapy with levothyroxine for solitary thyroid nodules: a double blind controlled clinical study and cumulative meta-analyses. J Clin Endocrinol Metab 1998;83:3881–3885.
26. Robbins J, Merino MJ, Boice JD, et al. Thyroid cancer: a lethal endocrine neoplasm. Ann Intern Med 1991;115:133–147.
27. Giuffrida D, Gharib H. Current diagnosis and management of medullary thyroid carcinoma. Ann Oncol 1998;9:695–701.
28. Spencer CA, Wang CC. Thyroglobulin measurement. Techniques, clinical benefits, and pitfalls. Endocrinol Metab Clin North Am 1995;24:841–863.
29. Juweid M, Sharkey RM, Behr T, et al. Improved detection of medullary thyroid cancer with radiolabeled antibodies to carcinoembryonic antigen. J Clin Oncol 1996;14:1209–1217.

14 Women's Oral Health Issues

Barbara J. Steinberg, DDS, *Laura Minsk,* DMD,
Joan I. Gluch, PhD, *and Susanne K. Giorgio,* RDH

CONTENTS

INTRODUCTION

Because oral health is an integral part of general health, oral problems specific to the female population have to be addressed. Women have special oral health needs and considerations that men do not have.

Hormonal fluctuations affect more than a woman's reproductive system. They have a surprisingly strong influence on the oral cavity. These changes are not necessarily the result of direct hormonal action on the tissue but are, perhaps, best explained as the effects of the local factors (e.g., bacterial plaque on tissues exacerbated by hormonal activity). Puberty, menses, pregnancy, and menopause all influence women's oral health and the way in which health care practitioners should approach their treatment. Similar influences may also be observed in women taking oral contraceptives. This chapter will lend itself to a discussion of these hormonal influences and also address the orofacial manifestations of certain conditions primarily affecting women, including eating disorders,

From: *Current Clinical Practice: Women's Health in Clinical Practice*
Edited by: Clouse and Sherif © Humana Press Inc., Totowa, NJ

temporomandibular disorders (TMD), osteoporosis, and those who are victims of domestic violence.

GINGIVAL TISSUE IN HEALTH

The gingival tissue is that part of the oral mucous membrane that covers the alveolar processes (bone) and the cervical (neck) portions of the teeth. The gingival surface is covered with a stratified squamous epithelium, normally of the keratinizing type. Clinically, the gingival tissue is pale pink or a coral color. This color may be modified by the presence of pigmentation, as observed in persons of dark complexion.

Gingival tissue in the anterior aspect of the mouth has a pyramid shape and the gingival tissue in the posterior aspect of the mouth has a more rounded appearance. The gingival margin (gumline) has a scalloped appearance and peaks to fill the space where adjacent teeth contact. Gingival tissue is tightly bound to the underlying hard tissues and, on palpation, feels firm. Mastication, routine tooth brushing, and flossing should not induce bleeding. Bleeding could be considered a sign of inflammation or trauma. However, it should be noted that absence of bleeding does not necessarily indicate good health (Fig. 1A).

PERIODONTAL DISEASES

Bacteria colonize the surface of a tooth, predominately around the gingival margin and the interdental spaces (between the teeth) creating a bacterial plaque biofilm. This developing bacterial plaque releases a variety of biologically active substances, including lipopolysaccharides, chemotactic peptides, protein toxins, and organic acids *(1)*. These products diffuse into the gingival tissues, initiating a host inflammatory response that eventually results in gingivitis. Clinically, gingivitis is characterized by a color change of pink to red, edema, and bleeding on probing by a dental professional. Patients may experience bleeding when brushing, as well sensitivity and tenderness (Fig. 1B).

Gingivitis may lead to periodontitis, which results in inflammation and progressive loss of the supporting structures of the teeth (tissue attachment and bone). If left untreated, periodontal disease could result in loosening of the teeth and eventual tooth loss. Pain may or may not accompany periodontal diseases.

Although bacterial plaque is the primary etiology of periodontal diseases, there are many factors that increase the risk of developing periodontal disease. These include but are not limited to:

- Smoking and chewing tobacco
- Systemic disease, such as diabetes, hematological disorders, and immunodeficiencies
- Medications, such as steroids, antiseizure medications, and calcium channel blockers

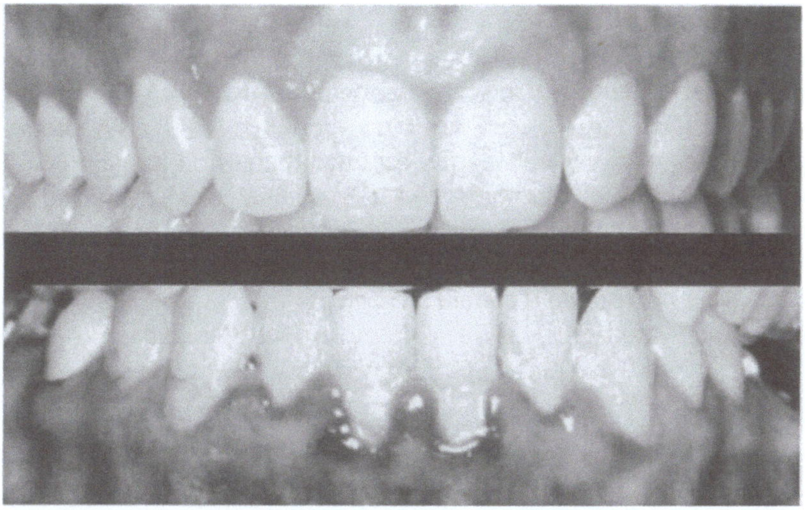

Fig. 1. Healthy and periodontal disease.

- Ill-fitting dental restorations and poorly aligned teeth
- Hormonal fluctuations
- Genetics
- Poor nutrition
- Stress

Tooth loss is not the only potential problem posed by periodontal diseases. Research suggest that there may be a link between periodontal diseases and other health concerns, such as diabetes, cardiovascular disease, stroke, bacterial pneumonia, and increased risk during pregnancy *(2)*.

Patients should be referred to a dental professional for a diagnostic workup and appropriate treatment. Periodontal treatment methods depend on the type and severity of the disease.

LIFE CYCLE CHANGES

Puberty and Menses

Estrogen and progesterone affect females throughout their lifecycles, beginning with puberty and continuing up to and even after menopause. Receptors for both estrogen and progesterone have been demonstrated in human gingiva *(3)*. It seems that the increase in circulating sex hormones during puberty has a modulatory effect in subgingival flora, favoring gram-negative anaerobic organisms associated with gingival inflammation *(4)*. Gingival tissues respond to the increased levels of circulating hormones and the related shift in subgingival flora with a greater degree of inflammation and gingival bleeding (*see* previous section, "Periodontal Diseases").

During puberty, young women may complain of increased gingival bleeding, sensitivity, and tenderness. Some women experience similar symptoms 3 to 4 days before menstruation, with resolution once the period has started *(5)*.

Intraoral recurrent aphthous ulcers and herpes labialis lesions may also present as a pattern during the menstrual cycle. These lesions appear during the luteal phase of the cycle and disappear after menstruation *(6)*.

Patients experiencing any of these symptoms or clinical findings should be referred to a dental professional for a diagnostic workup and appropriate treatment. Patients should be counseled to comply with the customized oral hygiene regimen recommended by the oral health professional.

Pregnancy

The oral changes that can occur during pregnancy have been recognized for many years. Pregnancy gingivitis is one of the most common findings, affecting 30 to 70% of all pregnant women *(7–9)*. It is characterized by erythema of the gingiva, edema, hyperplasia, and increased bleeding *(10–12)* (Fig. 2). Gingival inflammatory changes are generally observed in the second or third month of gestation, are maintained or increase in severity during the second trimester, and then decrease in the last month of pregnancy, eventually regressing after parturition *(11,12)*. Histologically, there are no differences between pregnancy gingivitis and other forms of gingivitis, but pregnancy gingivitis is characterized by an exaggerated response to local irritants (bacterial plaque and calculus).

The underlying mechanism for the enhanced inflammatory response during pregnancy is the result of the elevation in progesterone and estrogen. The severity of the response is attributed to the levels of these two hormones. Sex hormones also have an effect on the immune system. They depress neutrophil chemotaxis and phagocytosis, as well as T-cell and antibody responses *(13–15)*.

Specific estrogen receptors have been identified in gingival tissues *(3)*. Estrogen can increase cellular proliferation of gingival blood vessels, decreased gingival keratinization, and increased epithelial glycogen. These changes diminish the epithelial barrier function of the gingiva *(10,11,16)*.

Progesterone increases vascular membrane permeability, edema of the gingival tissues, gingival bleeding, and increased gingival crevicular fluid flow *(10,11,13,17)*. Progesterone also reduces the fibroblast proliferation rate, and alters the rate and pattern of collagen production, reducing the ability of the gingiva to repair *(16)*. Finally, the breakdown of folate, a requirement for the maintenance of healthy oral mucosa, is increased in the presence of increased levels of sex hormones *(18)*. This results in a folate

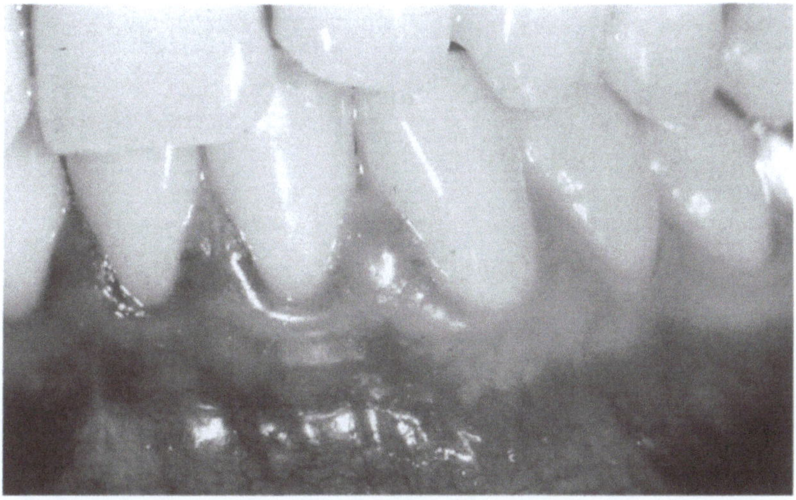

Fig. 2. Mild pregnancy gingivitis.

deficiency, which increases the inflammatory destruction of the oral tissue by inhibiting its repair.

Sex hormones can also affect gingival health during pregnancy, by allowing an increase in the anaerobic-to-aerobic subgingival plaque ratio, leading to higher concentration of periodontopathic bacteria *(19)*. A 55-fold increase in the levels of *Prevotella intermedia* has been shown in pregnant women compared with nonpregnant women *(20)*. *P. intermedia* is able to substitute progesterone and estrogen for vitamin K, an essential growth factor *(21)*.

To summarize, the increased levels of sex hormones found in pregnancy help depress the immune response, compromise the local defense mechanisms necessary for good oral health, and reduce the natural protection of the gingival environment. These changes, combined with the microbial shift favoring an anaerobic flora dominated by *P. intermedia*, are partly responsible for the exaggerated response to bacterial plaque in pregnancy.

Pyogenic granulomas which appear as hyperplastic, nodular, purple-red growths, are observed in 0.2% to 9.6% of pregnant patients, usually in the second or third trimester (Fig. 3) *(11,22)*. They may be more prevalent between the teeth, where there is usually less effective oral hygiene and, therefore, more bacterial plaque. These growths tend to enlarge rapidly and may bleed easily when injured. Pyogenic granulomas tend to regress after delivery and do not need to be removed unless they interfere with function or they present an esthetic concern to the patient.

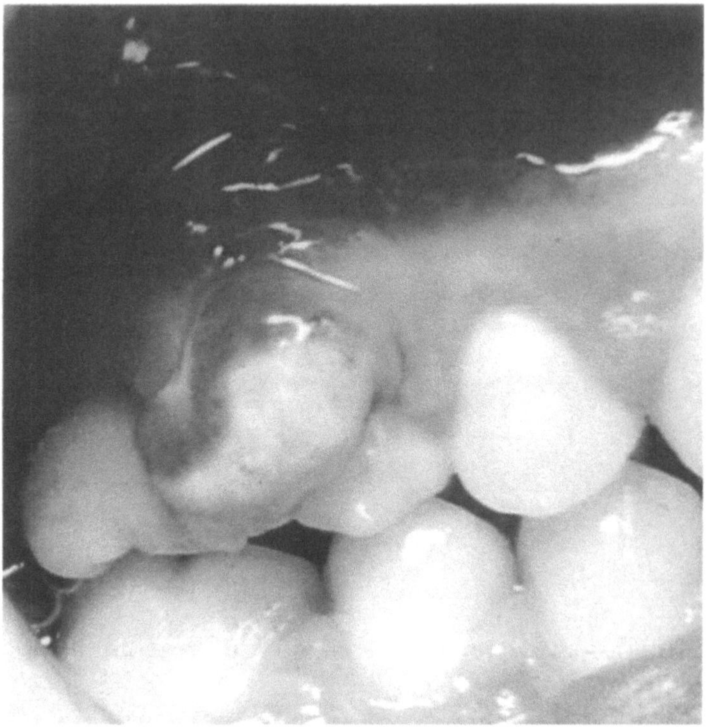

Fig. 3. Pregnancy granuloma.

In addition to the above-mentioned periodontal manifestations of pregnancy, 44% of pregnant women can experience some degree of xerostomia caused by hormonal alterations *(23)*. These symptoms can most easily be managed by increasing water consumption and other remedies (*see* Table 1). Care must be exercised to avoid an in increase tooth decay that could result from increased sugar consumption and/or lax oral hygiene. A rare finding associated with pregnancy is a temporary increase in tooth mobility *(24)*. This is transient and usually reverses after parturition, not requiring any treatment *(11,12)*.

Finally, although also rare, perimylosis (tooth erosion) can occur during pregnancy from repeated regurgitation associated with morning sickness or from esophageal reflux. It is recommended that patients rinse with water immediately after regurgitation and follow with a fluoride rinse to neutralize the acid and protect the surfaces of the teeth. Brushing immediately after regurgitation and before rinsing with water and fluoride may actually accelerate tooth erosion.

Oral infections may also contribute to the outcome of the pregnancy. Recent studies have linked periodontal infections during pregnancy with an increased

Table 1
Various Health Conditions and Concerns With Oral Manifestations Affecting Women

Health Condition/Disease	*Oral Manifestations*	*Dental Treatment Recommendations*
Dry mouth (xerostomia) (Could be the result of side effect of common medications, radiation treatment, Sjogren's syndrome, salivary gland disease, salivary gland obstruction and/or infection, and so on)	Mucositis	Use water, sugarless gum, or mints to hydrate mouth
	Glossitis, with coated, painful, and/or burning tongue	Use fluoride toothpaste, gels, and rinses to remineralize teeth to reduce dental decay avoid tobacco and caffeinated beverages
	Dental decay	Limit strongly flavored products and foods
	Breath malodor	Refer to dental professional for diagnostic work-up and more frequent dental care as appropriate
	Food, stains, and plaque bacteria biofilm retained on teeth	
	Angular cheilosis and/or candida infection in mouth	
Eating disorders	Perimylolysis (acid erosion of teeth from vomiting)	Avoid toothbrushing for at least 20 min after vomiting and rinse with water or baking soda rinses to neutralizeacids
	Trauma to oral mucosa, pharynx and/or soft palate	Use fluoride toothpaste, gels, and/or rinses to remineralize teeth and reduce dental decay

(Continued)

Table 1 (*Continued*)

Health Condition/Disease	*Oral Manifestations*	*Dental Treatment Recommendations*
	Dehydration	Evaluate for dry mouth and treat as needed
	Parotid salivary gland swelling	Refer to dental professional for diagnostic work-up and dental care as appropriate
	Dental decay	
	Gingivitis	
HIV/AIDS *(58)*	Oral lesions, including angular cheilosis, candidiasis, hairy leukoplakia, herpes simplex, herpes zoster, Kaposi's sarcoma	Careful and thorough oral hygiene
	Increased susceptibility to gingivitis, periodontitis, and/or necrotizing ulcerative gingivitis and periodontitis	Antimicrobial mouth rinse, such as chlorhexidine
	Dry mouth from medications	Anti-fungal agents
		See also treatment recommendations for dry mouth
		Refer to dental professional for diagnostic work-up and dental care as appropriate
Intimate partner and/or domestic violence	Lacerations, fractures and/or bruises around head and neck and in extraoral and intraoral tissue	Document injuries
	Evidence of repeated scarring in oral tissues	Refer for surgical treatment as indicated
	Loose or fractured teeth	Assist patient in referral for counseling and support

		Refer to dental professional for diagnostic work-up and dental care as appropriate
Lichen planus	White striated lesions on oral mucosa, gingiva, tongue, lip and palate	Topical steroids, anti-inflammatory agents, immunosuppressant agents
		Refer to dental professional for diagnostic work-up and dental care as appropriate
Menses, puberty	Gingivitis, with gingival bleeding, sensitivity and/or tenderness	Careful and thorough oral hygiene
	Aphthous ulcers	Refer to dental professional for diagnostic work-up and dental care as appropriate
	Herpes labialis lesions	
Menopause	Oral discomfort, altered taste perception, burning sensation and dry mouth	Careful and thorough oral hygiene
	Atrophy of oral mucosa	See also treatment recommendations for dry mouth
	Atrophic glossitis	Refer to dental professional for diagnostic work-up and dental care as appropriate
	Menopausal gingivostomatitis	
	Gingivitis	
	Dental decay	
	Osteoporosis and oral bone loss	
Oral contraceptives	Gingivitis	Careful and thorough oral hygiene
	Localized osteitis (dry socket) after dental extraction	Schedule dental extraction during placebo days of oral contraceptive

(*Continued*)

Table 1 (*Continued*)

Health Condition/Disease	*Oral Manifestations*	*Dental Treatment Recommendations*
		Refer to dental professional for diagnostic work-up and dental care as appropriate
Pemphigus	Desquamative gingival lesions	Topical and/or systemic steroids
		Refer to dental professional for diagnostic work-up and dental care as appropriate
Pregnancy	Pregnancy gingivitis, with exaggerated symptoms that may worsen throughout pregnancy	Careful oral hygiene
	Dry mouth	Excision of pyogenic granuloma if interferes with mastication,
bleeds,		
		or does not resolve after delivery
	Pyogenic granuloma	See also treatment recommendations for dry mouth
	Tooth decay	Refer to dental professional for diagnostic work-up and dental care as appropriate
	Increased tooth mobility	
	Perimylolysis (acid erosion of teeth)	
Rheumatoid arthritis	Temporomandibular joint dysfunction	Refer to dental professional for diagnostic work-up and dental care as appropriate
		See recommendations for temporomandibular joint disorders

Sjogren's syndrome	Dry mouth	Careful and thorough oral hygiene
	Painful, burning tongue with atrophied papilla	See also treatment recommendations for dry mouth
	Angular cheilosis	Refer to dental professional for diagnostic work-up and dental care as appropriate
	Dysgeusia, dysphagia	
	Mucositis	
	Parotid gland dysfunction	
	Increased dental decay rate caused by extreme dry mouth	
Systemic lupus erythematosis	Oral ulcerations and lesions	Refer to dental professional for diagnostic work-up and dental care as appropriate
	Noninfectious pharyngitis	Evaluate cardiac condition and consider antibiotic prophylaxis before dental treatment
	Characteristic butterfly rash across nose and cheeks	Evaluate systemic manifestations and hematologic profile before dental care
Temporomandibular disorders	Pain in muscles and/or joint	Refer to dental professional for diagnostic work-up and dental care as appropriate
	Facial, neck or shoulder pain	Moist heat
	Limited jaw movement	Anti-inflammatory, analgesic, and/or muscle relaxants
	Jaw locking	Physical therapy
	Clicking or popping sounds when opening or closing	

(*Continued*)

Table 1 (*Continued*)

Health Condition/Disease	*Oral Manifestations*	*Dental Treatment Recommendations*
	Headaches	
	Swelling on side of face	
	Change in the way teeth fit together	
Tobacco use	Increased susceptibility and severity of periodontal diseases and dental decay	Recommend and implement tobacco cessation counseling and nicotine replacement as needed
	Increased risk for cancer, most notably oral, pharyngeal, and lung cancer	Careful and thorough oral hygiene
	Dry mouth	Use fluoride gels or rinses to remineralize teeth and reduce dental decay
	Nicotine stomatitis	See also treatment recommendations for dry mouth
	Leukoplakia	Refer to dental professional for diagnostic work-up and dental care as appropriate

risk of having a preterm low-birth weight baby (PTLBW). In a 1996 study of 124 pregnant women or postpartum mothers, it was found that after controlling for other risk factors, periodontal diseases were a clinically significant risk factor for PTLBW, with an odds ratio of 7.9 *(25)*. The study found that periodontal infection caused an increase in prostaglandin E2 and tumor necrosis factor-α that may be sufficient to initiate the onset of premature labor.

An interventional pilot study published in 2003 evaluated whether periodontal treatment would reduce the risk of having a PTLBW *(26)*. Three hundred thirty-six pregnant women with at least three sites of clinical attachment loss of more than 3 mm were studied at 21 to 25 weeks of pregnancy. The greatest decrease in PTLBW was found in the group treated with scaling and root planing, with 4.1% of PTLBW, compared with 12.7% in the untreated group.

It is well-documented that without treatment directed at reduction of plaque levels, existing gingivitis may worsen considerably during pregnancy *(12,13)*. Studies suggest that pregnant patients or patients considering pregnancy maintain the highest level of oral health, and be encouraged to seek a professional evaluation and care as soon as possible. Pregnant women should be encouraged to continue regular dental visits. The majority of pregnant women can receive anti-infective and emergency dental treatment (including radiographs needed to evaluate problems) throughout the pregnancy. Communication among all health professionals may be necessary if special medical concerns exist. The health of the pregnant patient and the health of her baby depends on it.

Oral Contraceptive Use

Oral contraceptives contain combinations of progesterone and estrogen that after long-term, cumulative use can create the same effect in the gingiva as can be observed in the pregnant patient. The gingival effects can depend on the duration of use and the combination of hormones prescribed. Some patients complain of fiery red, enlarged, and hemorrhagic tissues.

There is a twofold to threefold increase in the incidence of painful, dry sockets (localized osteitis) after tooth extraction in women taking oral contraceptives *(27)*. A dry socket occurs after a tooth is extracted and a poor clot develops and the socket bone becomes exposed. To minimize the risk of a dry socket, it is recommended that women who take oral contraceptives schedule the extraction on the placebo days of their cycle (days 23–28) *(28)*. However, if this is not possible, the dentist can take additional precautions to minimize this occurrence.

Patients should be referred to a dental professional for evaluation and treatment. The treatment for gingivitis occurring with oral contraceptive use is similar to the treatment of gingivitis in other life cycles. Changing the oral contraceptive may also have an impact on lessening the inflammation. In extreme situations when inflammation persists, physicians may consider recommending another form of birth control.

Menopause

We also see changes in oral and periodontal tissues at the time of menopause, when production of sex hormones diminishes and ultimately ceases. Common findings among a significant number of postmenopausal women are occurrences of pain, burning sensation (burning mouth syndrome), altered taste perception, atrophic glossitis, chronic aphthous ulcers, and xerostomia. In addition, postmenopausal women have been found to have decreased unstimulated saliva flow, which has been associated with increased dental caries and alterations in taste *(29)*. It is not clear at this time if the saliva changes are related to reduction in estrogen or other systemic factors. Any of these findings should be further investigated.

Postmenopausal women may also experience changes in the oral mucosa varying from an atrophic and pale appearance to a condition known as menopausal gingivostomatitis. This condition is characterized by gingiva that is abnormally pale to deep red in color, dry, shiny, and smooth. The soft tissues may be thinner and the gingiva more likely to recede (Fig. 4). These findings can be the direct result of reduced estrogen levels, which help regulate cellular proliferation, differentiation, and keratinization of the gingival epithelium. Oral cytology of postmenopausal women demonstrated that oral mucosa is in many ways similar to vaginal mucosa *(30)*. Both are composed of stratified squamous epithelium and both demonstrate a desquamative growth pattern. The decrease in estrogen levels accompanying menopause results in a decrease in keratinization and atrophy of the vaginal and oral mucosa.

The loss of estrogen in menopause results in an increase of cytokines in the bone remodeling circuitry, increasing the risk for osteopenia and osteoporosis. The generalized bone loss from systemic osteoporosis may render the jaws more susceptible to accelerated alveolar bone resorption and decrease in the mean bone density of the mandible *(31)*.

A series of research articles have demonstrated a significant correlation between mandibular basal bone mineral density and systemic bone mineral density *(32–35)*. Data from the Women's Health Initiative Oral Health Ancillary Study confirmed these findings and found that image analysis of specially formatted intraoral radiographs could be used to determine whether basal mandibular bone mineral density correlated with hip bone mineral density determined by dual energy X-ray absorptiometry *(31)*. Although radiographs are often taken as part of the dental examination, they should

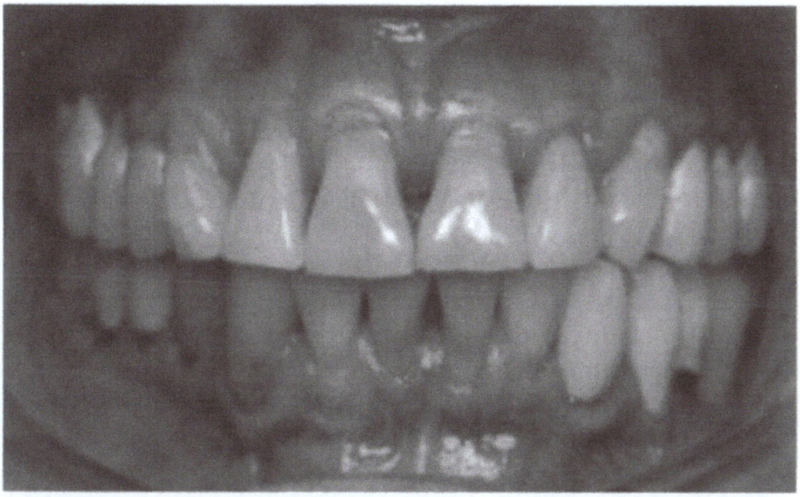

Fig. 4. Menopausal gingivostomatitis.

not be used as diagnostic, but rather to refer patients for appropriate evaluation and treatment.

Several studies have demonstrated a relationship between tooth loss and systemic osteoporosis. Women with low bone mineral density tend to have fewer teeth compared with controls *(36,37)*. After a 7-year longitudinal study showed that the rate of systemic bone loss was considered a predictor of tooth loss in postmenopausal women, researchers suggested that systemic bone loss may be a risk factor for tooth loss *(36,38)*. There is also evidence that estrogen replacement therapy is beneficial in reducing the risk of tooth loss in postmenopausal women *(39–41)*.

Unlike the clear relationship between osteoporosis and tooth loss, controversy still exists concerning the association between osteopenia/osteoporosis and periodontal disease. Several studies suggest that the incidence and rate of progression of periodontal disease increases after menopause, and that osteoporotic women present with greater periodontal attachment loss than non-osteoporotic women *(42–44)*. It is not clear whether there is a direct relationship between osteopenia/osteoporosis and periodontal disease, or whether the relationship may be explained, in part, by estrogen deficiency. This is demonstrated by the fact that women treated with supplemental estrogen experience less attachment loss and gingival bleeding compared with estrogen-deficient women *(32,45,46)*. Thus, estrogen deficiency is likely a factor in increasing the incidence and rate of progression of periodontal disease in women after menopause.

In view of the current trend of increasing and widespread use of chronic bisphosphonate therapy, the health care provider should be aware of reports of a risk of osteonecrosis of the jaw bones in patients being administered intravenous bisphosphonates. Knowledge of this should alert practitioners to monitor for this previously unrecognized potential complication. An early diagnosis might prevent or reduce the morbidity resulting from advanced destructive lesions of the jaw bone *(47)*.

At this time, there is no definitive evidence to support a decrease in the rate of dental implant success in osteoporotic patients. However, there is evidence that patients with poor quality bone and patients who are smokers have a decreased success rate of dental implants. Smoking may have an adverse effect on bone, and various mechanisms are being studied. Further research is necessary to support the claims that smoking may be associated with increased bone loss.

CONDITIONS AFFECTING WOMEN'S ORAL HEALTH

Eating Disorders

The most dramatic oral problems observed in eating-disordered individuals stem from self-induced vomiting. Although this symptom is more characteristic of the syndrome of bulimia nervosa, a subgroup of anorectic individuals also engage in self-induced vomiting with or without previous binge eating.

The most common and dramatic effect of chronic regurgitation of gastric contents is smooth erosion of enamel or perimylolysis. This manifests as a loss of enamel and dentin on the lingual surfaces of the teeth as a result of chemical and mechanical effects caused mainly by regurgitation of gastric contents and activated by movements of the tongue. This erosion typically is initially observed on the palatal surfaces of the maxillary anterior teeth and has a smooth, glassy appearance. There are few, if any, stains or lines in the teeth, and when the posterior teeth are affected, there is often a loss of occlusal anatomy. Perimylolysis is usually clinically observable after the patient has been binge eating and purging for at least 2 years *(48)*.

There seems to be a relationship, albeit not a perfect correlation, between the extent of tooth erosion and the frequency and degree of regurgitation, as well as with oral hygiene habits *(48)*. For example, some patients do not regurgitate all of the low pH stomach contents and, thereby, avoid severe enamel erosion.

Enlargement of the parotid glands and occasionally the sublingual glands are frequent oral manifestations of the binge–purge cycle in eating-disordered individuals *(49)*. The incidence of unilateral or bilateral parotid swelling in patients who frequently binge eat and purge has been estimated at between 10 and 50%. The occurrence and extent of parotid swelling is proportional to the duration and severity of the bulimic behavior *(48)*.

The etiology of this salivary gland swelling is still not identified, but most investigators have associated it with recurrent vomiting. The mechanisms, in this case, may be cholinergic stimulation of the glands during vomiting, or autonomic stimulation of the glands by activation of the taste buds *(49)*.

The oral mucosa membranes and the pharynx may also be traumatized in patients who binge eat and purge, both by the rapid ingestion of large amounts of food and by the force of regurgitation *(50)*. The soft palate may be injured by objects used to induce vomiting, such as fingers, combs, and pens. Dehydration, erythema, and angular cheilitis have also been observed *(50,51)*.

In light of the orofacial manifestations associated with bulimia nervosa, it is optimal for the dentist to be involved in the patient's comprehensive care.

It is widely recommended that dental treatment begin with a rigorous hygiene and fluoride regimen to prevent further destruction of tooth structures *(52)*.

Recommendations for the health care professional include:

- Rinsing with water immediately after vomiting and followed, if possible, by a 0.05% sodium fluoride rinse (available over the counter) to neutralize acids and protect tooth surfaces. It has been noted that tooth brushing at this time might accelerate the enamel erosion *(48,53)*.
- Use of artificial salivas for patients with severe xerostomia.

TMD

The National Institute of Dental and Craniofacial Research of the National Institutes of Health indicate that 10.8 million people in the United States suffer from TMD at any given time. Both men and women experience TMD, however, it affects women of childbearing age more than any other group *(54)*.

Some of the causes of TMD may include:

- Accidents or shock to the head and neck caused by a fall, sports injury, or car accident
- Health problems, such as arthritis or sinus and tooth infections
- Genetic or congenital abnormalities
- Poorly fitted dentures
- Bite problems in which upper and lower teeth do not fit properly
- Stress or parafunctional habits (clenching and grinding teeth) may be factors

Early detection of TMD is vital to a patient's successful treatment because it allows for more treatment options. TMD patients generally experience one or more of the following signs and symptoms:

- Facial pain
- Pain in the jaw joint and surrounding tissues including the ear
- Jaw locking open or closed
- Limited opening or inability to open the mouth
- Neck or shoulder pain

- Swelling on the side of the face
- Changes in the way the teeth fit together and/or occlusal (bite) discomfort
- Headaches
- Clicking or popping sounds (crepitus) when opening or closing mouth

Patients may unknowingly have signs or symptoms of TMD and the health history is a good way of identifying possible problems. A report of frequent migraines, headaches, or neck pain, may be the first indication of TMD. TMD symptoms are not easy to diagnose, because they are often similar to other disorders and many patients may have intermittent symptoms similar to TMD.

When TMD is suspected, referral to a dentist may be indicated. The following treatment may be recommended:

- Moist heat applied to painful areas
- Muscle relaxants, analgesics, or anti-inflammatory medications
- Soft diet
- Relaxation techniques
- Decreasing harmful clenching or grinding (bruxing) by wearing a special night guard or bite plate that prevents the teeth from touching while sleeping
- Fixing uneven or improper bites by adjusting or selectively grinding some teeth
- Orthodontic treatment may also be recommended to help reduce problems caused by poorly aligned teeth

If the jaw joints are affected and other treatments have been unsuccessful, surgery may be an option. It is usually reserved for advanced cases in which no other treatment plan has been successful *(54)*.

Intimate Partner Violence and Domestic Violence

Surveys suggest that 25% of women in the United States have reported partner violence at some time during their lives, creating a one in four lifetime chance for experiencing family violence *(55)*. The Centers for Disease Control and Prevention reports that approximately one in three female homicides is caused by intimate partner violence *(56)*. Contrary to commonly held beliefs, abuse happens to women of all ages, races, religions, income and education level, and sexual orientation.

Research has shown that the majority (68–94%) of these victims suffer head and neck trauma, including injuries to the orofacial structures *(57)*. These injuries may present as lacerations, fractures, and bruising. The physician and other health care providers have the responsibility to help identify women who may be in an abusive relationship. This can be very difficult because victims are reluctant to disclose abuse to their health care providers mainly because of the fear of their partner's retaliation, shame, humiliation, and denial regarding the seriousness of the abuse, and concern regarding confidentiality. The health care provider may need to refer victims to appropriate dental and/or medical specialists to address injuries sustained to the orofacial complex or head and neck region. In addition, most importantly, the health care provider must adhere to guidelines for screening, diagnosis, and treatment that have been developed and disseminated by numerous professional organizations.

CONCLUSION

In conclusion, we have addressed the hormonal effects on the oral cavity as well as other oral manifestations encountered during various stages in women's lives. Several conditions and concerns primarily affecting women, including eating disorders, TMD, and intimate partner/domestic violence with findings in the head and neck region including the orofacial complex, have also been discussed.

It was our intent to enlighten the healthcare provider of these sex-specific oral conditions, because oral health is an integral component of general health and will have a major impact on providing optimal care to female patients.

REFERENCES

1. Kornman K, Page R, Tonetti M. The host response to the microbial challenge in periodontitis: assembling the players. Periodontol 2000 1997;14:33–53.
2. American Dental Association. Periodontal diseases: preventing tooth loss. American Dental Association, Chicago, IL, 2003.
3. Vittek J, Hernandez M, Wenk E, Rappaport S, Southren A. Specific estrogen receptors in human gingiva. J Clin Endocrinol Metab 1982;54:608–612.
4. Mealey B, Rees T, Rose L, Grossi S. Systemic factors impacting the periodontium. In: Periodontics: Medicine, Surgery and Implants (Rose L, Mealey B, Genco R, Cohen D, eds.). Elsevier Mosby, St. Louis, 2004; pp. 790–845.
5. American Academy of Periodontology. Women and Periodontal Disease 21998. American Academy of Periodontology, Chicago, IL.
6. American Dental Association. Women and Gum Disease. Chicago, IL, 2002.
7. Loe H, Siness J. Periodontal disease in pregnancy: I. Prevalence and severity. Acta Odontol Scand 1963;21:533–551.
8. Loe H. Periodontal changes in pregnancy. J Periodontol 1965;36:209–216.
9. Cohen D, Shapiro J, Friedman L, Kyle G, Franklin S. A longitudinal investigation of the periodontal changes during pregnancy and fifteen months post-partum (Part II). J Periodontol 1971;42:653–657.
10. Sooriyamoorthy M, Gower D. Hormonal influences on gingival tissue: relationship to periodontal disease. J Clin Periodontol 1989;16:201–208.
11. Amar S, Chung K. Influence of hormonal variation on the periodontium in women. Periodontol 2000 1994;6:78–87.
12. Ferris G. Alteration in female sex hormones: their effect on oral tissues and dental treatment. Compend Contin Educ Dent 1993;14:1558–1570.
13. Zachariasen R. The effect of elevated ovarian hormones on periodontal health: oral contraceptives and pregnancy. Women Health 1993;20:21–30.
14. Raber-Durlacher J, Zeijlemaker W, Meinesz A, Abraham-Inpijn L. CD4 to CD8 ratio and invitro lymphoproliferative responses during experimental gingivitis in pregnancy and post-partum. J Periodontol 1991;62:663–667.

15. Raber-Durlacher J, Leene W, Palmer-Bouva C, Raber J, Abraham-Inpijn L. Experimental gingivitis during pregnancy and post-partum: Immunohistochemical aspects. J Periodontol 1993;64:211–218.
16. Mariotti A. Sex steroid hormones and cell dynamics in the periodontium. Crit Rev Oral Biol Med 1994;5:27–53.
17. O'Neil T. Plasma female sex-hormone levels and gingivitis in pregnancy. J Periodontol 1979;50:279–282.
18. Thomson M, Pack A. Effects of extended systemic and topical folate supplementation on gingivitis in pregnancy. J Clin Periodontol 1982;9:275–280.
19. Kornman K, Loesche W. The subgingival microflora during pregnancy. J Periodont Res 1980;15:111–122.
20. Jensen J, Liljemark W, Bloomquist C. The effect of female sex hormones on subgingival plaque. J Periodontol 1981;52:599–602.
21. Kornman K, Loesche W. Effects of estradiol and progesterone on *Bacterioides melaninogenicus*. Infect Immun 1982;35:256–263.
22. Arafat A. The prevalence of pyogenic granuloma in pregnant women. J Baltimore Coll Dent Surg 1974;29:64–70.
23. El-Ashiry GM, El-Kafrawy AH, Nasr MF, Younis N. Comparative study of the influence of pregnancy and oral contraceptives on the gingivae. Oral Surgery 1970;30:472–475.
24. Rateitschak K. Tooth mobility changes in pregnancy. J Periodontol 1967;2:199–206.
25. Offenbacher S, Katz V, Fertik G, et al. Periodontal disease as a possible risk factor for preterm low birth weight. J Periodontol 1996;67(Suppl):1103–1113.
26. Jeffcoat M, Hauth J, Geurs N, et al. Periodontal disease and preterm birth: results of a pilot intervention study. J Periodontol 2003;74:1214–1218.
27. Sweet J, Butler D. Increased incidence of postoperative localized osteitis in mandibular 3rd molar surgery associated with patients using oral contraceptives. Am J Obset Gynecol 1977;127(5):518–519.
28. Castellini J, Harvey D, Erickson S, Cherkin D. Effect of oral contraceptive cycle on dry socket (localized alveolar osteitis). J Am Dent Assoc 1980;101(5):777–780.
29. Lindquist L, Rockler B, Carlsson G. Bone resorption around fixtures in edentulous patients treated with mandibular fixed tissue-integrated prostheses. J Prosthet Dent 1988; 59:59–63.
30. Zachariasen R. Oral manifestations of menopause. Compend Contin Educ Dent 1993;14: 275–280.
31. Jeffcoat MK, Lewis C, Reddy M, et al. Post-menopausal bone loss and its relationship to oral bone loss. Periodontol 2000;23:94–102.
32. Jacobs R, Ghyselen J, Koninckx P, vanSteenberghe D. Long-term bone mass evaluation of mandible and lumbar spine in a group of women receiving hormone replacement therapy. Eur J Oral Sci 1996;104:10–16.
33. Kribbs P, Smith D, Chestnut C. Oral findings in osteoporosis. Part II. Relationship between residual ridge and alveolar bone resorption and generalized skeletal osteopenia. J Prosthet Dent 1983;50:719–724.
34. Kribbs P, Chesnut C, Ott S, Kilcyne R. Relationships between mandibular and skeletal bone in a population of normal women. J Prosthet Dent 1990;63:86–89.
35. Kribbs PJ. Comparison of mandibular bone in normal and osteoporotic women. J Prosthet Dent 1992;63:218–222.
36. Daniell HW. Postmenopausal tooth loss. Contributions to edentulism by osteoporosis and cigarette smoking. Arch Intern Med 1983;143:218–222.
37. Daniell H. Postmenopausal tooth loss. Contributions to edentulism by osteoporosis and cigarette smoking. Arch Intern Med 1983;143:1678–1682.

38. Krall E, Garcia R, Dawson-Hughes B. Increased risk of tooth loss is related to bone loss at the whole body, hip, and spine. Calcif Tisue Int 1996;59:433–437.
39. Grodstein F, Colditz G, Stamfer G. Post-menopausal hormone use and tooth loss: a prospective study. J Am Dent Assoc 1996;127:370–377.
40. Paganini-Hill A. Benefits of estrogen replacement therapy on oral health: the leisure world cohort. Arch Intern Med 1995;155:2325–2329.
41. Krall E, Dawson-Hughes B, Hannan M, et al. Post-menopausal estrogen replacement and tooth retention. Am J Med 1997;102:536–542.
42. Von Wowern N, Klausen B, Kollerup G. Osteoporosis: a risk factor in periodontal disease. J Periodontoly 1994;65:1134–1138.
43. Wactawski-Wende J, Grossi SG, Trevisan M, et al. The role of osteopenia in oral bone loss and periodontal disease. J Periodontol 1996;67(10):1076–1084.
44. Grossi S, Nishida M, Wactawski-Wende J, et al. Skeletal osteopenia increases the risk for periodontal disease. J Dent Res 1998;77.
45. Norderyd O, Grossi S, Machtei E, et al. Periodontal status of women taking post-menopausal estrogen supplementation. J Periodontol 1993;64:957–962.
46. Payne J, Zachs N, Reinhardt R, et al. The association between estrogen status and alveolar bone density changes in postmenopausal women with a history of periodontitis. J Periodontol 1997;68:24–31.
47. Ruggiero S, Mehrotra B, Rosenberg T, Engroff S. Osteonecrosis of the jaws associated with the use of bisphosphonates: a review of 63 cases. J Oral Maxillofac Surg 2004; 62(5):527–534.
48. Brown S, Bonifaz D. An overview of anorexia and bulimia nervosa and the impact of eating disorders on the oral cavity. Compend Contin Educ Dent 1993;14(12):1594–1608.
49. Mandel L, Kaynar A. Bulimia and parotid swelling: a review and case report. J Oral Maxillofac Surg 1992;50:1122–1125.
50. Ruff J, Koch M, Perkins S. Bulimia: dentomedical complications. Gen Dent 1992;40: 22–25.
51. Halmi K. Anorexia nervosa—recent investigations. Annu Rev Med 1970;29:137–148.
52. Steinberg B. Women's oral health issues. J Calif Dent Assoc 2000;28(9):663–667.
53. American Dental Association. Women's Oral Health Issue. Oral Health Care Series, 1995; pp. 22–25. American Dental Association, Chicago, IL.
54. American Dental Association. Temporomandibular Diorders. American Dental Association, Chicago, IL, 2003.
55. Tjaden P, Thoennes N. Prevalence, incidence and consequences of violence against women: findings from the National Violence Against Women Survey (Department of Justice, ed.). Research in Brief, Washington, DC, 1998.
56. Paulozzi L, Saltzman L, Thompson M, Holmgreen P. Surveillance for homicide among intimate partners—United States 1981–1998. MMWR CDC Surveillance Summary 2001;50(3):1–15.
57. Love C, Gerbert B, Caspers N. Dentists attitudes and behaviors regarding domestic violence. J Am Dent Assoc 2001;132:85–93.
58. Little J, Falace D, Miller C, Rhodus N. Dental Management of Medically Compromised Patients; 6th ed. CV Mosby Co, St. Louis, 2002.

15 Eating Disorders

Primary Care Assessment and Management

Amy L. Clouse, MD

Contents

INTRODUCTION

Eating disorders are among the most common psychiatric problems in the United States. Anorexia nervosa and bulimia nervosa in particular are associated with significant medical and psychiatric morbidity, with a mortality rate of 10%, the highest of all psychiatric disorders. Although primary care providers are often the first to identify patients with eating disorders, more than half of all cases go undiagnosed *(1)*. Primary care providers can learn to recognize eating disorders, manage the medical complications as they develop, and know when to refer patients for additional treatment.

From: *Current Clinical Practice: Women's Health in Clinical Practice*
Edited by: Clouse and Sherif © Humana Press Inc., Totowa, NJ

CLASSIFICATION

Anorexia nervosa is defined by the *Diagnostic and Statistical Manual, 4th edition (2)* as a refusal to maintain body weight at or above 85% of the expected weight for age and height, accompanied by an intense fear of gaining weight, an undue emphasis on body shape or weight, and amenorrhea for 3 consecutive months. Anorexia nervosa is further subdivided into restricting and purging subtypes. Those with the more common restricting type will severely restrict food intake and often overexercise, whereas those with the binge–purge subtype will also engage in purging behavior.

The same undue emphasis on body weight and shape is observed in bulimia nervosa. Additionally, bulimia nervosa is characterized by recurrent episodes of binge eating at least twice weekly for 3 months or more *(2)*. A binge is defined as eating an amount of food generally larger than what most people would eat during a defined time period, associated with a sense of lack of control over eating. There are also two subtypes of bulimia: the purging type and the non-purging type. In the purging type, binges are followed by some inappropriate compensatory behavior to avoid weight gain, such as self-induced vomiting, or the misuse of laxatives, diuretics, or enemas. Intermittent fasting or excessive exercise instead of purging compensates for binge eating in the nonpurging type.

The third eating disorder category is eating disorder not otherwise specified. This category includes all those that do not meet the strict criteria for either anorexia or bulimia and probably accounts for up to 50% of eating disorders overall *(2)*. Binge-eating disorder falls under this classification. Binge-eating disorder is similar to bulimia nervosa in that there is binge eating and loss of control over eating but not the compensatory behaviors to avoid weight gain. It is estimated that binge-eating disorder accounts for 30% of all medical obesity observed in the outpatient setting and is present in up to 50% of bariatric surgery candidates *(3)*.

Clinically, there is considerable overlap between the defined categories. It is not uncommon for patients to move to different points along the entire spectrum of eating and dieting disorders during the course of their lifetime *(4)*. Restricting anorexics may start to binge and purge when they no longer lose weight with caloric restriction alone or bulimics may add more anorexic type behavior whenever they have gained weight. The common theme however for all patients with eating disorders is the profound disturbance in perception of self-image.

EPIDEMIOLOGY

The estimated lifetime prevalence of anorexia nervosa is nearly 3%, whereas the lifetime prevalence for bulimia nervosa is reported as high as 5% *(5)*.

Women are 10 times more likely than men to suffer from eating disorders and young women and adolescents are more susceptible than older women. However, this gender difference is less pronounced in binge-eating disorder, with a 3:2 ratio of female to male patients *(6)*. Eating disorders occur across all racial and ethnic groups, but seem to be more common in white women than in African Americans. Anorexia is particularly rare in African Americans, who are more likely to have binging-type disorders such as bulimia or binge-eating disorder *(7)*.

ETIOLOGY

The etiology of an eating disorder is not well understood, though it is probably multifactorial, involving family history, personal psychology, and sociocultural factors. Multiple sources point to a cultural value on thinness to account for the recent increase in incidence of eating disorders in the United States and other Westernized countries. For example, the body mass index (BMI) of Miss America has steadily decreased since 1922, so much so that the majority of the pageant winners since 1970 fall below the World Health Organization's definition of undernutrition *(8)*. The media's depiction of an unrealistic female body image may also play a role in the development of eating disorders. Reading women's magazines and listening to the radio more than once per week was associated with a higher likelihood of developing an eating disorder in one prospective study of more than 2500 young girls *(9)*. Additionally, prolonged exposure to Western television was found to increase Fijian adolescent girls' weight concerns and vomiting for weight control *(10)*.

Any activity that promotes thinness or a particular weight classification, such as ballet dancing, modeling, gymnastics, or wrestling, can predispose someone to develop an eating disorder *(11)*. Certain personality traits, such as low self-esteem, difficulty expressing negative emotions, difficulty resolving conflict, and being a perfectionist are also contributing factors *(12)*. Diabetes mellitus type 1 may also be a risk factor for developing an eating disorder. Up to one-third of women with type 1 diabetes may have an eating disorder or at least have disordered eating behaviors not specifically meeting anorexia or bulimia diagnostic criteria *(13)*.

Family history can further contribute to developing an eating disorder. For anorexia, heritability has been estimated to be up to 70% *(14)* and for binge eating, this number is almost 50% *(15)*. Some twin studies also show a strong link, whereas others show no correlation *(16)*. Recent research has revealed that a mutation in one of the genes involved in appetite regulation, the melanocortin-4 receptor gene, is associated with binge eating in obese individuals *(17)*.

Although historical and cultural factors may predispose patients to develop an eating disorder, there is some evidence that there can be a precipitating event. These factors could include a significant stressor, either negative or positive, present in approx 60% of patients *(18)*. Sometimes a very specific event, such as weight-related comments by friends and family could trigger a predisposed person to develop an eating disorder *(19)*.

Once an eating disorder has developed, psychiatric comorbidity may contribute to its maintenance. Major depression is the most common psychiatric disorder, diagnosed in approx 60% of patients, with anxiety disorders and substance abuse observed in 30% of patients admitted to hospitals for their eating disorder *(4)*. Other psychiatric diagnoses observed in eating-disordered patients include posttraumatic stress syndrome and obsessive–compulsive disorders. Further sustaining factors could include social praise for weight loss, a sense of self-control leading to a rise in self-esteem, or physiological factors, such as the discomfort and bloating that may come with eating normally *(19)*.

SCREENING

Early detection and intervention may improve prognosis *(20)*, therefore, all patients at high risk for eating disorders should be screened at routine office visits. There are many comprehensive psychiatric inventories available for diagnosing eating disorders *(5)*, but these are too cumbersome in the primary care office setting. Table 1 reviews two screening questionnaires designed for use in a primary care setting *(21,22)*. Both have 100% sensitivity making them useful as rapid screening tools, however, their lower specificity, 87.5% for the SCOFF and 71% for the Eating Disorder Screen for Primary Care, make them unsuitable purely as diagnostic tests. A positive screen should be followed with more specific questions to define disordered-eating behaviors and body image perceptions.

INITIAL EVALUATION

Patients with eating disorders can present to their primary care providers in a variety of ways. Although some patients may have the classic symptoms of weight loss and refusal to gain weight, most patients will present with nonspecific complaints, such as fatigue, cold intolerance, dizziness, or lack of energy. Patients may also deny any symptoms, but their friends or family members might express concern regarding behavior changes, multiple empty laxative and/or diet pills boxes, or significant weight fluctuations. Amenorrhea is the most common presenting symptom for those who do seek treatment *(11)*.

The initial interview should focus on dietary intake, exercise, and body image perception. It is also important that an assessment include a full history of weight, dieting behaviors, and the use of diuretics, diet pills, syrup of ipecac, or laxatives. Establishing rapport with the patient is critical at this point, especially when the patient may not perceive a problem with her behaviors *(13)*.

Table 1
Screening Tools for Eating Disorders

SCOFF Questionnaire (21)
Do you make yourself **S**ick because you feel uncomfortably full?
Do you worry you have lost **C**ontrol over how much you eat?
Have you recently lost more that **O**ne stone (14 pounds) in a 3-mo period?
Do you believe yourself to be **F**at when others say you are too thin?
Would you say that **F**ood dominates your life?

One point for every "yes" answer. A score of 2 or more indicates an eating disorder with 100% sensitivity and 87.5% specificity.

ESP (Eating Disorder Screen for Primary Care) Questions (22)
Are you satisfied with your eating patterns?
Do you ever eat in secret?
Does your weight affect the way you feel about yourself?
Have any members of your family suffered with an eating disorder?
Do you currently suffer with or have you ever suffered in the past with an eating disorder?

One point for a "no" answer to first question and every "yes" answer to other questions. A score of 2 or more indicates an eating disorder with 100% sensitivity and 71% specificity.

The medical implications of anorexia and bulimia can impact nearly every organ system. However, aside from weight loss, many patients will have a completely normal exam on presentation, significantly contributing to a patient's denial. Table 2 compares important signs and symptoms for both anorexia and bulimia.

The physical exam should include measurement of weight and height. Scales should be in a private area and weigh-ins performed in a consistent manner. Some eating-disordered patients may attempt to distort their weight on the scale by drinking large amounts of fluid beforehand or by wearing weights *(13)*, so weighing patients in gowns could become necessary. Staff should be aware that discussions with patients regarding weight or appearance might be harmful to recovery.

A patient's weight should be expressed as a percent of her ideal body weight or with her BMI. Ideal body weight is traditionally calculated by the simple formula of allowing 100 lbs for the first five feet of height for a woman and 110 lb for the first 5 ft of height for a man and adding 5 lb for each additional inch. BMI, weight in kilograms divided by height in meters squared, can also be used to characterize an eating disordered patient's weight. Anorexia is typically defined by a BMI of 16 kg/m^2 or less.

Table 2
Important Signs and Symptoms of Anorexia Nervosa and Bulimia Nervosa[a]

Organ System	*Anorexia Nervosa*	*Bulimia Nervosa*
Body	Weakness, malnutrition	
Central nervous system	Decreased concentration, depressed irritable mood, cognitive impairment	
Cardiovascular	Palpitations, weakness, dizziness, bradycardia, shortness of breath, chest pain, cold intolerance, orthostatic hypotension	Palpitations, weakness, cardiac abnormalities (in ipecac abusers)
Endocrine, metabolic	Fatigue, cold intolerance, hypothermia	Weakness, poor skin turgor
Gastrointestinal	Abdominal pain and distension, bloating, constipation	Abdominal pain and distension, constipation, bloating, bowel irregularities, gastritis, gastroesophagoal reflux, hemaetemesis
Hematologic	Cold intolerance, bruising	
Integument	Hair loss, lanugo hair	Scarring on the dorsum of hand (Russell's sign)
Muscular	Muscle wasting	
Oropharyngeal	Dental decay, dental caries, enlarged salivary glands	
Reproductive	Amenorrhea, fertility problems	Menstrual irregularities, fertility problems

[a]Adapted from ref. *5*.

Initial laboratory work-up is geared toward identifying complications of eating disorders and excluding other causes or coexisting diseases. Testing should include a complete blood cell count and measurements of serum electrolytes, including magnesium, phosphorus, and calcium, blood urea nitrogen, creatinine, albumin, thyroid stimulating hormone, and liver function studies. All amenorrheic patients also deserve assessment with follicle-stimulating hormone, luteinizing hormone, and prolactin, and possibly a pregnancy test if they have been sexually active. Additional laboratory work is guided by the history and physical exam findings and used specifically to exclude other causes or complications of eating-disordered behaviors.

In addition to laboratory work, evaluation should include bone densitometry with a dual-energy X-ray absorptiometry (DXA) scan in all patients who have had a history of anorexia or 6 months of amenorrhea. An electrocardiogram is indicated to screen for potential cardiac complications.

DIFFERENTIAL DIAGNOSIS

A broad range of medical disorders, including hyperthyroidism, malignancy, inflammatory bowel disease, immunodeficiency, malabsorption, chronic infection, Addison's disease, and diabetes should at least be considered before making a diagnosis of an eating disorder *(13)*. Most women with eating disorders, however, will have a distorted body image and a desire to lose more weight, making a comprehensive work-up for other medical conditions unnecessary.

COMPLICATIONS

Laboratory Disturbances

Laboratory values are often normal despite significant weight loss or purging behavior. Occasionally, mild leukopenia or anemia may be present, reflecting bone marrow suppression from malnutrition; this generally will resolve with weight gain *(23)*. Serum electrolytes should routinely be followed in those with both anorexia and bulimia, although electrolyte abnormalities are more common with purging. Hypokalemia, hypochloremia, and a metabolic alkalosis often indicate vomiting *(24)*. Hypokalemia might also represent diuretic or laxative abuse, whereas hyponatremia could suggest excessive water ingestion. A rise in blood urea nitrogen out of proportion to creatinine signaling dehydration can be from diuretics, laxatives, or decreased fluid intake in anorexia. Hypoglycemia, thought to be from loss of liver glycogen and glucose stores, is a poor prognostic sign if the glucose value is less than 40 mg/dL *(19)*. Liver enzyme levels are often normal in the early stages of illness and, if abnormal, may provide clues to comorbid medical conditions, such as hepatitis or excessive alcohol intake. Increases in liver transaminases can also be observed when high-glucose foods are used in refeeding.

Starvation creates a euthyroid sick profile with a low thyroxine and triiodothyronine, an elevated reverse triiodothyronine (reverse T3) and a normal thyroid-stimulating hormone level *(25)*. Minimally low or high thyroid-stimulating hormone levels may also be observed. Generally, these will all resolve with weight restoration. Furthermore, clinicians should use caution in treating mild hypothyroidism in these patients, because thyroid hormone replacement abuse solely for weight manipulation has been reported *(19)*.

Hypophosphatemia is of particular concern, causing serious complications, such as congestive heart failure. This phenomenon, known as refeeding syndrome, is generally observed in the early stages of refeeding in the inpatient setting, and will be covered in the "Cardiac" section below.

Cardiac

Cardiac complications are common among patients with eating disorders. Although anorexia nervosa accounts for the most premature deaths of all the psychiatric diagnoses, half of these deaths are attributed to cardiac manifestations *(19)*. Cardiac-related deaths are less common in those with bulimia, but still can occur as the result of electrolyte abnormalities.

The most immediate and life-threatening complications for those with eating disorders are prolongation of the QT interval and cardiac arrhythmias *(26,27)*. Prolonged QT intervals have been noted in up to 40% of anorexic patients *(28)*. Other electrocardiographic abnormalities in patients with eating disorders include bradycardia, low voltage, and U waves from hypokalemia. Underweight patients may also develop mitral or tricuspid valve prolapse; as they lose weight, the heart muscle diminishes in size, yet the structural tissue of the valves remains unchanged. The resultant ventriculovalvular disproportion can cause typical symptoms of mitral valve prolapse, including palpitations and chest discomfort *(19,29)*. These symptoms could be treated with β-blockers if no bradycardia or hypotension are present. Prolonged or particularly severe eating disorders can lead to cardiomyopathy or congestive heart failure.

The speed and extent of weight loss, the nature of various purging methods and the existence of comorbid conditions all contribute to the potential for cardiac complications. Rapid or severe weight loss with subsequent acute electrolyte abnormalities, especially those augmented with vomiting or abuse of enemas, laxatives, or diuretics, can lead to fatal arrhythmias. Furthermore, the chronic use of ipecac to induce vomiting can lead to cardiomyopathy. One bottle of syrup of ipecac contains up to 32 mg of emetine and the heart must be exposed to a minimum of 1250 mg of emetine during a several months period for cardiotoxicity to occur *(19)*. Although this cardiotoxicity has been reportedly reversible with stopping the drug *(30)*, there are also multiple case reports of patients with either bulimia or anorexia nervosa who have died from the cardiac toxicity of ipecac *(31)*.

Other existing medical disorders may also increase the cardiac risks in patients with eating disorders. Diabetic patients already at increased cardiovascular risk may further complicate this with electrolyte abnormalities or rapid weight loss. Those with thyroid disease may manipulate their medications to hasten weight loss, resulting in thyroid storm and, potentially, congestive heart failure. Electrolyte disturbances can occur more readily in those with chronic diarrhea from inflammatory bowel disorders, such as Crohn's disease or ulcerative colitis.

Treatment of cardiac complications begins with electrolyte repletion and slow weight restoration. Typically, up to 2 lb per week can be gained safely without risk for congestive heart failure. Hospitalization is recommended in those with extremely low potassium (<3.0 mEq/L), magnesium, or phosphate levels. Those with a prolonged QT interval may need to be hospitalized in the early stages of refeeding *(32)*, and all medications with the potential to increase the QT interval should clearly be avoided. Because bradycardia is common and often asymptomatic, cardiac monitoring is only necessary in those with a resting heart rate below 30 beats per minute, symptomatic orthostasis, or arrhythmias *(19)*.

The refeeding syndrome, a potentially dangerous syndrome that can result in congestive heart failure, cardiopulmonary collapse, and sudden death, can occur during nutritional rehabilitation. This usually occurs in very low-weight individuals with a reduced heart mass who are unable to handle rapid increases in blood volume. An associated hypophosphatemia develops as an influx of glucose causes a shift of phosphate into the intracellular space. The resultant hypophosphatemia can impact heart contractility, further contributing to heart failure *(19)*. Prevention of this syndrome requires identifying and hospitalizing those very low-weight individuals for monitoring during refeeding and close attention to electrolytes during inpatient nutritional stabilization *(33,34)*.

Oral

Oral and dental complications are common both in bulimics and in anorexics who vomit for weight control. Oral and pharyngeal trauma may be present from various instruments used to induce vomiting. Chronic irritation from gastric acid can lead to dental erosions and sensitivity, gingivitis, and angular chelosis. Gastric acid causes deterioration of tooth enamel, particularly involving the occlusal surfaces of molars and the posterior surfaces of the maxillary incisors *(35)*. Dental caries are also more prevalent in both bulimics and other binge eaters secondary to high carbohydrate binges *(36)*.

Although dental erosion is irreversible, gentle brushing, using a fluoride mouth rinse *(37)*, or rinsing with a baking soda solution (1 tsp/1 qt of water) *(19)* after purging may help to limit caries. All those with dental complications should be referred for dental care, preferably with a dentist skilled at working with patients with eating disorders *(36)*.

Another common oral manifestation is sialadenosis, a noninflammatory and usually painless salivary gland enlargement observed in up to 50% of bulimics *(19)*. The etiology of this enlargement of the parotid and submandibular salivary glands is multifactorial, involving the direct stimulation from vomiting, consuming high-calorie foods, and chronic metabolic alkalosis. Sialendosis usually occurs within a few days of a vomiting cycle and is associated with an elevated serum amylase in 60% of cases *(38)*. Treatment options include abstinence from vomiting, warm compresses, and sialogogues, such as sour candies. If these conservative measures are not successful within a few weeks, 5.0 mg pilocarpine three times a day can be used until symptoms resolve *(39)*. Rarely, parotidectomy could be considered for cosmetic improvement *(40)*.

Gastrointestinal

In anorexia, gastroparesis and constipation are common, with their associated sensations of bloating and abdominal pain often perpetuating the syndrome. These symptoms are usually transient and improve with weight gain and return to normal eating patterns *(41–43)*. Small meals, liquid supplements, or motility agents, such as metoclopramide, may help to relieve bloating *(11)*. Cisapride has also been shown to be effective for this purpose *(44)*, but because of its arrhythmia risk, is only available under a restricted access program in the United States *(45)*. It should be used with great caution in eating-disordered patients at risk for a prolonged QT interval. Ensuring adequate water intake, low-dose fiber supplementation, and/or addition of a nonstimulant laxative, such as sorbitol, may help with constipation. Gastroesophageal reflux can occur from gastroparesis and should be treated with antacids, H2 antagonists, or proton pump inhibitors for symptom relief. Abnormal liver function test results have also been described as both a consequence of severe calorie restriction and with refeeding *(46)*.

Because of the frequent binging and purging associated with bulimia nervosa, these patients often experience more severe gastrointestinal symptoms compared with those who solely restrict food. Dyspepsia is a common complaint *(47)* and continued exposure to stomach acid could lead to esophagitis, dysphagia, and odonyphagia as well as Barrett's esophagus *(48)*. These patients generally will require a H2 blocker or a proton pump inhibitor to relieve symptoms. Refractory cases should be referred for an upper endoscopy. Gastroesophageal erosions and, rarely, Mallory-Weiss tears are also potential complications of chronic self-induced vomiting *(49)*.

Laxative abuse as a form of purging is often difficult to treat because patients develop laxative dependence and a cathartic colon. Although bowel function will return to normal a few weeks after cessation of the stimulant laxatives *(50)*, the refractory constipation can cause patients to resume their laxative use or replace it with another form of purging behavior. Adequate fluid intake, a high-fiber diet, and moderate amounts of exercise in those without a history of excessive exercise should be encouraged. If constipation persists, a glycerin suppository along with an osmotic laxative, such as sorbitol or lactulose, may be helpful, although stool softeners are often not useful *(51)*.

Endocrine

Secondary amenorrhea affects more than 90% of patients with anorexia nervosa *(11)* although those with bulimia may have normal menstrual cycles, oligomenorrhea, or amenorrhea, depending on their weight and binge/purge behaviors *(51)*. The exact cause of this resultant amenorrhea is not known, although low body weight, excessive exercise, and emotional distress all probably contribute to a state of hypogonadotropic hypogonadism. Levels of serum follicle-stimulating hormone and luteinizing hormone are low relative to estradiol. Furthermore, the normal pulsatile pattern of gonadotropin-releasing hormone is lost. Withdrawal bleeding with either progesterone or a combined progesterone plus estrogen regimen may not occur as a result of this interruption in gonadotropin-releasing hormone pulsatility *(11,52)*.

Early research suggested a "critical weight" or body fat percentage necessary for menarche *(53)* that was later confirmed at approx 90% of ideal body weight needed for menses to return *(54)*. Low body weight is not the only factor contributing to amenorrhea, however, because up to 20% of patients may lose their menstrual cycle before the onset of weight loss and an additional 50% could experience amenorrhea in the course of dieting *(19)*. Furthermore, some elite athletes have been recorded as maintaining their menstrual cycle with body fat as low as 4.7% *(55)*. Research that is more recent has focused on leptin, a hormone produced in fat cells that acts on the hypothalamus to control weight, appetite, and energy expenditure, as the link between nutritional status and reproductive function *(56)*. Leptin levels are high in those with obesity and are reduced in acute starvation and weight loss *(57,58)*. Leptin is initially low in those with anorexia in treatment programs but increases with refeeding, partial weight gain, and resumption of menses *(59,60)*.

A progestin challenge test with 10 mg medroxyprogesterone daily for 5 days can be used to assess adequate estrogen effect in those patients with amenorrhea thought to be secondary to anorexia nervosa. Some sources recommend estrogen–progesterone therapy in those who do not have a withdrawal bleed after this challenge *(19)*. However, resumption of normal body weight and nutritional status should remain the mainstay of treatment, because an artificial resumption of menstrual cycle may be overly reassuring to low-weight patients. Menses will generally resume within 6 months of reaching 90% of the ideal body weight *(11,54)*. A serum estradiol level greater than 110.1 pmol/L or a weight approx 5 lb greater than the weight at which menses was lost are good predictors of resumption of the menstrual cycle *(11,61)*. Fertility generally returns to normal in those who recover their menstrual cycle and maintain a normal body weight *(56)*. It should be noted, however, that even amenorrheic women with eating disorders can become pregnant and should be offered contraception if sexually active *(11)*.

Osteoporosis and osteopenia represent serious clinical complications associated with eating disorders, because adolescence is a critical period for peak bone mass acquisition. Anorexia nervosa is associated with markedly reduced bone mineral density (BMD), especially at the lumbar spine. One study has suggested an almost threefold increase in long-term fracture risk in anorexics compared with age-matched controls *(62)*.

The mechanism for this decrease in bone density and failure to reach peak bone mass is complex. Certainly, estrogen deficiency and its subsequent amenorrhea contribute to this, as many studies suggest that the longer the duration of the amenorrhea, the larger the reduction in BMD *(63,64)*. This is further complicated by research indicating that patients with anorexia nervosa have more severe bone loss than amenorrheic athletes without anorexia *(57)*. High serum cortisol levels and low levels of insulin-like growth factor *(65,66)* as well as low androgen levels and an increase in bone-remodeling cytokines *(19)* have all been implicated in the osteoporosis in eating-disordered patients. These factors, together with excessive exercise, malnutrition, and the low estrogen state described above lead to reduced bone formation and increased bone resorption. This results in a relatively low bone turnover state, differentiating this phenomenon from postmenopausal osteoporosis.

Unfortunately, research has not supported the use of estrogen and progestin for increasing bone mass in adolescents with anorexia-related osteoporosis *(67–70)*. One randomized controlled trial did suggest that estrogen protected against further bone loss in young osteopenic women who had initial ideal body weights less than 70% *(67)*. Another observational study of 65 anorexics found that those patients taking oral contraceptives had a higher BMD at the spine (but not the femur) compared with those not on hormones, although still less than that of controls *(71)*. Overall, resumption of normal body weight continues to be the best predictor of increased bone density *(72)* and bone formation does seem to increase as nutritional intake improves *(73)*.

Weight normalization along with calcium supplementation at 1500 mg/d and 800 IU/d of vitamin D are currently considered the foundations for treatment *(19)*. Zinc deficiency may also play a role in weight loss and amenorrhea and routine multivitamins are recommended *(74)*. Research on the role of dehydroepiandrosterone *(75)*, menatetrenone (vitamin K2) *(76)* and insulin-like growth factor-1 *(77)* in increasing bone density is ongoing. Moderate exercise, although protective against osteoporosis in healthy women, could contribute to low body weight and amenorrhea in anorexic women and is not routinely recommended.

Other potential treatment modalities include calcitonin, bisphosphonates, and selective estrogen receptor modulators. All are Food and Drug Administration (FDA)-approved for postmenopausal osteoporosis but lack data for use in adolescents or in anorexia-induced osteoporosis. Bisphosphonates, in particular, are just beginning to be studied for this purpose and could be cautiously considered in cases of severe osteoporosis not responding to standard care *(11)*. A small, randomized placebo-controlled trial of alendronate for osteopenia in adolescents with anorexia nervosa showed that although those treated with alendronate did have increased BMD at the femoral neck, weight restoration was still the most important determinant of BMD *(78)*.

Clinicians should screen for osteopenia and osteoporosis with a DXA scan in women with anorexia nervosa and other eating disorders when amenorrhea is present for longer than 6 months. When interpreting these results, it is important to look at both T-score and Z-score calculations, especially in adolescent patients because not all machines have appropriate control data for young women. Current consensus dictates regular DXA scans every 1 to 2 years until resumption of menses and sufficient weight restoration *(11,79)*. Bone resorption markers, such as N-telopeptide and urinary desoxypyridinoline, may also be used in the interim to assess stabilization of bone turnover *(79,80)*.

Neurological

Cerebral atrophy is the most serious neurological complication, specifically in anorexia nervosa. Enlarged ventricles and decreased gray and white matter volume have been described *(81,82)*. Studies have indicated that a normal ventricular size accompanies weight restoration, although it is not clear if any brain dysfunction is completely reversible *(83,84)*. Although a brain MRI study is not indicated in all patients with eating disorders, some patixents with atypical features may need brain imaging to exclude other diseases.

TREATMENT

Once a diagnosis of an eating disorder has been established, the treatment plan depends on the severity of illness. Options can range from outpatient care to an inpatient psychiatric or medical hospitalization. The American Psychiatric Association has created practice guidelines for site of treatment based on weight and extent of medical and psychiatric complications *(5)*. These recommendations can be found online at the American Psychiatric Association website at www.psych.org. Although no controlled trials have indicated when an inpatient hospitalization is necessary for either anorexia or bulimia, generally accepted guidelines suggest that those with a weight more than 25% to 30% below ideal body weight, rapid or severe disease refractory to outpatient treatment, symptomatic hypotension or syncope, severe hypokalemia (serum potassium less than 2.0 to 3.0 m*M*), bradycardia of less than 40 beats per minute, arrhythmias, or prolonged QT interval all deserve hospitalization *(11,51)*.

Those with mild illness or who are within 10 to 15% of their ideal body weight can often be managed as outpatients. Once the diagnosis of an eating disorder has been established, the challenge for the primary care provider is often to redirect patient focus away from weight and body image preoccupation and to interrupt destructive behaviors *(4)*. Goals of treatment also include restoration and maintenance of a healthy weight, detection and treatment of any physical complications, management of psychiatric symptoms, and prevention of relapse. To attain these goals, appropriate outpatient treatment requires a multidisciplinary approach with a team of clinicians including a psychotherapist or psychologist, nutritionist, medical care provider, and often a psychiatrist. Team members should agree on a target weight goal, usually at least 90% of ideal body weight, and expect an approx1 lb/wk weight gain in the outpatient setting. Exercise is typically discouraged until a patient reaches her target weight. Because of the complex and often chronic nature of an eating disorder, team members should be skilled in working with this population and should communicate regularly to assess goals and progress.

The primary care provider's role is to regularly ascertain the patient's body weight and medical status. Follow-up visits every 2 to 4 weeks during initial treatment is appropriate with this interval increasing as the patient improves. The primary care provider is also responsible for monitoring and treating medical complications as they arise and offering continued education regarding proper health and nutrition and the long-term consequences of eating disorders.

Pharmacological Therapy

Currently, no medications are approved by the FDA for the treatment of anorexia nervosa. Many medications could lead to further weight loss and most are thought not to be effective in the malnourished state. A few uncontrolled clinical trials suggest a role for fluoxetine in preventing relapse in weight-restored patients *(85,86)*, yet not in hastening weight restoration *(87)*. Furthermore, a recent retrospective study of selective serotonin reuptake inhibitor use in anorexia failed to demonstrate treatment efficacy *(88)*. The medications currently being most widely studied are the atypical antipsychotics, particularly olanzapine, with several promising open-label and pilot studies *(89–91)*. New evidence suggests that these neuroleptics may help the obsessionality and resistance to treatment observed in low-weight patients with anorexia *(92,93)*.

Alternately, pharmacological interventions have been proven useful in treating bulimia nervosa. A recent Cochrane database review concluded that multiple classes of antidepressants, including tricyclics, selective serotonin reuptake inhibitors, monoamine oxidase inhibitors, buproprion, and trazadone have demonstrated efficacy in placebo-controlled trials in reducing the symptoms of bulimia *(94)*. The only medication to date approved by the FDA for the treatment of bulimia is fluoxetine at a dose of 60 mg/d. In multiple double-blinded, placebo-controlled trials, fluoxetine has demonstrated up to a 50% reduction in the number of binge-purge episodes per week compared with a 21% reduction from placebo *(95,96)*.

Other medications have also proved useful in small trials, although large placebo-controlled randomized studies are still needed. Three small short-term trials suggest using the serotonin-3 receptor antagonist, ondansetron, to decrease binge eating and vomiting in bulimia nervosa *(97)*. Symptom improvement with ondansetron is postulated to result from correction of abnormal vagal stimulation *(98)*. Topiramate, an anticonvulsant, has also been suggested as a novel treatment for the symptoms of bulimia *(99)*. One small, randomized controlled trial indicated not only a reduction in binge and purge behaviors but also improvements in self-esteem, eating attitudes, anxiety, and body image *(100,101)*. Furthermore, open trials of the yet to be FDA approved selective noradrenergic receptor inhibitor, reboxetine, demonstrate efficacy in treating bulimia *(102,103)*. Inositol also has been shown effective for bulimia and binge-eating disorder in a double-blinded, placebo-controlled trial of 12 patients *(104)*.

Research on treatment for binge-eating disorder is still in its early stages. The selective serotonin reuptake inhibitors, fluoxetine, fluvoxamine, sertraline, and citalopram, have shown modest decreases in binge-eating frequency in double-blinded, placebo-controlled trials *(105)*. Randomized controlled trials of the anti-obesity drug, sibutramine *(106)*, and topiramate *(107)* and a small prospective trial of the anticonvulsant zonisamide *(108)* show a decrease in binge-eating behavior as well as a decrease in body weight.

Psychological Therapy

Although psychological therapy is part of the multifaceted approach to anorexia, little research is available to assess its effectiveness, and few randomized controlled trials exist *(109)*. Individual psychotherapy is considered helpful *(110)*, as is family therapy, especially in adolescents *(111)*. Cognitive–behavioral therapy (CBT), aimed at helping patients change underlying assumptions and body image misperceptions, may also be useful in recovery for patients with anorexia nervosa *(112,113)*.

CBT is much better studied in bulimia and binge-eating disorder. Although only a small number of randomized control led trials exist, a Cochrane database review supports the use of this modality at least in the short term *(114)*. For example, a 5-month study of 220 patients with bulimia showed a 30% remission rate (defined as purging less than twice per week) with CBT compared with only 6% in the individual psychotherapy group *(115)*.

A combination of antidepressants and CBT seems to be a more effective treatment strategy to reduce frequency of binging and purging than either treatment alone. A Cochrane metanalysis reviewing data from five trials comparing antidepressants vs the combination found a 42% remission rate for both modalities compared with 23% for antidepressants (desipramine, imipramine, or fluoxetine) *(116)*. Further review of the seven trials of psychological treatments vs a combination found a pooled remission rate of 49% for the combination of antidepressants and therapy compared with 36% for any single therapy alone *(116)*. As a single approach, psychotherapy was more effective than medication *(116)*. Whenever CBT fails to be useful, however, additional treatment with individual psychotherapy or with medication (fluoxetine or desipramine) yielded only 16% or 10% effectiveness, respectively, in one randomized trial *(117)*.

PROGNOSIS

Eating-disordered patients have a variable course and prognosis. Early age at diagnosis, quick initiation of treatment, good parent–child relationships, and healthy connections with friends or therapists all predict better outcomes *(118)*. The percentage of patients who actually fully recover is small. It may, therefore, be helpful to frame the eating disorder in terms of a chronic illness for patients discouraged by relapse or repeated hospitalizations.

A review of long-term follow-up studies of hospitalized patients with anorexia showed that approx 44% of the patients had "good" outcomes, in which weight was restored to within 15% of ideal body weight and regular menstrual cycles returned. Approximately 24% had "poor" outcomes, with weights never reaching 85% of their ideal body weight and sporadic or absent menses and approx 28% fell between the two extremes *(5,119)*. Many studies suggest that bulimia has a more favorable prognosis than anorexia, with recovery rates spanning from 30 to 70% of those treated in outpatient settings, with relapse rates as high as 50% after 6 months to 6 years of follow-up *(5)*. For hospitalized patients however, recovery rates are lower, ranging from 13 to 40% *(120)*. Although long-term outcome data for binge-eating disorder is not yet available, one community study suggests that symptoms may resolve spontaneously in many patients *(121)*.

CONCLUSION

Anorexia, bulimia, and other forms of disordered eating are associated with considerable morbidity and mortality. In the current culture of thinness in the United States, they have become an increasingly important health concern for women. Unfortunately, prevention is still an understudied concept and has yet to play a large role in shaping these illnesses. A multidisciplinary team remains the mainstay of outpatient treatment. Those with severely low weights or serious medical complications require inpatient hospitalization. Primary care providers can play an important role in detecting eating disorders, managing the medical complications as they arise and working within a treatment team to restore normal weight and body image awareness.

REFERENCES

1. Becker AE, Grinspoon SK, Klibanski A, Herzog DB. Eating disorders. N Engl J Med 1999;340:1092–1098.
2. American Psychiatric Association. Diagnostic and statistical manual of mental disorders. 4th ed., text revision. Washington, DC: American Psychiatric Association, 2000: pp. 583–594.
3. De Zwaan M. Binge eating disorder and obesity. Int J Obes Relat Metab Disord 2001;25 (Suppl 1):S51–S55.
4. Guarda AS, Redgrave GW. Eating disorders: detection, assessment, and treatment in primary care. Adv Stud Med 2004;4(9):468–475.
5. American Psychiatric Association Work Group on Eating Disorders. Practice guideline for the treatment of patients with eating disorders (revision). Am J Psychiatry 2000;157(Suppl 1):1–39.
6. Dingemans AE, Bruna MJ, van Furth EF. Binge eating disorder: a review. Int J Obes 2002;26:299–307.
7. Striegel-Moore RH, Dohm FA, Kraemer HC, et al. Eating disorders in white and black women. Am J Psychiatry 2003;160:1326–1331.
8. Rubinstein S, Caballero B. Is Miss America an undernourished role model? JAMA 2000;283(12):1569.
9. Martinez-Gonzalez MA, Gual P, Lahortiga F, et al. Parental factors, mass media influences, and the onset of eating disorders in a prospective population-based cohort. Pediatrics 2003;111:315–320.
10. Devlin MJ, Zhu AJ. Body image in the balance. JAMA 2001;286(17):2159.
11. Mehler PS. Diagnosis and care of patients with anorexia nervosa in primary care settings. Ann Intern Med 2001;134:1048–1059.
12. Bulik CM, Tozzi F, Anderson C, et al. The relation between eating disorders and components of perfectionism. Am J Psychiatry 2003;160:366–368.
13. Pritts, SD, Susman J. Diagnosis of eating disorders in primary care. Am Fam Physician 2003;67:297–304.
14. Gorwood P, Kipman A, Foulon C. The human genetics of anorexia nervosa. Eur J Pharmacol 2003;480:163–170.
15. Bulik CM, Sullivan PF. Kendler KS. Genetic and environmental contributions to obesity and binge eating. Int J Eat Disord 2003;33:293–298.
16. Fairburn CG, Cowen PJ, Harrison PJ. Twin studies and the etiology of eating disorders. Int J Eat Disord 1999;26:349–358.
17. Branson R, Potoczna N. Kral JG, et al. Binge eating as a major phenotype of melanocortin 4 receptior gene mutations. N Engl J Med 2003;348(12):1096–1103.
18. Schmidt U, Tiller J, Blanchard M, et al. Is there a specific trauma precipitating anorexia nervosa? Psychol Med 1997;27:523–530.
19. Mehler PS, Anderson AE, eds. Eating disorders: a guide to medical care and complications. Baltimore, MD. The Johns Hopkins University Press. 1999.
20. Herzog DB, Nussbaum KM, Marmor AK. Comorbidity and outcome in eating disorders. Psychiatr Clin North Am 1996;19(4):843–859.
21. Morgan JF, Reid F, Lacey JH. The Scoff questionnaire: assessment of a new screening tool for eating disorders. BMJ 1999;318:1467–1468.

22. Cotton MA, Ball C, Robinson P. Four simple questions can help screen for eating disorders. J Gen Intern Med 2003;18:53–56.
23. Devuyst O, Lambert M, Rodhain J, et al. Haematological changes and infectious complications in anorexia nervosa, a case control study. Q J Med 1993;86:791–799.
24. Mehler PS. Electrolyte disorders in bulimia. Eating disorders: The Journal of Treatment and Prevention 1998;6:65–68.
25. Croxson MS, Ibbertson HK. Low serum triiodothyronine (T3) and hypothyroidism in anorexia nervosa J Clin Endocrinol Metab 1977;44(1):167–174.
26. Durakovic Z, Durakovic A, Korsic M. Changes of the corrected Q-T interval in the electrocardiogram of patients with anorexia nervosa. Int J Cardiol 1994;45:115–120.
27. Fisler JS. Cardiac effects of starvation and semistarvation diets: safety and mechanisms of action. Am J Clin Nutr 1992;152:1073–1074.
28. Cooke RA, Chambers JB, Singh R, et al. QT interval in anorexia nervosa. British Heart J 1994;72:69–73.
29. Oka Y, Ito T, Matsumoto S, et al. Mitral valve prolapse in patients with anorexia nervosa. Two-dimensional echocardiographic study. Jpn Heart J 1987;28:873–882.
30. Ho PC, Dweik R, Cohen MC. Rapidly reversible cardiomyopathy associated with chronic ipecac ingestion. Clin Cardiol 1998;21(10):780–783.
31. Frideman EJ. Death from ipecac intoxication in a patient with anorexia nervosa. Am J Psychiatry 1984;141(5):702–703.
32. Swenne I. Heart risk associated with weight loss in anorexia nervosa and eating disorders. Acta Paediatr 2000;89(4):447–452.
33. Marinella MA. Refeeding syndrome and hypophosphatemia. J Intensive Care Med 2005;20(3):155–159.
34. Golden NH, Meyer W. Nutritional rehabilitation of anorexia nervosa. Goals and dangers. Int J Adolesc Med Health 2004;16(2):131–144.
35. McGilley BM, Pryor TL. Assessment and treatment of bulimia nervosa. Am Fam Phys 1998;57(11):2743–2750.
36. Little JW. Eating disorders: dental implications. Oral Surg Oral Med Oral Pathol Oral Radiol Endod 2002;93(2):138–143.
37. Milosevic A, Brodie DA, Slade PD. Dental erosion, oral hygiene, and nutrition in eating disorders. Int J Eat Disord 1997;21(2):195–199.
38. Kinzl J, Biebl W, Herold M. Significance of vomiting for hyperamylasemia and sialadenosis in patients with eating disorders. Int J Eat Disord 1993;13(1):117–124.
39. Mehler PS, Wallace JA. Sialadenosis in bulimia. A new treatment. Arch Otolaryngol Head Neck Surg 1993;119(7):787–788.
40. Coleman H, Altini M, Nayler S, et al. Sialadenosis: a presenting sign in bulimia. Head Neck 1998;20(8):758–762.
41. Benini L, Todesco T, Dalle Grave R, et al. Gastric emptying in patients with restricting and binge/purging subtypes of anorexia nervosa. Am J Gastroenterol 2004;99(8):1448–1454.
42. Hadley SJ, Walsh BT. Gastrointestinal disturbances in anorexia nervosa and bulimia nervosa. Curr Drug Targets CNS Neurol Disord 2003;2(1):1–9.
43. Chun AB, Sokol MS, Kaye WH, et al. Colonic and anorectal function in constipated patients with anorexia nervosa. Am J Gastroenterol 1997;92(10):1879–1883.
44. Szmukler GI, Young CP, Miller G, et al. A controlled trial of cisapride in anorexia nervosa. Int J Eat Disord 1995;17(4):347–357.
45. Richter JE. Cisapride: Limited access and alternatives. Cleve Clin J Med 2000;67:471–472.

46. Furuta S, Ozawa Y, Maejima K, et al. Anorexia nervosa with severe liver dysfunction and subsequent critical complications. Intern Med 1999;38(7):575–579.
47. Mendell DA, Logemann JA. Bulimia and swallowing: cause for concern. Int J Eat Disord 2001;30:252–258.
48. Anderson L, Shaw JM, McCargar L. Physiological effects of bulimia nervosa on the gastrointestinal tract. Can J Gstroenterol 1997;11(5):451–459.
49. Gowen GF, Stoldt HS, Rosato FE. Five risk factors identify patients with gastroesophageal intussusception. Arch Surg 1999;134(12):1394–1397.
50. Colton P, Woodside DB, Kaplan AS. Laxative withdrawal in eating disorders: treatment protocol and 3 to 20-month follow-up. Int J Eat Disord 1999;25(3):311–317.
51. Mehler PS. Bulimia nervosa. N Engl J Med 2003;349(9):875–881.
52. Golden NH, Shenker JR. Amenorrhea in anorexia nervosa. Neuroendocrine control of hypothalamic dysfunction. Int J Eat Disord 1994;16:53–60.
53. Frisch RE, McArthur JW. Menstrual cycle: fatness as a determinant of minimum weight for height necessary of maintenance or onset. Science 1974;185:949–951.
54. Golden NH, Jacobson MS, Schebendach J, et al. Resumption of menses in anorexia nervosa. Arch Pediatr Adolesc Med 1997;151:16–21.
55. Marcus R, Cann C, Madvig P, et al. Menstrual function and bone mass in elite women distance runners. Ann Int Med 1985;902:158–163.
56. Rome ES. Eating disorders. Obstet Gynecol Clin N Am 2003;30:353–377.
57. Grinspoon S, Gulick T, Askari H, et al. Serum leptin levels in women with anorexia nervosa. J Clin Endocrinol Metab 1996;81:3861–3863.
58. Mehler PS, Eckel RH, Donahoo WT. Leptin levels in restricting and purging anorectics. Int J Eat Disord 1999;26(2):189–194.
59. Eckert ED, Pomeroy C, Raymond N, et al. Leptin in anorexia nervosa. J Clin Endocrinol Metab 1998;83:791–795.
60. Kreitzer PM, Golden NH. Yoon DJ, et al. Leptin levels in amenorrheic versus normally menstruating nutritionally rehabilitated patients with anorexia nervosa. Ped Res 1997;21–6A.
61. Copeland PM, Sacks NR, Herzog DB. Longitudinal follow-up of amenorrhea in eating disorders. Psychosom Med 1995;57:121–126.
62. Lucas AR, Melton LJ 3rd, Crowson CS, et al. Long term fracture risk among women with anorexia nervosa: a population based cohort study. Mayo Clin Proc 1999;74:972–977.
63. Herzog, W, Minne H, Deter C, et al. Outcome of bone mineral density in anorexia nervosa patients 11.7 years after first admission. J Bone Min Res 1993;8:597–605.
64. Iketani T, Kiriike N, Nakanishi S, Nakasuji T. Effects of weight gain and resumption of menses on reduced bone density in patients with anorexia nervosa. Biol Psychiatry 1995;37(8):521–527.
65. Klibanski A, Biller BM, Schoenfeld DA, et al. The effects of estrogen administration on trabecular bone loss in young women with anorexia nervosa. J Clin Endocrinol Metab 1995;80:898–904.
66. Soyka LA, Grinspoon S, Levitsky LL, et al. The effects of anorexia nervosa on bone metabolism in female adolescents. J Clin Endocrinol Metab 1999;84:4489–4496.
67. Klibanski A, Biller BM, O'Fallon WM, et al. The effects of estrogen administration on trabecular bone loss in young women with anorexia nervosa. J Clin Endocrinol Metab 1995;80:898–904.
68. Ward A, Brown N, Treasure J. Persistent osteopenia after recovery from anorexia nervosa. Int J Eat Disord 1997;22:71–75.
69. Hergenroeder AC. Bone minieralization, hypothalamic amenorrhea, and sex steroid therapy in female adolescents and young adults. J Pediatr 1995;126:683–689.

70. Golden NH, Lanzkowsky L, Schebendach J, et al. The effect of estrogen-progestin treatment on bone mineral density in anorexia nervosa. J Pediatr Adolesc Gynecol 2002;15(3):135–143.
71. Seeman E, Szmukler GI, Formica C, et al. Osteoporosis in anorexia nervosa: the influence of peak bone density, bone loss, oral contraceptive use, and exercise. J Bone Miner Res 1992;7(12):1467–1474.
72. Goebel G, Schweiger U, Kruger R, et al. Predictors of bone mineral density in patients with eating disorders. Int J Eat Disord 1999;25:143–150.
73. Hotta M, Fukunda I, Sato K, et al. The relationship between bone turnover and body weight, serum insulin like growth factor and serum IGF-binding protein levels in patients with anorexia nervosa. J Clin Endocrinol Metab 2000;85(1):200–206.
74. Birmingham CL, Goldner EM, Bakan R. Controlled trial of zinc supplementation in anorexia nervosa. Int J Eat Disord 1994;15:251–255.
75. Gordon CM, Grace E, Emans SJ, et al. Effects of oral dehydroepiandrosterone on bone density in young women with anorexia nervosa: a randomized trial. J Clin Endocrinol Metab 2002;87(11):4935–4941.
76. Iketani T, Kiriike N, Murray, et al. Effect of menatetrenone (vitamin K2) treatment on bone loss in patients with anorexia nervosa. Psychiatry Res 2003;117(3):259–269.
77. Grinspoon S, Thomas L, Miller K, et al. Effects of recombinant human IGF-I and oral contraceptive administration on bone density in anorexia nervosa. J Clin Endocrinol Metab 2002;87(6):2883–2891.
78. Golden NH, Iglesias EA, Jacobson MS, et al. Alendronate for the treatment of osteopenia in anorexia nervosa: a randomized double-blind, placebo-controlled trial. J Clin Endocrinol Metab 2005;90(6):3279–3285.
79. Mehler PS. Osteoporosis in anorexia: prevention and treatment. Int J Eat Disord 2003;33: 113–126.
80. Zipfel S, Seibel MJ, Lowe B, et al. Osteoporosis in eating disorders: a follow up study of patients with anorexia and bulimia nervosa. J Clin Endocrinol Metab 2001;86(11):5227–5233.
81. Katzman DK, Lambe EK, Mikulis DJ, et al. Cerebral gray matter and white matter volume deficits in adolescent girls with anorexia nervosa. J Pediatr 1996;129:794–803.
82. Kornreich L, Shapira A, Horev G, et al. CT and MR evaluation of the brain in patients with anorexia nervosa. AJNR Am J Neuroradiol 1991;12:1213–1216.
83. Golden NH, Ashtari M, Kohn MR, et al. Reversibility of cerebral ventricular enlargement in anorexia nervosa demonstrated by quantitative magnetic resonance imaging. J Pediatr 1996;128:296–301.
84. Swayze VW II, Andersen A, Arndt S, et al. Reversibility of brain tissue loss in anorexia nervosa assessed with a computerized Talairach 3-D proportional grid. Psychol Med 1996;26:381–390.
85. Kaye WH, Nagata T, Weltzin TE, et al. Double-blind placebo-controlled administration of fluoxetine in restricting- and restricting-purging-type anorexia nervosa. Biol Psychiatry 2001;49(7):644–652.
86. Kaye WH, Weltzin TE, Hsu LK, Bulik CM. An open trial of fluoxetine in patients with anorexia nervosa. J Clin Psychiatry 1991;52(11):464–471.
87. Attia E, Haiman C, Walsh BT, Flater SR. Does fluoxetine augment the inpatient treatment of anorexia nervosa? Am J Psychiatry 1998;155(4):548–551.
88. Holtkamp K, Konrad K, Kaiser N, et al. A retrospective study of SSRI treatment in adolescent anorexia nervosa: insufficient evidence for efficacy. J Psychiatr Res 2005;39(3): 303–310.
89. Barbarich NC, McConaha CW, Gaskill J, et al. An open trial of olanzapine in anorexia nervosa. J Clin Psychiatry 2004;65(11):1480–1482.

90. Powers PS, Santana CA, Bannon YS. Olanzapine in the treatment of anorexia nervosa: an open label trial. Int J Eat Disord 2002;32(2):146–154.
91. Mondraty N, Birmingham CL, Touyz S, et al. Randomized controlled trial of olanzapine in the treatment of cognitions in anorexia nervosa. Australa Psychiatry 2005;13(1):72–75.
92. Mitchell JE, de Zwaan M, Roerig JL. Drug therapy for patients with eating disorders. Curr Drug Targets CNS Neurol Disord 2003;2(1):17–29.
93. Powers PS, Santana C. Available pharmacological treatments for anorexia nervosa. Expert Opin Pharmacother 2004;5(11):2287–2292.
94. Bacaltchuk J, Hay P. Antidepressants versus placebo for people with bulimia nervosa. Cochrane Database Syst Rev 2003;(4):CD003391.
95. Goldstein DJ, Wilson MG, Thompson VL, et al. Long-term fluoxetine treatment of bulimia nervosa. Fluoxetine Bulimia Nervosa Research Group. Br J Psychiatry 1995;166(5):660–666.
96. Fluoxetine Bulimia Nervosa Collaborative Study Group. Fluoxetine in the treatment of bulimia nervosa: a multicenter, placebo controlled, double-blind trial. Arch Gen Psychiatry 1992;49:139–147.
97. Fung SM, Ferrill MJ. Treatment of bulimia nervosa with ondansetron. Ann Pharmacother 2001;35(10):1270–1273.
98. Faris PL, Kim SW, Meller WH, et al. Effect of decreasing afferent vagal activity with ondansetron on symptoms of bulimia nervosa: a randomized, double-blind trial. Lancet 2000;355(9206):792–797.
99. Felstrom A, Blackshaw S. Topiramate for bulimia nervosa with bipolar II disorder. Am J Psychiatry 2002;159:1246–1247.
100. Hedges DW, Reimherr FW, Hoopes SP, et al. Treatment of bulimia nervosa with topiramate in a randomized, double-blind, placebo-controlled trial, part 2: improvement in psychiatric measures. J Clin Psychiatry 2003;64(12):1449–1454.
101. Hoopes SP, Reimherr FW, Hedges DW, et al. Treatment of bulimia nervosa with topiramate in a randomized, double-blind, placebo-controlled trial, part 1: improvement in binge and purge measures. J Clin Psychiatry 2003;64(11):1335–1341.
102. El Giamal N, de Zwaan M, Bailer U, et al. Reboxetine in the treatment of bulimia nervosa: a report of seven cases. Int Clin Psychopharmacol 2000;15(6):351–356.
103. Fassino S, Daga GA, Boggio S, et al. Use of reboxetine in bulimia nervosa: a pilot study. J Psychopharmacol 2004:18(3):423–428.
104. Gelber D, Levine J, Belmaker RH. Effect of inositol on bulimia nervosa and binge eating. Int J Eat Disord 2001;29(3):345–348.
105. Appolinario JC, McElroy SL. Pharmacological approaches in the treatment of binge eating disorder. Curr Drug Targets 2004;5(3):301–307.
106. Appolinario JC, Bacaltchuk J, Sichieri R, et al. A randomized, double blind, placebo-controlled study of sibutramine in the treatment of binge eating disorder. Arch Gen Psychiatry 2003;60(11):1109–1116.
107. McElroy SL, Shapira NA, Arnold LM, et al. Topiramate in the long-term treatment of binge-eating disorder associated with obesity. J Clin Psychiatry 2004;65(11):1463–1469.
108. McElroy SL, Kotwal R, Hudson JI, et al. Zonisamide in the treatment of binge-eating disorder: an open-label, prospective trial. J Clin Psychiatry 2004;65(1):50–56.
109. Hay P, Bacaltchuk J, Claudino A, et al. Individual psychotherapy in the outpatient treatment of adults with anorexia nervosa. Cochrane Database Syst Rev 2003;(4):CD003909.
110. Eisler I, Dare C, Russell GF, et al. Family and individual therapy in anorexia nervosa. A 5-year follow-up. Arch Gen Psychiatry 1997;54(11):1025–1030.
111. Robin AL, Siegel PT, Moye AW, et al. A controlled comparison of family versus individual therapy for adolescents with anorexia nervosa. J Am Acad Child Adolesc Psychiatry 1999;38(12):1482–1489.

112. Kleifield EI, Wagner S, Halmi KA. Cognitive-behavioral treatment of anorexia nervosa. Psychiatr Clin North Am 1996;19(4):715–737.
113. Pike KM, Walsh BT, Vitousek K, et al. Cognitive behavior therapy in the posthopitalization treatment of anorexia nervosa. Am J Psychiatry 2003;160(11):2046–2049.
114. Hay PJ, Bacaltchuk J, Stefano S. Psychotherapy for bulimia nervosa and binging. Cochrane Database Syst Rev 2004;(3):CD000562.
115. Agras WS, Walsh T, Fairburn CG, et al. A multicenter comparison of cognitive-behavioral therapy and interpersonal psychotherapy for bulimia nervosa. Arch Gen Psychiatry 2000;57:459–466.
116. Bacaltchuk J, Hay P, Trefigli R. Antidepressants versus psychological treatments and their combination for bulimia nervosa. Cochrane Database Syst Rev 2001;(4):CD003385.
117. Mitchell JE, Halmi K, Wilson GT, et al. A randomized secondary treatment study of women with bulimia nervosa who fail to respond to CBT. Int J Eat Disord 2002;32(3): 271–281.
118. Herzog DB, Nussbaum KM, Marmor AK. Comorbidity and outcome in eating disorders. Psychiatr Clin North Am 1996;19:843–859.
119. Steinhausen HC, Rauss-Mason C, Seidel R. Follow-up studies of anorexia nervosa: a review of four decades of outcome research. Psychol Med 1991;21:447–454.
120. Herzog D, Keller M, Lavori P, Sacks N. The course and outcome of bulimia nervosa. J Clin Psychiatry 1991;52(Suppl):4–8.
121. Fairburn CG, Cooper Z, Doll HA. The natural course of bulimia nervosa and binge eating disorder in young women. Arch Gen Psychiatry 2000;57:659–665.

16 Psychiatric Disorders in Women

Brenda J. Butler, MD

CONTENTS

INTRODUCTION

Engel proposed the biopsychosocial model for patient care in 1977, which called on physicians to care for patients in an integrated manner. Despite the longstanding adaptation of this theory in the training of physicians, mental disorders remain underdiagnosed in primary care settings *(1–3)*. Strategies to improve detection and treatment of mental disorders are imperative to the mental and physical health of a striking number of individuals worldwide. The World Health Organization's (WHO) 2001 report on mental health revealed a significant "treatment gap," claiming that, of the 450 million people suffering from a mental or behavioral disorder, only a small minority were receiving treatment. A Needs Study found that two-thirds to three-quarters of all people were identified as suffering from mental health symptoms, and did not report receiving treatment *(4)*. This further highlights the gap between epidemiology and service use. An epidemic of untreated and poorly treated mental disorders

From: *Current Clinical Practice: Women's Health in Clinical Practice*
Edited by: Clouse and Sherif © Humana Press Inc., Totowa, NJ

exists in the United States, especially among vulnerable groups and the underinsured *(5)*. Patients' race, sex, and coexisting medical conditions affect physicians' awareness of mental health issues. This calls for improved strategies of detection and intervention *(6)*.

In 1993, the Harvard School of Public Health in collaboration with the World Bank and the WHO assessed the Global Burden of Disease. The DALY, a health cap measure, was used to quantify the burden of disease. It combined information regarding the impact of premature death and of disability and other nonfatal health outcomes. In the original estimate developed for 1990, mental and neurological disorders accounted for 10.5% of the total DALYs lost caused by all diseases and injuries. The estimate for 2000 is 12.3%. Projections indicate that it will increase to 15% in the year 2020. During the course of time, psychiatric prevalence increased in all sociodemographic categories, despite improved socioeconomic conditions in certain populations. The increasing complexity of life takes its toll, even of the socially best equipped *(7)*. A prospective study examining the association of psychiatric disorders with health care use revealed that behavioral health disorders (including additive, depressive, and anxiety disorders) make an independent contribution to nonpsychiatric health care use *(8)*. Mental illness affects one in five people in the United States *(9)*. Approximately 50% of all patient visits for mental health concerns and symptoms and their resulting complications are to primary care physicians. Twenty-four percent of all patients seen in primary health practices have one or more mental disorders (WHO 2001). Further increases in the number of sufferers are likely in view of the aging of the population, worsening social problems, and civil unrest (WHO 2001). The positive evolution toward decreasing stigma and de-institutionalization of treatment for mental illness creates a further challenge for primary care providers who must also function with limited community and insurance resources.

Primary care patients will often present with physical symptoms but not often with complaints related to their emotions, thinking, or behavior. It has been estimated that 38% of primary care patients present with physical symptoms that have no discernable medical basis *(10)*. Psychiatric problems are frequently manifested in somatic form and as noncompliance with primary care physicians' recommendations. Psychiatric disorders are prevalent and commonly known to cause serious impairment, suffering, complications of medical treatment and recovery, and even mortality. Even subthreshold psychiatric disorders identified in primary care settings have been associated with significant psychological distress, disability, and poor health perception *(11)*. Research has pointed to two main pathways through which mental and physical health mutually influence each other with time (WHO 2001). The first key pathway is directly through physiological systems, such as neuroendocrine and immune functioning. Anxious and depressed moods initiate a cascade of adverse changes in endocrine and immune functioning, and create increased susceptibility to a range of physical illnesses. It is know for instance, that stress is related to the development of the common cold, and that stress delays wound healing (WHO 2001). The second primary pathway is through health behavior. The term health behavior covers a range of activities, such as eating sensibly, regular exercising, adequate sleep, avoiding smoking, engaging in safe sexual practices, wearing safety belts in vehicles, and adhering to medical therapies. The health behaviors of an individual are highly dependent on the state of one's mental health. Enhancing primary and general health care practitioners' abilities in the detection and treatment of common mental and behavioral disorders is an important public health measure. When investigating common mental, behavioral, and social problems in a wide range of communities, women were found to be more likely than men to be adversely affected by specific mental disorders (WHO 2001).

Prevalence rates of depressive disorders, common anxiety disorders, and somatization disorders are found to be higher is women. These findings are consistent across a range of studies undertaken in a variety of countries and settings. Women are also more likely to suffer from the effects of domestic violence, sexual violence, and childhood sexual abuse. There is a concerning escalation of rates of substance abuse among women, which increases the risk for comorbid conditions and co-occurring trauma. Explanations for sex differences in mental disorders have been discussed in relation to the help-seeking behaviors of the sexes, biological differences, and social causes, and in the different ways that women and men acknowledge and deal with stress (WHO 2001).

Artifact theories postulated that women tended to seek help and report psychiatric symptoms more frequently than men *(12)*. Differences in symptom reporting or differential recall suggested a diagnostic biased by sex *(13)*. However, higher rates in community-based surveys and studies that varied method of evaluation and symptom threshold found that such factors do not account for the sex differences found *(14)*.

Biological differences in explaining sex differences in common mental disorders have focused on hormonal factors. Factors related to the reproductive cycle may play a role in women's vulnerability to depression *(15)*. Estrogen and progesterone affect neurotransmitter, neuroendocrine, and circadian systems implicated in mood disorders *(16)*. Oxytocin increases fivefold in puberty and seems related to both sexual behavior and pair bonding in females. During this time, girls are at risk, because of increased desire for interpersonal and romantic interactions, which can lead to disappointments *(17,18)*. Puberty marks the beginning of increased risk for depression in women. Most women report emotional symptoms premenstrually. Women transitioning through perimenopause, particularly those with past psychiatric histories, report depressive symptoms *(19)*.

The American Association of University Women's study of 1990 looked at 3000 young girls and boys aged 9 to 15 years *(20)*. Preadolescent girls begin to retreat from academic and athletic excellence and descend into feelings of low self-esteem, decreased self-assertion and self-confidence, depression, hopelessness, increased self-criticism, vulnerability, and a negative attitude toward their body. Despite the fact that women are entering higher education settings in higher numbers, they still do not have equal pay or leadership in jobs or professions. Their occupations tend to be more stressful because of a higher degree of responsibility compared with their level of autonomy *(21)*. Across socioeconomic levels, the multiple roles that women fulfill in society put them at greater risk of experiencing mental and behavioral disorders. Women continue to bear the burden of responsibility associated with being wives, mothers, educators, and caretakers of others, while they increasingly become an essential part of the labor force. In one-quarter to one-third of households, women are the prime source of income (WHO 2001). In addition to the pressures placed on women because of their expanding and often conflicting roles, they face significant sex discrimination and associated poverty, hunger, malnutrition, overwork, and domestic and sexual violence (WHO 2001).

Sex-specific socialization and coping skills have also been investigated. Examination of PET studies indicated sex differences in processing emotional stimuli, which is postulated to contribute to longer and more severe depressive episodes in women *(22)*. Coping styles have been found to differ, with women tending to adapt a self-focused ruminative style in response to sadness, as compared with men, who apply distracting strategies in response to sadness *(23)*. Girls are socialized by parents and teachers to be more nurturing and concerned with evaluations of others, whereas boys demonstrate a greater sense of mastery and independence *(24)*. A Cognitive Vulnerability–Transactional Stress Theory has been elaborated as an explanation for the development of sex differences in depression *(25)*. It postulates that negative events contribute to the initial elevations of general negative mood and, with generic cognitive vulnerability factors, moderate the likelihood that the initial negative affect will progress to full-blown depression. This increases depression and can lead transactionally to more self-generated negative life events, and, thus, begins the chain. Scientific evidence indicates that mental and behavioral disorders are the result of the interaction of biology along with social and psychological factors. Primary health care providers play a crucial role with the integration of mental play health care into primary health care settings.

Primary care providers must be familiar with the criteria for diagnosing common psychiatric disorders, possess astute interviewing skills, and understand psychosocial issues and their implications to identify, diagnose, and treat psychiatric disorders. They also play a key role in helping patients acknowledge their symptoms. They can provide counseling and make an effective referral to mental health care professionals. A correct objective diagnosis is fundamental for the planning of individual care, and for the choice of appropriate treatment. Mental and behavioral disorders can be diagnosed with a high level of reliability. There are an extensive number of diagnostic and research assessment tools used in detecting psychiatric disorders. Many of them have been used for substantial periods of time and have, therefore, established historical precedence warranting their continued use (e.g., Beck Depression and Anxiety, or Hamilton Depression and Anxiety). It is, however, important to consider the primary care setting when determining which assessment tool would be more helpful in routine practice. In 1995, psychiatrist Dr. Robert Spitzer, developed a tool called the Primary Care Evaluation of Mental Disorders (PRIME-MD). Although reliable, the PRIME-MD's administration time limited its clinical usefulness. The revised PRIME-MD Patient Health Questionnaire was developed to correct for this issue and make the assessment tool more useful in clinical practice. Studies have shown the PRIME-MD Patient Health Questionnaire to be a useful instrument in a busy clinical practice, in assessing for mental disorders, functional impairments, and psychosocial stressors *(26,27)*.

Because different treatments are indicated for different diseases, diagnosis is an important starting point of any intervention (WHO 2001). Early intervention is fundamental in preventing progression to a full-blown disease, in controlling symptoms, and in improving outcomes. The earlier the institution of a proper course of treatment is in place, the better the prognosis. The appropriate treatment of mental disorders implies the rational use of pharmacological, psychological, and psychosocial interventions in a clinically meaningful, balanced, and well-integrated way (WHO 2001). It is also imperative to maintain close follow-up and to encourage a healthy doctor–patient relationship, because this will enhance both detection and treatment of mental disorders. Primary care providers can frame their patients' appointments to provide for the time and atmosphere to facilitate detection and treatment of mental disorders. As has often been taught, open-ended questions tend to encourage the greatest disclosure. While comfortably listening to your patients, you may also make important observations regarding their thoughts, emotions, and behaviors. Topics such as sexual history, domestic violence, childhood abuse, suicidal and homicidal thoughts, as well as thoughts not based in reality, are important in the process of making an appropriate diagnosis. Patients are generally accustomed to talking about sensitive topics in the office, and expect intimate questions from their doctors. It is also important to elicit the patient's perceptions regarding their illness and to address their concerns. The following sections will provide a template for diagnosis and treatment of some of the most prevalent mental disorders that are observed in primary care settings. Issues related to women's mental health will be highlighted.

AFFECTIVE OR MOOD DISORDERS

Affective or Mood Disorders include Major Depressive Disorder, Dysthymic Disorder, Bipolar Disorder Types I and II, Cyclothymic Disorder, and Mood Disorders related to hormone status in women. Depression is a major health concern for women, who are affected two or three times more frequently than men. There are increased rates for women of Major Depression, Dysthymic Depression, Major Depression with a Seasonal Component, and Mood Disorders related to the reproductive status of women. Bipolar Type II Disorder may be more common in women than in men. Women with Bipolar Type II Disorder may be at increased risk of developing subsequent episodes in the immediate postpartum period. Bipolar Type I Disorder presents equally in men and women, as does Cyclothymic Disorder, although women with Cyclothymic Disorder may present for treatment more frequently than men. Mood Disorders are among the most common afflictions that bring patients to doctors. Almost 20% of adults will have a mood disorder requiring treatment in their lifetime *(8)*.

Depression

The 2001 WHO report indicates that an estimated 121 million people currently suffer from Depression. An estimated 5.8% of men and 9.5% of women will experience an episode of Depression in any given year. Women are at an increased risk for first-onset Major Depression from early adolescence until their mid-50s. There is conflicting evidence regarding what happens with the rates of depression after midlife *(28–30)*. Lifetime rates of major depression are 1.7 to 2 .7 times greater for women than for men *(19)*. Lifetime prevalence for Major Depression in women is 21.3%, compared with 12.7% for men. For Dysthymic Depression, the lifetime prevalence is 8% for women compared with 4.8% for men *(31)*. Longitudinal studies demonstrate the sex difference emerging at age 13 years and extending into midlife *(18)*. Risk factors for women include, but are not limited to, marriage, no occupation outside of the home, three or more children younger than 11 years of age, a history of childhood abuse, and family history of Depression, Alcoholism, and Substance Abuse *(32)*. The risk affect of marriage can be ameliorated if the woman is working by choice and has adequate supports. A multilevel analysis from

The Harvard School of Public Health reported that, with the exception of political participation, the indicators of women's status in society (employment and earnings, economic autonomy, and reproductive rights) were significantly linked to women's depressive symptoms. The risk of a major depression increases 1.5 to 3.0 times if the illness is present in a first-degree relative as compared with no such illness in a first-degree relative *(33,34)*. Depressive illnesses carry significant risks of death and disability. Approximately 15 to 20% of patients with a mood disorder die by their own hand *(35,36)*, and at least 66% of all suicides are preceded by depression. The rates of suicide are higher in lesbian youth than in their heterosexual counterparts. Depressive Disorders are associated with poor work productivity, and increased rates of death and disability from cardiovascular disease. Depressive illnesses also affect family members and care givers *(37)*. There is increasing evidence that children of women with depression have increased rates of problems in school and with behavior. They have lower levels of social competence and self-esteem than their classmates with mothers who do not have depression *(38)*. Depression is the leading cause of disability and premature death among people aged 18 to 44 years, and it is expected to be the second leading cause of disability for people of all ages by 2020 *(39,40)*. Despite the devastating consequences of depression and its high prevalence, only one-third of all patients with depression receive adequate treatment *(41)*.

The criteria of a Major Depressive episode are at least five of the following symptoms, which must have been present most of the day, every day, for at least 2 weeks. The symptoms must include either one or two, and this must represent a change from previous functioning and not be caused by another medical or psychiatric condition. Severe Depression can present with psychotic symptoms associated with the mood episode, which remit when the depressive episode is adequately treated.

1. Depressed (sad) or irritable mood.
2. Anhedonia or marked diminished interest or pleasure in all of almost activities.
3. Significant weight loss or weight gain.
4. Insomnia or hypersomnia nearly every day.
5. Psychomotor agitation or retardation.
6. Fatigue or loss of energy.
7. Feelings of worthlessness or excessive or inappropriate guilt.
8. Diminished ability to think or concentrate or indecisiveness.
9. Recurrent thoughts of death or suicidal ideation.

Atypical Depression is more common in late adolescent girls. Two independent studies undertaken in Australia and North America support a theory for primacy of personality style (rather than mood reactivity) and for certain expressions of anxiety in Atypical Depression *(42)*. The individual must have two or more of the following features: significant weight gain or increase in appetite (frequently craving sweets and carbohydrates), hypersomnia, leaden paralysis, and a long-standing pattern of interpersonal rejection sensitivity (not limited to episodes of mood symptoms). Seasonal Affective Disorders occur more frequently in women than men *(43)*. Seasonal Affective Disorders implies a regular temporal pattern of mood symptoms established during a 2-year period. The seasonal episodes must predominate over nonseasonal episodes. A recent study compared two questionnaires for Seasonal Affective Disorder in primary care settings and found that the Seasonal Health Questionnaire was more sensitive and specific than the Seasonal Pattern Assessment Questionnaire. It also had higher positive and negative predictive values in screening for Seasonal Affective Disorder *(44)*. Light therapy is a viable treatment specifically aimed at patients with Seasonal Affective Disorder and should be explored. Postpartum depression occurs at concerning rates. The Diagnostic and Statistical Manual (DSM) IV reports that postpartum mood episodes occur in from 1 in 500 to 1 in 1000 deliveries. Postpartum episodes can present as depression, mania, or a mixed episode (meeting criteria for both depression and mania). The onset of the episode must be within 4 weeks postpartum. Recent studies have reported prevalence rates of 10 to 15% for postpartum depression *(45–47)*. A large cross-sectional prevalence study conducted in Europe in 2004 showed increasing rates of postpartum depression during the course of time from delivery. Rates were extremely high and increased from 29% at 0 to 2 months to 42.7% at longer than 13 months postpartum *(48)*. Approximately 4 to 7% of menstruating women suffer from Premenstrual Dysphoric Disorder (PDD). Women with previous episodes of depression are at increased risk, and PDD and postpartum depression are related. There have been some methodological difficulties in studying PDD, which placed it in a category for further study in DSM IV. A variety of treatments has also been attempted, including dietary and vitamin supplements, exercise, psychotrophic medications, and hormones. The current diagnostic criteria call for at least five of the following symptoms to have been present most of the time during the last week of the luteal phase, with at least one of the symptoms included in one of the first four:

1. Feeling sad, hopeless, or self-deprecating.
2. Feeling tense, anxious or "on edge."
3. Marked lability of mood interspersed with frequent tearfulness.
4. Persistent irritability, anger, and increased interpersonal conflicts.
5. Decreased interest in usual activities.
6. Difficulty concentrating.
7. Feeling fatigued, lethargic, or lacking in energy.

8. Marked changes in appetite, which might be associated with binge eating or food cravings.
9. Hypersomnia or insomnia.
10. A subjective feeling of being overwhelmed or out of control.
11. Physical symptoms, such as breast tenderness, headaches, "bloating."

Dysthymic Disorder is a chronically depressed mood that occurs for most of the day, more days than not, for at least 2 years. Individuals must also have two or more of the following:

1. Poor appetite.
2. Insomnia or hypersomnia.
3. Low energy or fatigue.
4. Low self-esteem.
5. Poor concentration or difficulty making decisions.
6. Feelings of hopelessness.

Despite the specifically outlined diagnostic criteria and reliability of diagnosing Depressive Disorders, approximately two-thirds of the 6 million women with Major Depression or Dysthymic Depression remained undiagnosed. In addition to familiarity with the diagnostic criteria, primary care practitioners must understand the nuance of Mood Disorders. This problem is furthered by the fact that women have higher rates of comorbidity than men. Comorbid conditions include specific phobias, Generalized Anxiety Disorder (GAD), Panic Disorder, eating disorders, and alcohol abuse, as well as several medical conditions that include thyroid disease, migraines, irritable bowel syndrome, chronic fatigue, chronic pelvic pain, and fibromyalgia *(49,50)*. Some reasons associated with failure to detect and treat depression include insufficient questioning, failure to consult a family member, or failure to start treatment for depression despite adequate diagnostic criteria *(8)*. The best tool for diagnosing depression is listening. Allow time for open-ended discussion following data related to sleep, mood, activities, energy, concentration, appetite, guilt, and themes of hopelessness. Patients will often present with vague physical complaints and complain of feeling "tired." They may become tearful and report feeling overwhelmed or "not caring." Do not avoid uncomfortable topics, such as suicide, homicide, disturbances in thought, sexual histories, and abuse histories. These are important contributors to the diagnosis and will help to establish the appropriate treatment course. Begin by presenting a clear definition of depression to the patient. Include the factors that contribute to the onset of depression. Assure your patient that depression is not a reflection of personal weakness and review the course you will follow. It is fitting to emphasize the toll that their depression has had on them, but remain hopeful and optimistic for treatment success. You should then review the treatment options. First assess your patient for safety and evaluate whether there is a need for hospitalization or referral to a specialist. Some factors pointing to the need for hospitalization include suicide, psychotic symptoms, and regression to the point of your patient not being able to care for herself. You will want to treat medical conditions that could contribute to depression and eliminate medications that can exacerbate mood. You must also address comorbid conditions, especially substance use. The most affective treatment regimen includes psychotropic medications in combination with psychotherapeutic techniques.

Antidepressants work with equal efficacy, leaving the decision regarding which to choose to several contributing factors. It is useful to take a history of the patients' or the patients' family experience with antidepressants. This can often provide data useful to consider in your choice. If a patient has had a positive experience with a medication in the past, you should consider that medication again. Equally, if the patient has a first-degree family member with a positive response to certain medication, that medication should be considered. The next consideration is the side effect profile. Certain antidepressants might be more sedating and should be considered in more agitated patients who are having difficulty sleeping at night. Others might be more elevating and can be administered to patients who are feeling lethargic and chronically tired. Familiarize yourself with one or two medications in each class and use those medications with which you are most familiar. The current classes of medications include tricyclic antidepressants (TCAs) (e.g., imipramine, nortriptyline, amitriptyline, and desipramine), monoamine oxidase inhibitors (phenelzine and tranylcypromine), selective serotonin reuptake inhibitors (SSRIs) (fluoxetine, sertraline, paroxetine, citalopram, and escitalopram), combined serotonin and neuradrenergic agents (venlafaxine, duloxetine), and bupropion, which works primarily in the dopamine system. Since the emergence of SSRIs, they have become first-line treatment because of their safety and ease of administration. Recent concern regarding the possibility of induction of suicide in patients taking SSRIs has prompted much debate. It is likely that a significant amount of research will be performed to fully investigate this concern. One recent study looking at an Analysis of National Vital Statistics from the Centers for Disease Control and Prevention found that the overall relationship between antidepressant medication prescriptions and suicide rates was not significant *(51)*. Higher suicide rates in rural areas are associated with fewer antidepressant prescriptions, lower income, and relatively more prescriptions for TCAs. By contrast, increases in prescriptions for SSRIs and other new-generation non-SSRIs are associated with lower suicide rates. Because of an increase of difficulty in stabilizing and episode, it is most important to initiate psychotropic medications as quickly as possible once a diagnosis is made. Kindling also occurs; meaning that patients are at increased risk for further episodes when current episodes are not stabilized quickly. Medication choice can also be made based on cost, half-life, and convenience. Medications can take 6 to 8 weeks to reach full effect, during which time, patients should be seen frequently to monitor symptoms and side effects. Women may metabolize medications differently because of several factors. Hormones may alter drug levels, women have slower gastric emptying, lower gastric acid secretion, more body fat, slower hepatic metabolism, and lower renal clearance *(52)*. This can lead to increased plasma levels of medications, a longer half-life, and increased sensitivity to side effects. These factors should be taken into consideration when dosing medications. Major Depressive episodes can last from 3 to 18 months, on average lasting 9 months. Therefore, medication treatment should be continued throughout the course of the illness and somewhat longer in patients with recurrent episodes. Vegetative signs of depression will improve before the subjective sense of the depression improves. Doses of medications should be adjusted early in the course of the treatment to maximize benefit while considering minimizing side effects. Be sure to achieve a therapeutic dose and allow the medication the appropriate length of time to show its effectiveness. The doctor–patient relationship can encourage medication compliance. This connection remains one of the most important factors in success.

Primary care providers can offer a great deal of counseling. Their patients should be advised to increase physical activity (exercise has been shown to have clear benefit), increase daily routine and structure, enhance problem solving skills, and increase social contacts. In the office, some cognitive counseling can be instituted to help patients decrease harsh and punishing thoughts and underlying assumptions, which influence the development of depression. The WHO 2001 report stated that 20 years of research found several forms of time-limited psychotherapy as effective as drugs in mild-to-moderate depressions. These include cognitive behavioral therapy and interpersonal therapy. Some recent studies confirm these findings, which have been long established *(53–55)*. Patients with more complex syndromes should be referred to psychotherapy outside the primary care office. Depressive episodes can be complicated by psychodynamic precursors to the depression, early childhood effects on the current condition, length of illness, personality factors that contribute to illness, and psychiatric comorbidity. Primary care providers play an important role in helping patients become comfortable with the concept of seeing a therapist. Become familiar with good psychotherapists in your area. Make the referral process as streamlined as possible.

Bipolar Disorders

Bipolar Disorder is an episodic Mood Disorder that is lifelong and has a variable course. The first episode of Bipolar Disorder may be manic, hypomanic, depressed, or mixed (meeting criteria for both depression and mania) in nature. Most patients have a Depressive episode, which predates any form of Mania, and Bipolar Disorder should always be considered when a patient presents with a Depressive episode. Patterns vary among patients; some patients can very predictably plan for their episodes and other find no pattern. Before the initiation of lithium therapy, individuals suffered, on average, with approximately four episodes a year. With time, the episodes lengthened and inter-episode periods were shorter. Family history is very important. First-degree biological relatives of individuals with Bipolar Type I Disorder and Bipolar Type II Disorder have elevated rates of Bipolar Type I Disorder, Bipolar Type II Disorder, and Major Depressive Disorder. There may also be an increased familial risk of substance abuse in patients with Cyclothymic Disorder. Bipolar Type I Disorder has a lifetime prevalence of 0.4 to 1.6%, with men being equally affected as women. Bipolar Type II Disorder affects approximately 0.5% of the population, but is more common in women. Women are more prone to a depressive diathesis of the disorder, have a later onset, and are more likely to manifest a seasonal pattern *(56,57)*. Women also have higher rates of mixed episodes and rapid cycling, and their episodes can be more resistant to treatment. Women also have higher rates of comorbidity, leading to a poorer prognosis. Conditions frequently comorbid with Bipolar Disorder include Substance Use Disorders, Anxiety Disorders, and Eating Disorders. Women with Bipolar Disorder may be more inclined than men with Bipolar Disorder to have difficulties with migraine headaches and thyroid disease. Cyclothymic Disorder often begins earlier in life and is sometimes thought to reflect a premorbid personality, which may be an attenuated expression of an affective illness. In other cases of Bipolar Disorder, the illness emerges as discrete episodes. There may be hormonal affects on the expression of Bipolar Disorder. Studies have shown that 66% of women with Bipolar Disorder demonstrate menstrual or premenstrual exacerbation of their disorder *(58)*. Postpartum women have an increased risk of onset (36%) or relapse (25–50%) and can present with a postpartum psychosis as part of their Bipolar Disorder. Treating women with Bipolar Disorder during pregnancy and lactation can be challenging, because mood stabilizers carry teratogenic risks. Electroconvulsive therapy (ECT) is sometimes used as a substitute for traditional medications. Certain medications can sometimes stabilize a woman's symptoms and pose less of a risk to her infant. These include some of the antipsychotic medications and antianxiety medications. Although the course of Bipolar Disorder is variable, it is a serious illness with potentially devastating affects. It is written that 19 to 25% of patients with Bipolar Disorder will attempt suicide during a 30-year course of illness, and 1 in 10 will die from suicide.

Bipolar Type I Disorder is defined by the presence of at least one Manic episode. After the occurrence of the first Manic episode, each episode that follows will be defined as Bipolar Type I Disorder, with the current episode being specified (e.g., depressive, mixed, hypomanic, or manic).

Manic episodes are defined as follows:

1. A distinct period of abnormally and persistently elevated, expansive, or irritable mood, lasting at least 1 week (or any duration if hospitalization is necessary).
2. During the period of mood disturbance, at least three of the following symptoms have persisted (four if the mood is only irritable) and have been present to a significant degree:
   a. Inflated self-esteem or grandiosity.
   b. Decreased need for sleep (feels rested after only 3 hours of sleep).
   c. More talkative than usual or pressured to keep talking.
   d. Flight of ideas or subjective experience that thoughts are racing.
   e. Distractibility.
   f. Increase in goal-directed activity or psychomotor agitation.
   g. Excessive involvement in pleasurable activities that have a high potential for painful consequences (e.g., engaging in unrestrained buying sprees, sexual indiscretions, or foolish business investments).

The symptoms do not meet criteria for a Mixed episode (meeting criteria for both Mania and Major Depression, except for length of episode of depression), cause marked impairment in functioning and are not caused by any direct physiological effects of a substance or medical condition. Secondary Mania or Mania arising from another cause, must be identified and could occur from a toxic metabolic state, an infectious process, trauma, stroke, prescribed or over-the-counter medications, as well as substances of abuse. Nonetheless, these episodes may be difficult to discern and treat. A psychiatrist could be consulted.

Bipolar Type II Disorder is defined by episodes of Major Depression and at least one Hypomanic episode. There can be no history of a Manic episode. There are no other conditions that would better account for the episode. There is clinical distress or impairment in social, occupational, or other important areas of functioning.

Hypomanic episodes are as follows:

1. A distinct period of persistently elevated, expansive, or irritable mood, lasting at least 4 days, that is clearly different from the usual nondepressed mood.
2. During the period of mood disturbance, at least three of the following symptoms have persisted (four if the mood is only irritable) and have been present to a significant degree:
   a. Inflated self-esteem or grandiosity.
   b. Decreased need for sleep (feels rested after 3 hours of sleep).

c. More talkative than usual or pressure to keep talking.
d. Flight of ideas or subjective experience that thoughts are racing.
e. Distractibility.
f. Increase in goal-directed activity.
g. Excessive involvement in pleasurable activities that have a high potential for painful consequences.

The episode is associated with an unequivocal change in functioning that is uncharacteristic of the person when not symptomatic. The disturbance in mood and the change in functioning are observable by others but not severe enough to cause marked impairment in functioning. As always, the episode is not caused by the direct physiological effects of a substance or a general medical condition.

Cyclothymic Disorder is a chronic, fluctuating mood disturbance involving numerous periods of hypomanic symptoms and numerous periods of depressive symptoms. The hypomanic symptoms are of insufficient number, severity, pervasiveness, or duration to meet full criteria for a Manic episode, and the depressive symptoms are of insufficient number, severity, pervasiveness, or duration to meet full criteria for a Major Depressive episode (DSM IV). The symptoms must last for at least 2 years and, during that period, the person must not be without symptoms for more than 2 months. Cyclothymic Disorder usually begins in adolescence or early adult life; later onset may indicate a mood disorder secondary to a medical cause (e.g., Multiple Sclerosis). It often has an insidious onset and a chronic course, and 15 to 50% of individuals with Cyclothymic Disorder will subsequently develop Bipolar Type I or II Disorder. The differential diagnosis for Cyclothymic Disorder includes Borderline Personality Disorder, which will be discussed later in this chapter.

The primary care provider can play a pivotal role in the treatment of patients with Bipolar Disorders. These patients should be referred to psychiatrists to follow the psychopharmacological treatment. Psychotherapy should be used in combination with medications. Because of the challenging nature of this illness, the primary care provider may want to aid in the differential by excluding secondary Manias and help to make the accurate diagnosis. They can offer many psychosocial interventions with the patient and her family while in the office setting. Becoming educated regarding Bipolar Disorder is extremely important not only as it relates to treatment compliance, but also for women in considering aspects of conception, pregnancy, and during postpartum periods. There are several lifestyle adjustments recommended that can be very useful in maintaining stability of mood. These include reducing stress and emotional reactivity. Patients should be cautioned regarding substance use and should abstain as much as possible from using substances. Sleep hygiene is essential, because becoming overly tired or sleep deprived can trigger episodes. Patients should be encouraged to become experts on their moods and report any observations to their clinicians. Patients should be cautioned that suicidal or self-destructive feelings can emerge quickly. Nonetheless, the primary care provider can help patients remain optimistic, maintain their self-esteem, and talk to people they trust so that they do not feel isolated. Dr. Kay Jamison's book, An Unquiet Mind: A memoir of moods and madness by Kay Redfield Jamison. First Vintage Books Editor. (1995), is often comforting and is a good recommendation for patients.

Psychopharmacology for Bipolar Disorders is more often managed by a psychiatrist. The following information comes from the latest Practice Guidelines from the April 2002 *American Journal of Psychiatry*. First-line pharmacological treatment for more severe acute manic or mixed episodes is the initiation of either lithium plus an antipsychotic or valproate plus an antipsychotic. Most studies still find lithium superior to valproate for manic episodes. For less ill patients, monotherapy with lithium or valproate, or an antipsychotic such as olanzapine may be sufficient. Short-term adjunctive treatment with a benzodiazepine may also be helpful. Baseline laboratory values should be obtained, including thyroid function studies (when using lithium), liver function studies (when using valproate), and renal function studies (creatinine and blood urea nitrogen) when using lithium. These should be followed during the course of treatment for any emerging abnormalities. Blood levels of lithium and valproate should guide the dosing of these medications, with specific levels identified for acute and maintenance management of symptoms. Antidepressants may need to be withdrawn during manic or mixed episodes. First-line pharmacological treatment for Bipolar Depression is the initiation of either lithium or lamotrigine. Antidepressant monotherapy is not recommended. For individuals who are more severely depressed, a combination of lithium and an antidepressant (preferably a newer-generation medication, such as a SSRI) is recommended. After remission of an acute episode, patients remain at high risk of relapse for a period of up to 6 months. The patients' mood stabilizer should be continued. If an antipsychotic was used during the acute treatment, it can be slowly tapered off, depending on the patient's history. ECT may also be considered for patients with severe or treatment-resistant mania or mixed episodes, or for pregnant patients experiencing manic or mixed episodes. ECT is also a reasonable option in severe Depressive episodes, treatment-resistant Depression, or Psychotic Depression. If ECT is used to stabilize an acute episode, it can be administered on a maintenance schedule. Primary care providers should maintain communication with the patient and their patient's treating specialists.

ANXIETY DISORDERS

Anxiety Disorders are the most prevalent psychiatric disorders. Women have a two to three times higher rate of Anxiety Disorders. The Epidemiologic Catchment Area study and National Comorbidity Survey report lifetime prevalence rates comparing female with male patients as Panic Disorder (3.4% vs 0.9%), Agoraphobia (9% vs 3%), Social Phobia (16.4% vs 11.2%), Specific Phobia (13.9% vs 7.2%), GAD (7.7% vs 2.9%), Posttraumatic Stress Disorder (PTSD; 11.3% vs 6%), and Obsessive Compulsive Disorder (3.1% vs 2.1%). Anxiety is also a normal part of human development, and a sensation most people can understand when they are given guidance. One of the earliest experiences with anxiety occurs in our toddler years as separation anxiety. This emotion can propel us toward our ultimate goal of autonomy with comfortable attachment, or, for subtle reasons, can result in excessive, chronic, and inappropriate fears. Anxiety is often experienced as somatic symptoms, such as heart palpitations, shortness of breath, shaking, sweating, numbness, headaches, stomach aches, and chest pain. Other, more difficult symptoms, include difficulty concentrating, irritability, low frustration tolerance, insomnia, cognitive defects, and avoidance. Anxiety is elusive and pervasive. It can occur as many different symptoms and can change its presentation just as you begin to zero in on managing the initial manifestation. It seems to be a coalescing of genetic predisposition, early childhood developmental experiences, and specific life events, which leave an impact and the current stresses in an individual's life. Despite anxiety's universality, it is frequently not recognized in primary care settings, placing an obstacle to appropriate treatment. Primary care practitioners must recognize the overt and veiled manifestations of the illness, exclude a potential medical cause, and begin to use treatment modalities, knowing that chasing down anxiety will be extremely difficult. Analyses of large prevalence studies of psychiatric illnesses in the United States find that Anxiety Disorders afflict 15.7 million people in the United States each year, and 30 million people in the United States at some point in their lives. Compared with other psychiatric disorders, people with anxiety disorders are high care users who present to general practitioners more frequently than to psychiatric professionals *(59)*. These statistics further emphasize the importance of recognition and management of Anxiety Disorders in primary care settings.

Patients with Anxiety Disorders often feel embarrassed about their symptoms and feel that their symptoms represent a personal weakness. They have struggled with many disappointments in their personal and professional lives, stemming from low self-esteem and a lack of sense of mastery *(60)*. It is important to empathize with the misery they experience as a result of their symptoms. Primary care providers can also present an accurate conceptualization of patient's disorders, referring to the commonality of these disorders in an effort to address misperceptions and assure them regarding treatment options.

Anxiety Disorders also have high rates of comorbidity with other Anxiety Disorders, Substance Abuse Disorders, and Mood Disorders. We can start by appropriately recognizing the symptoms of anxiety. Patients can be advised on the affects of stimulants on anxiety (alcohol, cigarettes, and caffeine) and be encouraged to begin the process of making a mind and body connection. It is helpful to hold off on prescribing medications, despite the fact that you, as a clinician, may be feeling anxious in the face of the patient's extreme alarm, worry, and frustration. Benzodiazepines are affective in treating anxiety and are, therefore, among the most common prescriptions written. However, the message to the patient is of concern, it reinforces a sense of helplessness, which is exacerbated by the fact that they may eventually develop tolerance to these medications. Patients have been successfully treated with psychotherapy without medications and will show the same physiological changes as those patients treated with medications. Listening to your patients can be extremely powerful coupled with certain lifestyle recommendations, such as exercise and yoga. Meditation can help patients understand the importance of the state of relaxation. It is useful for patients to "tune in" more to their emotional states and begin to identify what situations, thoughts, feelings, and experiences are triggering their anxiety. There are some basic psychotherapeutic techniques that are known to be helpful interventions in anxiety disorders. Progressive Muscle Relaxation, Deep Breathing Techniques, Exposure, Guided Imagery, and Self-Hypnosis all have specific protocols that your patient can practice on a daily basis. If patients do not respond to these interventions, they can be referred to Cognitive Behavioral Therapists or Clinics devoted to treating Anxiety Disorders. Certain individuals might be better referred to more Psychodynamic (insight oriented) Psychotherapists. They might be identified as individuals with residuals from early life experiences, difficulty identifying or experiencing emotions, personality or interpersonal difficulties, and unconscious conflicts. If medications are chosen or necessary, there are certain guidelines that may be useful. Patients with acute, brief, and occasional symptoms of anxiety can be treated with benzodiazepines as needed, with careful monitoring of tolerance and abuse. Patients with performance anxiety sometimes benefit from β-blockers. Some of the more selective agents are less sedating. Chronic anxiety symptoms should be treated either with antidepressants with an antianxiety indication and spectrum or with buspirone (an azapirone), which is a partial serotonin agonist. The serotonin reuptake inhibitors are typically first-line treatments, and each has an indication for anxiety. Fluoxetine has an indication for Obsessive Compulsive Disorder, paroxetine has indications for GAD and Social Anxiety, sertraline has indications for Panic Disorder and Obsessive Compulsive Disorder, fluvoxamine is indicated for Obsessive Compulsive Disorder, and escitalopram was recently granted indication for GAD. Tricyclic antidepressants and monoamine oxidase inhibitors have been used to treat anxiety, but are not as frequently prescribed because of their side effect profiles. The following section outlines the clinical manifestations of each of the anxiety disorders.

Panic Attack

A discrete period of intense fear or discomfort, in which at least four of the following symptoms develop abruptly and reached a peak within 10 minutes:

1. Palpitations, pounding heart, or accelerated heart rate.
2. Sweating.
3. Trembling or Shaking.
4. Sensations of shortness of breath or smothering.
5. Feeling of choking.
6. Chest pain or discomfort.
7. Nausea or abdominal distress.
8. Feeling dizzy, unsteady, lightheaded, or faint.
9. Derealization (feelings of unreality) or Depersonlization (being detached from oneself).
10. Fear of losing control or going crazy.
11. Fear of dying.
12. Paresthesias.
13. Chills or hot flashes.

Panic Disorder

Panic Disorder is defined by recurrent unexpected Panic Attacks followed by at least one of the attacks being followed by at least 1 month of at least one of the following symptoms:

1. Persistent concern about having additional attacks.
2. Worry about the implications of the attack or its consequences.
3. A significant change in behavior related to the attacks.

Panic Disorder can occur with or without Agoraphobia.

Agoraphobia

Anxiety about being in places or situations from which escape might be difficult (or embarrassing), or where help may not be available in the event of having an unexpected or situationally predisposed Panic Attack of panic-like symptoms. Agoraphobic fears typically involve characteristic clusters of situations that include being outside the home alone, being in a crowd or standing in a line, being on a bridge, and traveling in a bus, train, or automobile. The situations are avoided or are otherwise endured with marked distress or with anxiety about having a Panic Attack or panic-like symptoms. The presence of a companion is often required.

A Specific Phobia is a marked and persistent fear that is excessive or unreasonable, cued by the presence or anticipation of a specific object or situation. Exposure to the phobic stimulus almost invariably provokes an immediate anxiety response, which may take the form of a situationally bound or situationally predisposed Panic Attack. Although the person recognizes that the fear is excessive or unreasonable, the phobic situations are avoided or else endured with intense anxiety or distress.

Social Phobia (Social Anxiety Disorder) is a marked and persistent fear of one or more social or performance situations in which the person is exposed to unfamiliar people or to possible scrutiny by others. The individual fears that she will act in a way (or show anxiety symptoms) that will be humiliating or embarrassing. Exposure to the feared social situation almost invariably provokes anxiety, which may take the form of a situationally bound or situationally predisposed Panic Attack. The person recognizes that the fear is excessive or unreasonable and social or performance situations are avoided or else are endured with intense anxiety or distress. Social Anxiety is very prevalent and cause enormous distress in peoples' lives. It can manifest itself by causing the person to feel self-conscious walking across a courtyard, making telephone calls, having dinner with friends, or giving a presentation.

Obsessive Compulsive Disorder

Obsessive Compulsive Disorder (not to be confused with Obsessive Compulsive Personality Disorder) consists of either Obsessions or Compulsions.

Obsessions:

1. Recurrent and persistent thoughts, impulses, or images that are experienced, at some time during the disturbance, as intrusive and inappropriate and that cause marked anxiety or distress.
2. The thoughts, impulses, or images are not simply excessive worries about real-life problems.
3. The person attempts to ignore or suppress such thoughts, impulses, or images, or to neutralize them with some other thought or action.
4. The person recognizes that the obsessional thoughts, impulses, or images are a product of their own mind (not imposed from without, as in though insertion).

Compulsions:

1. Repetitive behaviors or mental acts that the person feels driven to perform in response to an obsession, or according to rules that must be applied rigidly.

2. The behaviors or mental acts are aimed at preventing or reducing distress or preventing some dreaded event or situation; however, these behaviors or mental acts either are not connected in a realistic way with what they are designed to neutralize or prevent, or are clearly excessive.

GAD

GAD is characterized as excessive anxiety and worry (apprehensive expectation), occurring more days than not for at least 6 months, about a number of events or activities. The person finds it difficult to control the worry and the anxiety or worry are associated with at least three of the following symptoms:

1. Restlessness or feeling keyed up or on edge.
2. Being easily fatigued.
3. Difficulty concentrating or mind going blank.
4. Irritability.
5. Muscle tension.
6. Sleep disturbance.

Clinical presentation of GAD is very similar in men and women in terms of severity, severity of concomitant depressive symptoms, duration of GAD, and quality-of-life impairment in physical health; however, women have been found to present at an earlier age and to have higher somatic factor scores compared with men *(61)*.

PTSD and Acute Stress Disorder

PTSD and Acute Stress Disorder (ASD) present certain specific treatment needs. As with all other anxiety disorders, PTSD and ASD are best treated with a combination of supportive interventions, psychoeducation, psychotherapy, and psychopharmacology. The nature of the pathophysiology of PTSD and ASD warrants some additional guidelines. The essential features of PTSD and ASD are the development of characteristic symptoms after exposure to the following events: an extreme traumatic stressor involving direct personal experience of an event that involves actual or threatened death, serious injury, or other threat to one's physical integrity; witnessing an event that involves death, injury, or a threat to physical integrity of another person; learning about the unexpected or violent death, serious harm, or threat of death or injury experienced by a family member or other close associate. The definition of trauma has been expanded with time, and the diagnostic criteria provide for acute (<3 mo), chronic (≥3 mo), and delayed onset (≥6 mo have passed between the traumatic event and the onset of the symptoms) specifiers allowing for identification of patients with the diagnoses and in need of treatment. The DSM IV diagnostic criteria are as follows:

PTSD

1. The person has been exposed to a traumatic event in which both of the following were present:
   a. The person experienced, witnessed, or was confronted with an event or events that involved actual or threatened death, serious injury, or a threat to physical integrity of self or others.
   b. The person's response involved intense fear, helplessness, or horror.
2. The traumatic event is persistently reexperienced in at least one of the following ways:
   a. Recurrent and intrusive distressing recollections of the event, including images, thoughts, and perceptions.
   b. Recurrent distressing dreams of the event.
   c. Acting or feeling as if the traumatic event were recurring.
   d. Intense psychological distress at exposure to internal or external cues that symbolize or resemble an aspect of the traumatic event.
   e. Physiological reactivity on exposure to internal or external cues that symbolize or resemble an aspect of the traumatic event.
3. Persistent avoidance of stimuli associated with the trauma or numbing of general responsiveness (not present before the trauma), as indicated by at least three of the following:
   a. Efforts to avoid thoughts, feelings, or conversations associated with the trauma.
   b. Efforts to avoid activities, places, or people that arouse recollections of the trauma.
   c. Inability to recall an important aspect of the trauma.
   d. Markedly diminished interest or participation in significant activities.
   e. Feeling of detachment or estrangement from others.
   f. Restricted range of affect.
   g. Sense of a foreshortened future.
4. Persistent symptoms of increased arousal (not present before the trauma), as indicated by at least two of the following:
   a. Difficulty falling or staying asleep.
   b. Irritability or outbursts of anger.
   c. Difficulty concentrating.
   d. Hypervigilance.
   e. Exaggerated startle response.

ASD

1. The person has been exposed to a traumatic event in which both of the following were present:
   a. The person experienced, witnessed, or was confronted with an event or events that involved actual or threatened death or serious injury, or a threat to the physical integrity of self or others.

   b. The person's response involved intense fear, helplessness, or horror.

2. Either while experiencing or after experiencing the distressing event, the individual has at least three of the following dissociative symptoms:
   a. A subjective sense of numbing, detachment, or absence of emotional responsiveness.
   b. Reduction in awareness of their surroundings.
   c. Derealization.
   d. Depersonalization.
   e. Dissociative amnesia.

3. The traumatic event is persistently reexperienced in at least one of the following ways:
   a. Recurrent images, thoughts, dreams, illusions, or flashback episodes.
   b. A sense of reliving the experience.
   c. Distress on exposure to reminders of the traumatic event.

4. Marked avoidance of stimuli that arouse recollections of the trauma.
5. Marked symptoms of anxiety or increased arousal.

Community-based studies reveal lifetime prevalence for PTSD ranging from 1 to 14%, with a variability related to methods of ascertainment and the population sampled. Studies of at-risk individuals (combat veterans, victims of natural disasters, or criminal violence) have yielded prevalence rates ranging from 3 to 58% (DSM IV). Women have higher lifetime prevalence rates and longer duration of illness. A recent small study found that 16% of patients with Multiple Sclerosis sampled in the study met criteria for PTSD, and 75% reported intrusions related to future-oriented concerns regarding their prognosis *(62)*. Primary care providers may want to consider PTSD in their patients with chronic debilitating illnesses. Exposure to previous trauma may affect vulnerability to subsequent trauma, influence the development of PTSD, and complicate treatment and recovery. Recent loss, particularly if sudden and unexpected, is also associated with an increased prevalence of PTSD and may also complicate treatment *(63)*. An acute episode of PTSD or ASD may be precipitated by a recent trauma but may be related to more remote traumatic experiences. Practice Guidelines, therefore, recommend that psychotherapeutic interventions aimed at the acute trauma must also target the remote trauma to diminish symptoms *(63)*. Differences in trauma exposures between women and men may also affect treatment considerations. Men are more likely to be exposed to combat and physical violence, whereas women are more likely to be exposed to rape and sexual assault. Women also have a higher incidence of childhood sexual abuse, creating increased vulnerability to the development of PTSD in adulthood.

Treatment of PTSD and ASD requires the initial step of identifying individuals by screening for recent or remote trauma exposure. The first interventions in the aftermath of an acute trauma consist of stabilizing and supportive medical care coupled with supportive psychiatric care and assessment. Once a safe physical and psychological environment has been established, a complete diagnostic evaluation can be performed. Assess for the symptoms of PTSD and ASD and establish the chronology of events. Individuals who have suffered acute trauma with no predisposing factors and have good supports will generally do well with psychoeducation and supportive psychotherapy. It is helpful for them to understand the symptoms of PTSD and ASD, and that the symptoms are usually short lived (<3 mo), and are expected under the circumstances. It is important to encourage the victims of trauma to use their own inherent strengths and social and family supports to assure their sense of safety. The goals of treatment are to reduce symptoms, prevent comorbid conditions from emerging, improve adaptive functioning, and to restore a psychological sense of safety and trust. Encourage patients to maintain healthy living habits (sleep, exercise, and healthy eating), because they realign the individual with their daily routine. Benzodiazepines may be useful in reducing anxiety and improving sleep for a short-term course of treatment. The patient should reintegrate into their routine (work, school, and so on) as quickly, yet as comfortably, as possible. It is helpful to use friends or family to help in this reintegration (e.g., having support people walk to and from work with the patient, have someone stay with the patient for a while, and so on). Although it has been hypothesized that pharmacological treatment soon after trauma may prevent development of ASD or PTSD, existing evidence is limited and preliminary *(63)*. SSRIs are recommended as first-line treatment for PTSD, and provide relief of core symptoms in all three symptom clusters. Patients with chronic or delayed-onset PTSD may require psychotherapy that is more intensive and should be referred to a specialist.

SOMATOFORM DISORDERS

Somatoform Disorders are characterized by the presence of physical symptoms that suggest a general medical condition but are not fully explained by one, or by the direct effects of a substance, or by another psychiatric disorder. The symptoms cause clinically significant distress or impairment in social, occupational, and other areas of functioning. Most importantly, the symptoms are not in voluntary control. This is in contrast with Factitious Disorders and Malingering, when the physical symptoms are in voluntary control and aimed at assuming a sick role or related to environmental circumstances, respectively. Patients with Somatoform Disorders are very high users of health care, seeing multiple physicians and obtaining multiple evaluations and treatments. It has been estimated that Somatoform Disorders account for 50% of American health care costs. Somatoform Disorders have a much higher prevalence in women than men. Physicians can become frustrated with patients with Somatoform Disorders. Certain interventions can reduce the frustration, cost, iatrogenic sequella, and impairment of these disorders. Providers should keep office visits brief but regular (every 4 to 6 weeks) and should only allow for appointed times for visits or communication. A brief physical examination targeted to the site of complaint can reassure the patient and physician that the complaint is not the result of a significant medical illness. The physician can validate the patient's symptoms and continue to monitor them in follow-up visits. The physician can interpret and relieve these symptoms rather than cure them. The physician will want to avoid extensive diagnostic studies, laboratory studies, surgery, hospitalization, and addictive medications. In addition, avoid terms that imply a disability, while keeping in mind that the goal is to reduce impairment. It is helpful to keep the individual in one practice and involve her family and other social supports. Encourage continued work and social functioning and make your expectations explicit, while stressing increased responsibility on the patient's part. It is recommended to gradually transition patients with Somatoform Disorders to specialists for psychiatric treatment while maintaining a relationship with the patients for continued medical consultation. DSM IV describes the following diagnostic categories of Somatoform Disorders.

Somatization Disorder

Studies have reported widely variable lifetime prevalence rates of Somatization Disorder, ranging from 0.2 to 2% among women and less than 0.2% in men. A 10-to-1 female–to-male ratio of the lifetime prevalence was found in the Epidemiologic Catchment Area Study, and most patients were treated in somatic health services. A familial pattern is observed in 10 to 20% of cases. Full remission is rare. There are no specific pharmacological recommendations, unless there is a comorbid psychiatric disorder.

Somatization Disorder consists of:

1. A history of many physical complaints beginning before age 30 years that occur during a period of several years and result in treatment being sought or significant impairment in social, occupational, or other important areas of functioning.
2. Each of the following criteria must have been met, with individual symptoms occurring at any time during the course of the disturbance:
   a. Four pain symptoms: a history of pain related to at least four different sites or functions.
   b. Two gastrointestinal symptoms: a history of at least two gastrointestinal symptoms other than pain.

c. One sexual symptom: at history of at lease one sexual or reproductive symptom other than pain.
d. One pseudoneurological symptom.

Conversion Disorder

Conversion Disorder typically begins in late childhood or early adulthood, but rarely before 10 years of age or after age 35 years. It affects women much more frequently than men. Conversion symptoms are very common in medically ill patients and in postpartum women. Typically, individual conversion symptoms are of short duration. Recurrence is common occurring in one-fifth to one-quarter of individuals within 1 year. A single recurrence predicts future episodes. Factors associated with good prognosis include acute onset, presence of clearly identifiable stress at the time of onset, a short interval between onset and the institution of treatment, and above average intelligence. Symptoms of paralysis, aphonia, and blindness are associated with a good prognosis, whereas tremor and seizures are not. Limited data suggest that conversion symptoms are more frequent in relatives of individuals with Conversion Disorder. Treatment techniques include hypnosis, cognitive–behavioral therapy, psychodynamic therapy, and biofeedback. Pharmacology is not recommended unless there is a comorbid psychiatric disorder.

Conversion Disorder consists of:

1. One or more symptoms or deficits affecting voluntary motor or sensory function that suggest a neurological or other general medical condition.
2. Psychological factors are judged to be associated with the symptom or deficit because the initiation or exacerbation of the symptom or deficit is preceded by conflicts or other stressors.

Pain Disorder

Pain Disorder seems to be relatively common. It is estimated that in any given year, 10 to 15% of adults in the United States have some form of work disability caused by back pain alone. Most acute pain resolves in relatively short periods. There is a wide range of variability in the onset of chronic pain. Important factors that seem to influence recovery from Pain Disorder are the individual's participation in regularly scheduled activities despite the pain and resistance to allowing the pain to become the determining factor in her lifestyle. Psychological factors play a significant role in etiology, but the illness is not feigned. Nonsteroidal antiinflammatory agents, in combination with some of the antidepressants (e.g., TCAs) may be helpful. Alternative nonpharmacological measures, such as acupuncture and massage, have a useful role in shortening the disability.

Pain Disorder consists of:

1. Pain in at least one anatomical sites is the predominant focus of the clinical presentation and is of sufficient severity to warrant clinical attention.
2. The pain causes clinically significant distress or impairment in social, occupational, or other important areas of functioning.
3. Psychological factors are judged to have an important role in the onset, severity, exacerbation, or maintenance of the pain.

Hypochondriasis

The prevalence of Hypochondriasis in the general population is unknown and is equal in both men and women. The prevalence in general medical practice has been reported to be between 4 and 9%. It can begin at any age but is observed most commonly early adulthood. The course is usually chronic, with waxing and waning symptoms, although recovery sometimes occurs. A link to other disorders of serotonin dysregulation (anxiety and depression) leads to some benefit from SSRIs in certain cases. Supportive psychotherapy is helpful.

Hypochondriasis consists of:

1. Preoccupation with fears of having, or the idea that one has, a serious disease based on the misinterpretation of bodily symptoms.
2. The preoccupation persists despite appropriate medical evaluation and reassurance.
3. The belief in criterion 1 is not of delusional intensity.
4. The duration of the disturbance is at least 6 months.
5. The preoccupation causes clinically significant distress or impairment in social, occupational, or other important areas of functioning.

Body Dysmorphic Disorder

Body Dysmorphic Disorder (BDD) is common in women (estimates of 49–76% of BDD cases), but remains underdiagnosed, and is sometimes difficult to treat. Prevalence rates are unclear. Community studies from the United States have reported rates of 2.3% and 1.1% BDD, usually beginning during adolescence, but possibly taking years to be diagnosed. The onset can be either gradual or abrupt. The disorder has a fairly continuous course, with few symptom-free intervals, although the intensity of symptoms may wax and wane. Most women with BDD seek nonpsychiatric treatments, which are often costly (dermatological and surgical treatments). Cognitive–behavioral treatment may be effective for BDD, and SSRIs have been studied and found to be helpful. Fluoxetine at doses similar to Obsessive Compulsive Disorder is recommended (60–80 mg).

BDD consists of:

1. Preoccupation with an imagined defect in appearance. If a slight physical anomaly is present, the person's concern is markedly excessive.

2. The preoccupation causes clinically significant distress or impairment in social, occupational, or other important areas of functioning.
3. The preoccupation is not better accounted for by any other mental disorder (e.g., Anorexia Nervosa).

PSYCHOTIC ILLNESSES

Psychotic illnesses are characterized by having psychotic symptoms as their defining feature. The term psychotic has historically received a number of different definitions, none of which has achieved universal acceptance (DSM IV). Definitions have ranged from restrictive, such as having hallucinations or delusions, to broader definitions, including other positive symptoms, such as disorganized speech and behavior, to earlier inclusive definitions, which stated that psychosis was related to a severe degree of functional impairment. Finally, the term has been defined conceptually as a loss of ego boundaries or a gross impairment in reality testing. Psychotic illnesses include Schizophrenia, Schizophreniform Disorder, Schizoaffective Disorder, Delusional Disorder, Brief Reactive Psychosis, and Shared Psychotic Disorder. Psychosis can also occur secondary to a medical condition, can be induced by substances, and can occur during an episode of Depression or Mania. This section will focus on Schizophrenia and some of the sex-specific issues present among women with Schizophrenia or Postpartum Psychosis.

Stigma remains a problem despite advances made in understanding psychotic illnesses and treatment. Because of inadequacies in insurance coverage and social support systems, patients with Psychotic illnesses often lack appropriate medical and psychiatric treatment. Psychotic illnesses often coexist with general medical and gynecological illnesses, increasing the need for care. Patients with Schizophrenia have high rates of suicide (10–30%). Women with Schizophrenia are vulnerable to become victims of sexual and physical violence. They may also begin to abuse alcohol and other substances early in life, making them at increased risk of substance-related health problems. According to the Centers for Disease Control and Prevention, in 1995, women with Schizophrenia are at higher risk of contracting HIV and Hepatitis C than men with Schizophrenia. These findings emphasize the vital role the primary care practitioner plays in helping to minimize the morbidity and mortality of these devastating illnesses. Although psychotic symptoms are striking, they are frequently missed in the hurried, medically focused setting of a primary care practice. In 1996, psychiatrist Roberta J. Apfel addressed the issue, focused on the fact that severe mental illness was frequently missed because physicians fail to take note of the obvious. Identifying Psychosis does not necessarily match the characteristic role of the primary care physician *(64)*. Apfel stated "making the diagnosis of psychosis—a break with reality frequently accompanied by delusions, hallucinations, incoherent speech, or bizarre actions—begins with brief, matter of fact interchanges that can reveal something unusual." Open-ended questions are sometimes effective in eliciting psychotic symptoms. Patients can develop symptoms acutely or after a prodromal period of social withdrawal, impaired functioning, peculiar behavior, and neglect of personal hygiene. The characteristic symptoms of Schizophrenia include at least two of the following, each present for a significant portion of time during a 1-month period (or shorter, if successfully treated):

1. Delusions.
2. Hallucinations.
3. Disorganized speech.
4. Grossly disorganized or catatonic behavior.
5. Negative symptoms (affective flattening, alogia, or avolition).

Patients with Schizophrenia have significant social and occupational impairment, well below the level achieved before the onset of illness. They generally have continuous signs of disturbance for at least 6 months. They may also suffer from neurocognitive decline, such as a decrease in verbal and arithmetic IQ, memory deficits, slowed reaction time, and decreased executive functioning (planning, organization, and problem solving). Although the lifetime prevalence for Schizophrenia is approximately equal for men and women, there are certain characteristics that differ. Women are likely to have a later onset of illness with more mood symptoms (dysphoria), less aggression, and lower rates of suicide. They present more with positive symptoms of paranoia and prosecutory delusions compared with men, who present more commonly with negative symptoms. Women will more likely marry, maintain some degree of work functioning, and parent children. Treatment of Schizophrenia requires continuous medication management with periodic hospitalization for acute exacerbations. Newer atypical antipsychotics (clozaril, risperdone, olanzapine, quietiapine, zisprasidone, and ariprazole) are thought to have lower incidence of some of the serious long-term side effects (tardive dyskinesia) of the older typical antipsychotics (haloperisol, fluphenazine, and chlorpromazine). They do however, pose some concerns specifically related to metabolism and hormone changes. Treatment is often incomplete, leaving residual symptoms. Studies have shown that women may respond to lower doses of antipsychotic medication because of their lipophilic nature and decreased gastric emptying. Women are also sensitive to some specific side effects that could affect compliance. They may develop antipsychotic-induced hyperprolactinemia, leading to galactorrhea and irregular menses. Antipsychotic medications may also influence the development of osteoporosis and can cause sexual dysfunction and affect fertility. Primary care practitioners involved in treating women with Schizophrenia can provide the important support needed to assure continuity of treatment for medical conditions and ongoing management of psychiatric illness with a specialist. Keeping family involved and maintaining open communication with your patient can enhance your relationship. There are certain psychosocial interventions that are always helpful, including, but not limited to, decreasing stigmatization. The physician should encourage individuals to keep their stress levels to a minimum and to maintain a hopeful attitude regarding maximizing treatment.

Postpartum Psychosis is not currently addressed in the DSM IV. Continued study is strongly suggested because the devastating consequences of this condition are not fully understood or addressed. There is debate regarding whether this condition is related to childbirth or an episodic presentation of a psychotic illness. It is thought to occur in 1 to 2 of 1000 postpartum women. The risk of symptoms is highest during the first month after delivery and declines after that period. Women with Bipolar Type I Disorder seem to be at particular risk, and Postpartum Depression can occur with or without psychotic features. Women with Psychotic Depression are often tearful, experience psychomotor retardation, sleep and appetite disturbance, are preoccupied with feelings of guilt and worthlessness, develop delusions that their infant is dead or defective, may deny having given birth, and experience hallucinations commanding them to harm their baby. Women with Manic Psychosis are more irritable, excited, euphoric, hyperactive, have decreased sleep and insight, and grandiose delusions that interfere with their infant's safety either directly (delusions leading to harming their baby) or indirectly (unable to care for their baby). A more Schizophreniform diathesis would present with thought disorder, delusions, inappropriate affect, agitation, motor retardation, bizarre delusional ideas, and decreased insight. It is imperative to recognize this syndrome because of its potential harm and because 95% of women who are treated improve within 2 to 3 months.

SUBSTANCE MISUSE

Although substance abuse and dependence is more common in men, rates in women have been increasing dramatically. One in three alcoholics in the United States are women, accounting for 6 million women in the United States. Women may also progress more rapidly into the illness and the complications of substance use. On college campuses, a higher proportion of rapes occur when women are intoxicated, indicating a need for prevention programs *(65)*. There are very high rates of comorbidity of psychiatric disorders in women with substance use disorders. Co-occurring psychiatric illness and substance misuse among primary care patients has been increasing approx 10% each year, and comorbid cases are becoming younger *(66)*. The health consequences of substance abuse must be considered. There has also been a large range of medical health conditions that are related to alcohol and other substance abuses, such as hypertension, coronary artery disease, HIV infection, hepatitis, liver disease, congestive heart failure, pancreatic disease, asthma, and acid-related peptic disorders *(67)*. Deaths from addictive disorders are estimated to account for one-quarter to one-third of all deaths in the United States. Risk factors for the development of substance misuse in women include Depression, Bipolar Disorder, Anxiety Disorders, Eating Disorders, family history of substance abuse, stressful life events, avoidant coping style, partner abuses, and physical or sexual victimization in childhood. Alcoholism among elderly women is on the rise because of isolation, loss of spouse, and decreased social supports. Lesbian patients pose an especially high risk of substance abuse problems compared with heterosexual women (alcoholism, 23% vs 8%; marijuana abuse, 67% vs 7%; cocaine abuse, 23% vs 2%; and nicotine abuse, 27% vs 13%). Lesbians have higher rates of histories of sexual assault, incest, and other victimization. This makes them at increased risk of not only substance misuse disorders but other comorbid psychiatric conditions. Diagnosis of illness in lesbians may be delayed because of their perception that the health care system is hostile, combined with their need to counter the assumption of heterosexuality. The fact is that they are more likely to be uninsured than heterosexual women. Women of other special populations that should be screened include women with socioeconomic stress, minorities, and athletes, who may abuse narcotics, stimulants, and steroids. Once substance misuse is identified, women can be referred to 12-step programs. It might be best to find a particular group for women because they can benefit from other women role models and may have complicated histories with men. Women are more likely to have a spouse with a substance abuse problem, further complicating their attempts at abstinence. Family therapy and psychotherapy are useful at addressing many of the confounding factors related to substance abuse in women. Comorbid psychiatric conditions should be treated, avoiding medications of abuse. There are specific pharmacotherapies that are used depending on the substance of abuse (disulfuram and naltrexone), with new medications being studied. There are times when inpatient treatment is needed; consenting patients should be referred. Education is extremely important. Issues related to the effects of children raised by addictive mothers, risks during pregnancy, medical complications, psychiatric comorbidities, and other consequences should be emphasized.

PERSONALITY DISORDERS

Although it will be unusual for primary care providers to treat patients personality disorders, it is very useful to have a broad understanding of the disorders that exist. This knowledge may help in maintaining a healthy and appropriate doctor–patient relationship and in predicting what barriers to treatment may be encountered. The DSM-IV (American Psychiatric Association, 1994) defines a Personality Disorder as a stable, durable pattern of behavior and internal experience that differs sharply from cultural expectations, is rigid and pervasive, begins in adolescence or early adulthood, and results in impairments or distress. There are 10 specific personality disorders classified, divided into three clusters. Often, patients manifest characteristics of more than one personality disorder or cluster. The clusters are as follows:

The "odd" Cluster A, generally more common in men than women, consists of:

1. Paranoid Personality Disorder, at least four of the following:
   a. Suspects, without sufficient basis, that others are exploiting, harming, or deceiving.
   b. Preoccupied with unjustified doubts regarding the loyalty or trustworthiness of others.
   c. Is reluctant to confide in others for fear that the information will be misused.
   d. Reads hidden demeaning or threatening meanings into benign remarks or events.
   e. Persistently bears grudges.
   f. Perceives attacks on his or her character or reputation and is quick to react.
   g. Recurrent suspicions regarding fidelity of spouse or sexual partner.
2. Schizoid Personality Disorder, at least four of the following:
   a. Neither desires no enjoys close relationships (including family).
   b. Almost always chooses solitary activities.
   c. Has little, if any, interest in have sexual experiences with another person.
   d. Takes pleasure in few, if any activities.
   e. Lacks close friends or confidants other than first-degree relatives.
   f. Seems indifferent to the praise or criticism of others.
   g. Shows emotional coldness, detachment, or flattened affectivity.
3. Schizotypal Personality Disorder, at least five of the following:
   a. Ideas of reference (excluding delusions).
   b. Odd beliefs or magical thinking that influences behavior and is not the norm.
   c. Unusual perceptual experiences, including bodily illusions.
   d. Odd thinking and speech.
   e. Suspiciousness or paranoid ideation.
   f. Inappropriate or constricted affect.
   g. Behavior or appearance that is odd, eccentric, or peculiar.
   h. Lack of close friend or confidants other than first-degree relatives.
   i. Excessive social anxiety associated with paranoid fears.

The "dramatic" Cluster B consists of:

1. Antisocial Personality Disorder (3% men vs 1% women), occurring since age 15 years, at least three of the following:
   a. Failure to conform to social norms with respect to lawful behaviors.

b. Deceitfulness, repeated lying, use of aliases, conning others.
c. Impulsivity or failure to plan ahead.
d. Irritability and aggressiveness.
e. Reckless disregard for safety of self or others.
f. Consistent irresponsibility.
g. Lack of remorse.

2. Borderline Personality Disorder (75% of cases are women, high association with sexual and physical abuse), at least five of the following:
   a. Frantic efforts of avoid real or imagined abandonment.
   b. A pattern of unstable and intense interpersonal relationships characterized by alternating between extremes of idealization and devaluation.
   c. Identity disturbance; markedly and persistently unstable self-image.
   d. Impulsivity in at least two potentially harmful areas (spending, sex, recklessness).
   e. Recurrent suicidal behavior, gestures, or threats; self-mutilation.
   f. Affective instability, marked reactivity of mood.
   g. Chronic feelings of emptiness.
   h. Inappropriate, intense anger or difficulty controlling anger.
   i. Transient, stress-related paranoid ideation or dissociative symptoms.
3. Histrionic Personality Disorder (more common in women), at least five of the following:
   a. Uncomfortable if not the center of attention.
   b. Interacts frequently in sexually seductive or provocative ways.
   c. Displays rapidly shifting and shallow expressions of emotions.
   d. Consistently uses physical appearance to draw attention to self.
   e. Style of speech is excessively impressionistic and lacking in detail.
   f. Shows self-dramatization, theatricality, and exaggerated expression of emotion.
   g. Is suggestible.
   h. Considers relationships to be more intimate than they actually are.
4. Narcissistic Personality Disorder (50–75% men), at least five of the following:
   a. Grandiose sense of self-importance.
   b. Preoccupied with fantasies of unlimited success, power, brilliance, or ideal love.
   c. Believes they are "special" and unique, only understood by high-status people.
   d. Requires excessive admiration.
   e. Has a sense of entitlement.
   f. Is interpersonally exploitative.
   g. Lacks empathy.
   h. Is often envious of others or believes they are envious.
   i. Shows arrogant, haughty behaviors or attitudes.

The "anxious" Cluster C consists of:

1. Avoidant Personality Disorder, at least four of the following:
   a. Avoids occupational activities that involve interpersonal contact.

   b. Unwilling to get involved with people unless certain of being liked.
   c. Shows restraints within intimate relationships fearing being shamed or ridiculed.
   d. Preoccupied with being criticized or rejected in social situations.
   e. Inhibited in new interpersonal situations, feeling inadequate.
   f. Views self as socially inept, personally unappealing, or inferior to others.
   g. Is unusually reluctant to take personal risks or engage in new activities.

2. Dependent Personality Disorder, at least five of the following:
   a. Difficulty making everyday decisions without excessive advice or reassurance.
   b. Needs others to assume responsibility for most major areas of life.
   c. Difficulty expressing disagreement with others fearing loss of support or approval.
   d. Difficulty initiating projects or doing things on his or her own.
   e. Goes to excessive lengths to obtain nurturance and support of others.
   f. Feels uncomfortable or helpless when alone.
   g. Urgently seeks another relationship when a close relationship ends.
   h. Unrealistically preoccupied with fears of being left to care for self.

3. Obsessive–Compulsive Personality Disorder (twice as common in men), at least four of the following:
   a. Preoccupied with details, rules, lists, order, organization, to the extent that the major point of the activity is lost.
   b. Shows perfectionism that interferes with task completion.
   c. Is excessively devoted to work and productivity to the exclusion of leisure.
   d. Overly conscientious, scrupulous, and inflexible regarding matters of morality, ethics, or values.
   e. Unable to discard worn-out or worthless objects.
   f. Reluctant to delegate tasks or to work with others unless they submit.
   g. Adopts a miserly spending style toward self and others.
   h. Shows rigidity and stubbornness.

The sex distribution of Personality Disorders is confounded by multiple determinants. One must consider the comorbid Axis I Disorders, differential environmental exposure, and impact of risk factors, social role training, biological influences, adaptive styles, diagnostic biases, and a differential threshold to seek treatment. Treatment studies have focused mostly on Borderline Personality Disorder because this particular Personality Disorder is most likely to come to the attention of health care providers. Treatments encompass a range of options, including Cognitive–Behavioral Therapy, Psychodynamic Psychotherapy, Dialectical Behavioral Therapy, and Psychopharmacology. The primary psychopharmacological agents found to be beneficial in Borderline Personality Disorder are the SSRIs ,although virtually every class of medication has been tried. It is best to refer these patients to specialized care.

SUMMARY

The scope of mental health needs and mental disorders worldwide is dramatic and growing. In both developed and developing countries, 25% of individuals develop one or more mental or behavioral disorders at some stage in life (WHO 2001). Despite the gravity of these numbers, we are still lagging behind in adequately diagnosing and treating these disorders. The consequences of inadequate detection and treatment are well-known, beginning from lack of fulfillment of potential progressing to the most devastating morbidities and mortality. Psychiatric Disorders account for an overwhelming majority of the number of reported suicides. Women are among the groups identified as being most vulnerable to some of the most prevalent Psychiatric Disorders. Management and treatment of Psychiatric Disorders in primary care is a fundamental step, enabling the largest number of people to obtain easier and faster access to services. The integration of mental health care into primary health care services has many potential advantages. These include a decrease in stigmatization, improved detection rates for patients presenting with vague somatic complaints, improved treatment for physical problems in those suffering from Mental Illness, and better management of the mental aspects of "physical problems." Additionally, services for women need to include an enhanced, unbiased understanding of the factors influencing the development of Psychiatric Disorders as they relate to gender. Primary Care Providers must be able to elicit the patients' story, listen thoughtfully and nonjudgmentally, and to tolerate sensitive topics and powerful emotions. These approaches are essential to accurate diagnosis, leading to patient trust and compliance with treatment. The integration of mental health care into primary health care also requires careful analysis of what is and what is not possible to treat in a primary care setting. If there is need for specialized care for Psychiatric Disorders, the process of referral can be facilitated if the primary care provider has already established a network and pattern of referral as part of his or her practice. Most importantly, informed treatment by the primary care provider alone or in concert with a specialist can almost always alleviate the patients' symptoms and improve her state of health.

REFERENCES

1. Kahn LS, Halbreich U, Bloom MS, et al. Screening for mental illness in primary care clinics. Int J Psychiatry Med 2004;34(4):345–362.
2. Dilts SL Jr., Mann N, Dilts JG. Accuracy of referring psychiatric diagnosis on a consultation-liaison service. Psychosomatics 2003;44(5):407–411.
3. Lynge I, Munk-Jorgensen P, Pedarsen Al, et al. Common Mental Disorders among patients in primary healthcare in Greenland. Int J Circumpolar Health 2004;63(2):377–383.

4. Aoun S, Pennebaker D, Wood C. Assessing population need for mental health care: a review of approaches and predictors. Ment Health Serv Res 2004;6(1):33–46.
5. Wang PS, Berglund P, Kessler RC. Recent care of common mental disorders in the United States: prevalence and conformance with evidence-based recommendations. J Gen Intern Med 2000;15(5):284–292.
6. Borowsky SJ, Rubenstein LV, Meredith LS, et al. Who is at risk of non-detection of mental health problems in primary care? J Gen Intern Med 2000;15(6):381–188.
7. Hodiamont PPG, Rijnder CATH, Mulder J, Furer JW. Psychiatric disorders in a Dutch health care area: a repeated cross-sectional survey. J Affect Disord 2005;84(1):77–83.
8. Murphy JM, Laid NM, Monson RR, et al. A 40-year perspective on the prevalence of depression: the Stirling County study. Arch Gen Psychiatry 2000;57:209–215.
9. Mental Health: A report of the Surgeon General, Epidemiology of Mental Illness. Rockville, MD: US Department of Health and Human services, substance tox and mental Health Services Administration, Center for Mental Health Services. (2001).
10. Calabrese LV. Approach to the patient with multiple physical complaints. In: the MGH Guide to Psychiatry in Primary Care (Stern TA, Herman JB, Slavin PL, eds.). McGraw-Hill, New York, 1998; pp. 89–98.
11. Rucci P, Gherardi S, Tansella M, et al. Subthreshold psychiatric disorders in primary care: prevalence and associated characteristics. J Affect Disord 2003;76(1-3):171–181.
12. Kessler RC, Brown RL, Broman CL. Sex differences in psychiatric help-seeking: evidence from four large-scale surveys. J Health Soc Behav 1981;22:49–64.
13. Angst J, Dubler-Mikola A. Do the diagnostic criteria determine the sex ratio is depression? J Affect Disord 1984;7:189–198.
14. Kessler RC. Gender differences in major depression: epidemiological findings. In: Gender and its Effects on Psychopathology (Frank E, ed.). American Psychiatric Press, Washington DC, 2000; pp. 61–84.
15. Parry BL. Hormonal basis of mood disorders in women. In: Gender and its Effects on Psychopathology (Frank E, ed.). American Psychiatric Press, Washington DC, 2000; pp. 61–84.
16. Young MA, Scheftner WA, Fawcett J, et al. Gender differences in the clinical features of unipolar depressive disorder. J Nerv Ment Dis 1990;178:200–203.
17. Frank E, Young E. Pubertal changes and adolescent changes: who do rates of depression rise precipitously for girls between ages 10 and 15 years? In: Gender and its Effects on Psychopathology (Frank E. ed.). American Psychiatric Press, Washington DC, 2000; pp. 85–101.
18. Cyranowski JM, Frank E, Young E, et al. Adolescent onset of the gender difference in lifetime rates of major depression: a theoretical model. Arch Gen Psychiatry 2000;57:21–27.
19. Burk VK, Stein K. Epidemiology of depression throughout the female life cycle. J Clin Psychiatry 2002;63(7):9–15.
20. American Association of University Women. Shortchanging Girls, Shortchanging America. American Association of University Women, Washington DC, 1991.
21. Stotland NL. Psychiatric and psychosocial issues in primary care for women. In, Women's Primary Health Care (Seltzer VL, Pearce WH, eds.). 2nd ed., McGraw-Hill, 2000; pp. 575–611.
22. George MS, Ketter TA, Parekh PI, et al. Gender differences in regional cerebral blood flow during transient self-induced sadness or happiness. Biol Psychol 1996;40:859–871.
23. Nolen-Hoeksema S. Gender differences in coping with depression across the lifespan. Depression 1995;3:81–90.
24. Ruble DN, Greulich F, Pomerantz EM, et al. The role of gender-related processes in the development of sex differences in self-evaluation and depression. J Affect Disord 1993;29: 97–128.
25. Hankin BL, Abramson LY. Development of gender differences in depression: an elaborated cognitive vulnerability—transactional stress theory. Psychol Bull 2001;127(6):773–796.

26. Spitzer RL, Kroenke K, Williams JB. Validation and utility of a self-report version of PRIME-MD: the PHQ primary care study Primary Care Evaluation of Mental Disorders. Patient Health Questionnaire. JAMA 1999;282(18):1737–1744.
27. Spitzer RL, Williams JB, Kroenke K, et al. Validity and utility of the PRIME-MD Patient Health Questionnaire in assessment of 3000 obstetric-gynecologic patients: The PRIME-MD Patient Health Questionnaire Obstetrics-Gynecology Study. Am J Obstet Gynecol 2000; 183(3):759–769.
28. Jogenelis K, Pot AM, Eisses AMH, et al. Prevalence and risk indicators of depression in elderly nursing home patients: the AGED study. J Affect Disord 2004;83(2–3):135–142.
29. Zunzunegui MV, Beland F, Llacer A, et al. Gender Differences in depressive symptoms among Spanish elderly. Soc Psychiatry Psychiatr Epidemiol 1998;33:195–205.
30. Meller I, Fichter MM, Schroppel H. Risk factors and psychosocial consequences of octo and nonagenerians: results of an epidemiological study. Eur Arch Psychiatry Clin Neurosci 1997;247:278–287.
31. Kessler RC, McGonagle KA, Swartz M, et al. Sex and depression in the national comorbidity survey: lifetime prevalence, chronicity and recurrence. J Affect Disord 1993;29:85–96.
32. Larson Mark. Depression. In: Women's Health Care Handbook (Johnson B, Johnson C, Murray J, Apgar B, eds.). 2nd ed. Harley and Belfus, Philadelphia, 2000;381–394.
33. Bland RC. Epidemiology of affective disorders: a review. Can J Psychiatry 1997;42(4): 367–377.
34. Sadovnick AD, Remick RA, Lam RW, et al. Mood Disorder Service Genetic Database: morbidity risks for mood disorders in 3,942 first-degree relatives of 671 index cases with single depression, recurrent depression, bipolar I, or bipolar II. Am J Med Genet 1994; 54:132–140.
35. Bostwick JM, Pankratz VS. Affective Disorders and suicide risk: a re-examination. Am J Psychiatry 2000;157:1925–1932.
36. O'Donnell L, O'Donnell C, Wardlaw DM, Stueve A. Risk and resiliency factors influencing suicidality among urban African American and Latino youth. Am J Community Psychol 2004;33(1–2):37–39.
37. Denihan A, Bruce I, Coakley D, Lawlor BA. Psychiatric morbidity in cohabitants of community-dwelling elderly depressives. J Geriatr Psychiatry 1998;13:691–694.
38. Goodman SH, Gotlib IH. Risk for psychopathology in the children of depressed mothers: a developmental model for understanding mechanisms of transmission. Psychol Rev 1999;106:458–490.
39. Murray CJ, Lopez AD. Alternative projections of mortality and disability by cause 1990–2020: Global Burden of Disease Study. Lancet 2001;349:1498–1504.
40. Gredon JF. The burden of disease in treatment-resistant depression. J Clin Psychiatry 2001;62:26–31.
41. Remick RA. Diagnosis and management of depression in primary care: a clinical update and review. Can Med Assoc J 2002;167(11):1253–1260.
42. Parker G, Parker K, Mitchell P, Wilhelm K. Atypical depression: Australian and US studies in accord. Curr Opin Psychiatry 2005;18(1):1–5.
43. Choutoi J, Smedh D, Johansson C, et al. An epidemiological study of gender differences in self-reported seasonal changes in mood and behavior in a general population of Nothern Sweden. Nord J Psychiatry 2004;58(6):429–437.
44. Thompson C, Thompson S, Smith R. Prevalence of seasonal affective disorder in primary care: a comparison of the seasonal health questionnaire and the seasonal questionnaire. J Affect Disord 2004;78(3):219–229.
45. Crotty F, Sheehan J. Prevalence and detection in an Irish community sample. Ir J Psychol Med 2004;21(4):117–121.

46. Gale S, Harlow BL. Postpartum mood disorders: a review of clinical and epidemiological factors. J Psychosom Obstet Gynaecol 2003;24(4):257–266.
47. Adewuya AO, Eegunranti AB, Lawal AM. Prevalence of postnatal depression in Western Nigerian women: a controlled study. Int J Psychiatry Clin Practice 2005;9(1):60–64.
48. Bugdayci R, Sasmaz CT, Tezan H, et al. A cross-sectional prevalence study of depression at various times after delivery in Mersin Province in Turkey. J Womens Health 2004;18(1): 63–68.
49. Franko DL, Thompson D, Barton BA, et al. Prevalence and comorbidity of major depressive disorder in young black and white women. J Psychiatr Res 2005;39(3):275–283.
50. Kessler RC, McGonagle KA, Zhao S, et al. Lifetime and 12 month prevalence of DSM-III-R psychiatric disorders in the United States: results from the National Comorbidity Study. Arch Gen Psychiatry 1994;51(1):8–19.
51. Gibbons RD, Hur K, Bhaumik DK, Mann JJ. The relationship between antidepressant medication use and rate of suicide. Arch Gen Psychiatry 2005;62(2):165–172.
52. Rosenfeld JA. Singular health care of women. In: Handbook of Women's Health: An Evidence Based Approach (Rosenfeld JA, ed.). Cambridge University Press, Cambridge, New York, 2001; pp. 1–12.
53. Bower P, Rowland N, Handy R. The clinical effectiveness of counseling in primary care: a systematic review and metaanalysis. Psychol Med 2003;33:203–215.
54. Proudfood J, Goldberg D, Mann A, et al. Computerized, interactive, multimedia cognitive-behavioral therapy for anxiety and depression in general practice. Psychol Med 2003;33: 217–227.
55. Gabbay M, Shiels C, Bower P, et al. Patient-practitioner agreement: does it matter? Psychol Med 2003;33:241–251.
56. Liebenluft E. Women with bipolar illness: clinical and research issues. Am J Psychiatry 1996;153:163–173.
57. Kennedy N, Boydell J, Kalidindi S, et al. Gender differences in incidence and age at onset of mania and bipolar disorder over a 35-year period in Camberwell, England. Am J Psychiatry 2005;162(2):257–262.
58. Blehar MC, Depaulo JR Jr., Gershon ES, et al. Women with Bipolar Disorder: Findings from the NIMH genetics initiative sample. Psychopharmacol Bull 1998;34:239–243.
59. Lepaine JP. The epidemiology of anxiety disorders: prevelence and societal costs. J Clin Psychiatry 2002;63(14):4–8.
60. Shear MK, Mammen O. Anxiety disorders in primary care: a life-span perspective. Bull Menninger Clin 1997;61(A):37–53.
61. Steiner M, Allugulander C, Ravindram A, et al. Gender differences in clinical presentation and response to sertraline treatment of generalized anxiety disorder. Hum Psychopharmacol: Clin Experiment 2005;20(1):3–13.
62. Chalfant AM, Bryant RA, Fulcher G. Posttraumatic stress disorder following diagnosis of multiple sclerosis. J Trauma Stress 2004;17(5):423–428.
63. Phillips KA. Body dysmorphic disorder. In: Women's Mental Health: A Comprehensive Textbook (Kornstein SG, Clayton AH, eds.). Guilford, New York, 2002; pp. 295–306.
64. Zerbe KJ. Women's Mental Health in Primary Care. W.B. Saunders, Philadelphia, 1999: p. 273.
65. Mohler-Kuo M, Dowdall GW, Koss MP, Wechsler H. Correlates of rape while intoxicated in a national sample of college women. J Stud Alcohol 2004;65(1):37–45.
66. Frisher M, Collins J, Millson D, et al. Prevalence of comorbid psychiatric illness and substance misuse in primary care in England and Wales. J Epidemiol Community Health 2004;58:1036–1041.
67. Mertens JR, Yun WL, Parthasarathy S, et al. Medical and psychiatric conditions of alcohol in drug treatment patients in an HMO. Arch Int Med 2003;163(20):2511–2517.

17 Intimate Partner Violence

How It Harms Your Patients and Impacts Your Practice

Connie Mitchell, MD, MPH
and Deirdre Anglin, MD, MPH

CONTENTS

INTRODUCTION

Prevalence studies of intimate partner violence (IPV) victimization in primary care indicate that 5.5% of adult female patients in an outpatient clinic setting had experienced physical abuse by an intimate partner in the year before their doctor's visit. If these patients are asked whether they had experienced abuse by an intimate partner at some time in their life, the number rises to 21.4% *(1)*.

From: *Current Clinical Practice: Women's Health in Clinical Practice*
Edited by: Clouse and Sherif © Humana Press Inc., Totowa, NJ

Partner violence directly harms the physical and emotional well-being of patients and is linked as a comorbid factor with numerous other physical and mental health problems, thus, complicating care plans and imposing liability to health care providers if not diagnosed and appropriately addressed. Numerous studies have shown that many victims of IPV are not identified in the health care setting, and, in a study by Sharps, 50% of femicide victims sought medical care in the year before being murdered by their abusers *(2)*. In addition, Wisner found that victims of IPV cost their health plan an additional $1,775 during 1 year compared with non-abused women *(3)*. It has been estimated that, in the United States, the cost from IPV totals an astounding $8.3 billion annually in 2003 dollars *(4)*. Therefore, health care providers need to become more proficient and more comfortable in identifying and addressing IPV in their practices.

DEFINITION

IPV has been perceived as a social justice and criminal justice issue for many years. Numerous terms have been used to refer to IPV, including domestic violence, spouse abuse, wife beating, and battered woman. IPV has been defined by the Family Violence Prevention Fund, a major national advocacy organization as: "A pattern of assaultive and coercive behaviors that may include physical injury, psychological abuse, sexual assault, progressive social isolation, stalking, deprivation, intimidation and threats that adults or adolescents use against their intimate partners" *(5)*. In 1999, the Centers for Disease Control and Prevention (CDC) issued their publication "Intimate Partner Violence Surveillance—Uniform Definitions and Recommended Data Elements" and indicated preference in all future research and funding for the term "intimate partner violence." They defined IPV as the threat or infliction of physical or sexual violence, or psychological or emotional abuse by current or former intimate partners *(6)*. In the International Classification of Diseases (ICD), the preferred diagnostic term is "Adult Maltreatment" *(7)*.

By any definition, intimate partners or dating couples manifest abuse in different ways, either singly or in combination, for short periods, or during many years (Table 1).

EPIDEMIOLOGY

IPV is a stigmatized health issue and, thus, has been hidden, underrecognized, underreported, and underappreciated as a major public health issue. Some of the barriers perceived by health care provides leading to underrecognition of IPV include lack of professional education, time constraints, unproven interventions, fear of offending the patient, and low disclosure rates by the patient *(8)*. Patient barriers to disclosure include fear of further abuse by the batterer, lack

Table 1
Types of Abuse in Intimate Partner Violence

Physical abuse	Hitting, slapping, pushing, shoving, punching, kicking, biting, strangulation, burning, use of weapons such as knives or firearms, and preventing access to medicines or medical care
Sexual abuse	Coerced sexual activity, sexual assault, forced unprotected sex, forced sex with or in front of others, and forced sex involving violence and the use of objects
Psychological abuse	Berates, ridicules, intimidates, degrades, humiliates, emotionally isolates from friends or family, or stalks; threats of violence against the victim, the victim's family, or pets; threatens suicide or homicide, or purchasing and/or displaying a firearm; uses children (threatens to hurt or take children away or withhold support)
Economic abuse	Limiting access to work, education or resources; incurring crippling debt; threatening to withhold access to insurance; threatening to imperil immigration status

of self-esteem, fear of losing her children, economic dependency, apprehension regarding the response of the clinician, cultural and religious values, and fear of being deported.

Numerous studies and databases provide some information regarding the prevalence of IPV. However, substantial variability in prevalence is noted. This is largely because of differences in the definitions of IPV being used, the types of abuse being measured, the period of time during which the abuse occurred (1 yr vs lifetime prevalence), the clinical setting, and the population being studied.

According to several studies conducted in primary care settings, the prevalence of current IPV among women presenting for medical care ranged from 8 to 29%. Between 21 and 39% of women had experienced IPV at some point during their lives (lifetime prevalence) *(9)*. At least 85% of victims of IPV are women, with most being abused by male partners *(10)*. The remainder of victims are in same-sex relationships, or are male victims abused by a female partner. There have been very few studies that have measured IPV against men. The tools used to identify IPV have not been validated in men. In addition, studies that have questioned men have not determined the degree of injury, or whether the violence was in self-defense, retaliation, or retribution. In a primary care-based study by Gin, 4% of males reported current IPV and 12% reported lifetime IPV *(11)*. There is also limited data on IPV among individuals is same-sex relationships. The National Violence Against Women Survey, a community-based survey, reported lower rates of IPV among women in same-sex relationships (11%) than in opposite-sex relationships (20%); whereas men in same-sex relationships reported increased rates of IPV (23%) compared with men with female partners (8%) *(12)*.

Numerous studies have been conducted to measure the prevalence of IPV during pregnancy. In a review by Gazmararian of 13 studies, the prevalence of IPV during pregnancy ranged from 1 to 20% *(13)*. Higher rates of IPV were detected in studies in which women were asked about IPV on more than one occasion during their pregnancy, and when in-depth, in-person interviews were conducted with the women.

Prevalence rates seem to be higher among lower socioeconomic groups, but may just be more hidden in upper socioeconomic families with access to private resources. Couples younger than age 30 years seem to be at highest risk, along with those who become parents at a young age *(14)*. The National Center on Elder Abuse commissioned a review of domestic violence in the elderly and, although in most of the cases the adult child is the perpetrator, the next most common perpetrator of abuse is the spouse *(15)*. Prevalence rates seem generally consistent across racial groups, although African American women seem more willing to disclose violence in some survey studies.

DYNAMICS

How do couples, who at one point were attracted to and loved or appreciated one another, become violent and abusive? There are several theories, each with some foundation and research, that provide insight into a phenomenon that has intrigued experts in violence and abuse for many years. Is it learned behavior? Is it culturally based? Does it result from flawed relationship dynamics with both persons participating in some way? Why do people stay in abusive relationships once recognized?

It would be highly unlikely that one theory could explain such a complex phenomena. In 1998, Heise proposed that theories regarding the etiology of IPV could be arranged within the context of a social ecology model that had been used for other complex social issues *(16)*. Some theorize that IPV is an individual issue that can be related to a personal history of previous exposure to learning experiences with violence, drug exposure, mental illness, traumatic brain injury, or individual psychopathology. Other researchers have examined the dynamics of the couple or the families, their ability to resolve conflict, communicate, and maintain an operating family system. These theories are lumped under the category called “Family Unit” or “Microsystem.” The role of the community as an etiological agent has also been evaluated. How do economics, employment, neighborhood safety issues, and access to drugs and alcohol within a neighborhood influence the occurrence of IPV? This is the “Community” or “Exosystem” category. Finally, the culture, be it ethnic, religious, political, or philosophical, creates a set of rules that can condone or condemn violence and gender equity in terms of access to resources and tools of empowerment. Although no culture condones abusive behaviors of an intimate partner, some cultures may characterize physical and verbal chastisement as a means of discipline necessary to maintain a certain order to the family structure and do not perceive it as abuse. Asymmetrical power structures between intimate partners seem to be a risk for physical violence and abuse in cases of conflict and if both partner do not agree with the power arrangement. This is the “Culture” or “Macrosystem,” and plays a role in the etiology of IPV.

Johnson, in 1995, challenged the notion that all violence between couples is the same and suggested that there may be two forms of violence, one he termed “true battering” and the other “common couple violence” *(17)*. He differentiates the two mostly in the ways that power is distributed. In “battering” there is clearly a power imbalance with one person dominating the other through fear, and who is able to maintain control in the relationship using a variety of tactics over time that can include acts of violence and other forms of intimidation. On the other hand, “couple violence” is physical assault that results as a culmination of deteriorating communication skills, such that the violent act is the expression of ultimate frustration, anger, and hurt. The violence is an expression of the one partner’s inability to cope as opposed to their need to control. Some would argue that, in battering relationships, the violence occurs as other means of control seem to be insufficient to maintain the degree of dominance desired by the perpetrator, and can become increasingly desperate and deadly.

Many researchers have asked whether there is a certain type of person or personality characteristics that are more likely to manifest abuse to another through physical or emotional aggression. As domestic violence was criminalized and men, more so than women, were referred to intervention programs, typologies on male batterers were formulated based on psychological and demographic data. Studies of psychological traits of men who batter generally reveal three main types of batterers *(18,19)*:

1. Negativistic/borderline/dependent.
2. Antisocial/narcissistic/generally violent.
3. The nonpsychopathological/family-only violent batterers.

In very broad terms, each of these groups is described below *(20)*.

Negativistic/Borderline/Dependent Batterers

These men appear as brooding, emotionally intense men who can simultaneously seem lost and dependent on their partner in their search for their true selves. However, this dependence, in turn, creates a huge internal conflict with their fear of being engulfed by their partner. Partners of such men describe them as "Dr. Jekyll and Mr. Hyde," in that they can be engaging and sensitive in one minute and angry and controlling in the next. These men seem to be the most depressed, have higher rates of drug and alcohol abuse, and commit more serious violence than nonpsychopathological/family-only violent men.

Antisocial/Narcissistic/Generally Violent Batterers

These men seem extremely self-centered, lacking in empathy, and incapable of relationship reciprocity. They may appear confident, flamboyant, and exciting, which may be attractive to a more withdrawn or vulnerable partner. However, the lack of reciprocity means that the partner must also acquiesce to his rules, values, and perceptions of reality while being blamed as the source of these problems. These men commit severe battery and the most severe sexual abuse and battery of the three types. They have a history of more arrests and more violent crime than family-only batterers.

Nonpsychopathological/Family-Only Batterers

These men are less likely to show signs of psychopathology and seem to live very conventional lives. They tend to be either passively dependent with outbursts of rebellious aggression, or obsessive compulsive and react violently when their partners violate their rules of conduct. The violence is generally confined within the family and is of lesser frequency and severity than the other two groups.

Although helpful, these typologies are limited in that the studies have consisted primarily of white, heterosexual men. Only recently have populations of cultural minority, gay/lesbian batterers, or heterosexual female batterers been addressed, but these results are beyond the limits of this chapter.

IDENTIFICATION

The clinical goals for identifying IPV in primary care are to:

1. Identify IPV among symptomatic patients presenting with illnesses or injuries secondary to abuse.
2. Identify IPV among asymptomatic patients who are in abusive intimate relationships.

Identification of victims of IPV in the health care setting may occur through patient disclosure or may be suspected based on pattern recognition.

Patient disclosure regarding IPV may be spontaneous or prompted in the clinical setting. Spontaneous disclosure usually occurs during the triage process or while the health care provider is obtaining the medical history or performing the physical exam and asks, "What happened?" Prompted disclosure occurs either through routine inquiry (scan) or specific inquiry in the history of present illness (search).

Routine Inquiry

Because of the varied presentations of IPV, numerous professional health care organizations, including the American Medical Association *(21)*, the American Academy of Family Physicians *(22)*, the American College of Physicians *(23)*, the American College of Obstetrics and Gynecology *(24)*, the American Academy of Pediatrics *(25)*, and the American Academy of Nurse Practitioners *(26)*, have supported routine inquiry of all patients regarding IPV. In surveys, victims of IPV have responded that they think that health care providers should inquire about IPV. Research has found that both abused and non-abused women favor routine inquiry regarding IPV by their physicians *(27–30)*. Further, patients also report feeling comfortable when asked about IPV by their health care providers *(28,31)*.

The National Consensus Guidelines recommend that routine inquiry should be performed at all new patient visits, annual visits, during each trimester of pregnancy, and when other factors in the patient's history or physical examination result in a suspicion of IPV on the part of the health care provider *(5)*. In addition, routine inquiry should be incorporated into pediatric visits as part of general safety assessment and violence prevention promotion. Routine inquiry regarding violence victimization may be included within the social history. Routine inquiry may be conducted within the context of empathic dialog between patient and practitioner or using a verbal tool, a written questionnaire, or a computer-based questionnaire *(32)*. When written or computer-based questionnaires are used, additional assistance should be available for patients who need translation, are not able to read, or who may feel uncomfortable using a computer. Before inquiring about IPV, the health care provider should inform the patient of the limits of confidentiality, particularly if the health care provider has a legal mandate to report IPV when it is disclosed.

There are several brief tools for the identification of IPV that may be used in the primary care setting. These include the Abuse Assessment Screen (*see* Table 2) *(33)*, the Hits screen (Hurt, Insulted, Threatened, or Screamed) *(34)*, the Women's Experience with Battering (WEB) *(35)*, and the Woman Abuse Screening Tool (WAST) *(36)*. These have all been found to have good-to-fair quality when compared with longer, validated instruments *(37)*. These screens

Table 2
The Abuse Assessment Screen for the Identification of Intimate Partner Violence Among Female Patients *(33)*

Abuse Assessment Screen (AAS)

1. Have you ever been emotionally or physically abused by your partner or someone important to you? Yes No
2. Within the last year, have you been hit, slapped, kicked, or otherwise physically hurt by someone? Yes No
   If yes, by whom? ______________________________
   Total number of times? ___________
   Mark the area of injury on a body map.
3. Since you have been pregnant, have you been hit, slapped, kicked, or otherwise physically hurt by someone? Yes No
   If yes, by whom?___________________________________
   How many times? ___________
   Mark the area of injury on a body map.
   Score the most severe incident according to the following scale:
   1 = Threats of abuse, including use of weapon.
   2 = Slapping, pushing; no injuries and/or lasting pain.
   3 = Punching, kicking, bruises, cuts, and/or continuing pain.
   4 = Beaten up, severe contusions, burns, broken bones.
   5 = Head, internal or permanent injury.
   6 = Use of weapon; wound from weapon.
4. Within the last year, has anyone forced you to have sexual activities?
   If yes, who?____________________________
   Number of times:__________
5. Are you afraid of your partner or anyone listed above? Yes No

have been tested on female patients in the primary care setting. To date, there are no screening tools developed and validated for use with male patients. When using a tool that does not ask about sexual abuse or strangulation, it is wise to add additional questions that specifically address these forms of abuse. Between one-third and one-half of patients who are physically abused are also sexually abused by their partners *(38)*. Yet women may be reluctant to divulge this abuse to their health care provider. When asking about sexual abuse, refrain from asking about "rape," but rather whether they have been forced or coerced to have sexual activities by their partner. Likewise, when asking patients whether they have ever been strangled by their partner, it is preferable to use the term "choked," because this is a lay term that patients are more likely to understand. Questions regarding IPV may also be included in a more extensive health risk assessment that is administered to patients during their medical visit. Prompts on patient charts have been shown to increase routine inquiry by heath care providers *(39)*. Additional guidelines to foster patient disclosure are in Table 3.

Recently the United States Preventive Services Task Force reviewed the literature regarding screening for IPV and came to the recommendation that there was insufficient evidence to recommend for or against routine screening of women for IPV *(40)*. This recommendation was based on an analysis of 14 studies that were reviewed based on specific criteria, with a randomized clinical trial being the most desirable study design. These studies did not show an effect of screening in reducing harm from IPV, nor did they show adverse effects caused by the screening. Health care providers should not be dissuaded from routinely inquiring of their patients regarding IPV. Its prevalence and negative impact on the physical and mental health of patients is substantial. A failure to routinely inquire about IPV may result in misdiagnoses, inappropriate workups and excessive costs, and increasing morbidity and mortality for victims, their families, and other members of society *(41)*.

Although routine inquiry is described as a means of identification, it may also serve as a means of prevention. Routine inquiry may increase patients' awareness of the impact IPV may have on their health, decrease subsequent violence if patients receive appropriate referrals to interventions, and lessen the impact of the violence by receiving referrals for the mental and physical sequelae of IPV.

Pattern Recognition

Pattern recognition is the process of gathering a constellation of clues from the medical history, physical examination, and patient presentation that are suggestive of a specific diagnosis. Clinicians use pattern recognition on a daily basis in arriving at differential diagnoses. The same process is used in identifying IPV, because research has shown that there are diagnostic patterns consistent with IPV.

Medical History

When health care providers are eliciting a medical history from a patient, they should pay careful attention to responses that may indicate IPV (Table 4). When this occurs, additional questions should be asked to further explore the possibility of IPV. If the patient discloses abuse, additional assessment questions should be asked regarding alcohol and substance abuse, past medical history, child abuse, and the access of the abuser to a firearm.

Physical Examination

When victims of IPV present to the health care setting, their medical presentations may be obvious (i.e., injuries) or subtle (i.e., headaches caused by repetitive traumatic brain injury). Most often, patients seek care for medical complaints other than acute injuries (Table 5). While performing a physical examination,

Table 3
Guidelines to Foster Patient Disclosure

Use a "framing" statement before questioning the patient to put both the patient and health care provider more at ease, and convey that the questions are routine and not prejudicial. For example, "Because of the impact of intimate partner violence on women's health, I ask all my female patients these questions."
Use all-inclusive phrases such as "boyfriend, husband, or partner."
Patients should be asked about IPV in as private an environment as possible. Partners and family members should be asked to leave the examination room. If patients are given written or computer-based questionnaires regarding IPV to complete, they should also be provided with a private, safe place to do so.
Occasionally, a patient's partner may not be willing to leave the examination room, such as in the situation of a controlling abuser. In this case, a health care provider may need to create another opportunity to question the patient in private, for example, by accompanying the patient to radiology without the partner.
Preferably, patients should be questioned in their primary language. If a translator is needed, an individual other than the patient's partner, a family member, child, or a friend should be used. Patients may not feel comfortable disclosing abuse in front someone they know.

Table 4
Clues in the Medical History That May Indicate Intimate Partner Violence

Frequent medical visits
Use of alcohol or of abuse drugs
Noncompliance with medications or health care appointments
"Accident prone" patient
Past history of injuries
Delay in seeking medical attention
A changing history related to the mechanism of injury
A medical history inconsistent with the injuries

the health care provider may detect injuries caused by IPV. The most common locations of injuries are the head, face, and neck *(42)*. Locations of intentional injuries are also more likely to be central, bilateral, and defensive (i.e., bruising on the backs of the hands from protecting her face with her hands). When injuries are observed, additional questions should be posed regarding the mechanism of the injuries. Injuries frequently observed in victims of IPV should make the health care provider more alert to the possibility of IPV as the underlying etiology (Table 6). When injuries are detected, each one should be assessed for location, tenderness, swelling, size, evidence of healing, discoloration, and

Table 5
Medical Presentations Commonly Observed in Intimate Partner Violence

Cardiorespiratory	Palpitations, chest pain, shortness of breath, exacerbation of asthma, and hyperventilation
Gastrointestinal	Functional bowel disorder
Gynecological	Chronic pelvic pain, dyspareunia, sexually transmitted diseases, HIV, urinary tract infections
Neurological	Headaches, vertigo, migraines
Constitutional symptoms	Weakness, fatigue, dizziness, weight gain or loss, chronic pain, and loss of appetite
Psychiatric	Alcohol or substance abuse, depression, suicidal ideation, homicidal ideation, posttraumatic stress disorder, anxiety, insomnia, and eating disorders

whether a pattern is present (i.e., a patterned burn from contact with a hot iron). Document the color of bruises but avoid judgments about specific ages of injuries, because this varies greatly by individual and the degree of force. Health care providers may document that a specific injury is consistent with the patient's history.

Strangulation is increasingly being recognized as a frequent mechanism of injury in IPV assaults. Strangulation is a form of asphyxia resulting from compression of veins or arteries in the neck, or the trachea. Strangulation may be performed with one or two hands, or a ligature, such as a chain worn around the victim's neck. Patients who have been strangled may have complaints of voice changes, difficulty swallowing, shortness of breath, a loss of consciousness, or confusion. Physical findings may include hoarseness of the voice, erythema of the neck, petecchiae on the face, subconjunctival hemorrhages, marks on the front or back of the neck from a ligature, ecchymoses on the neck, stridor, respiratory changes, and altered mental status. The results of the patient's physical examination may also be entirely normal. Further examinations, such as direct laryngoscopy, CT, or MRI may be needed to determine the full extent of the injuries *(43–45)*.

As part of the physical examination, the health care provider should perform a neurological examination to assess for sequelae of blunt head trauma, or hypoxia caused by strangulation.

Other Medical Presentations

Victims of IPV also present to health care providers for multiple nontraumatic complaints. These complaints may be neurological, cardiorespiratory, gastrointestinal, pain, constitutional medical symptoms, and obstetrical and gynecological. These problems may be acute, chronic, or stress related. Diaz-Olavarrieta found

Table 6
Injuries Commonly Observed in Intimate Partner Violence

Injuries to the Head and Face
Facial contusions and lacerations
Facial fractures
Petecchiae
Traumatic alopecia
Concussion
Skull fractures
Intracranial hemorrhages
Injuries to the Eye
Subconjunctival hemorrhages
Corneal abrasions
Hyphema
Retinal detachment
Ruptured globe
Orbital floor fracture
Injuries to the Ear
Ruptured tympanic membrane
Hearing loss
Dental/Oral Injuries
Chipped, fractured, or avulsed teeth
Contusions and lacerations to the mouth and tongue
Injuries to the Neck
Erythema, contusions, abrasions
Patterned marks from ligatures
Laryngeal edema
Fractured hyoid
Injuries to the Extremities
Contusions, abrasions, lacerations,
Fingertip contusions ("grab" marks) to upper arms
Fractures, dislocations
Injuries to Other Parts of the Body
Ano-genital injuries
Burns
Abdominal injuries in pregnancy
Stab wounds, firearm injuries

that 35% of women with neurological disorders, including migraines, epilepsy, trigeminal neuralgia, and headaches were victims of IPV *(46)*. Patients may also experience exacerbations of chronic medical conditions, such as asthma or coronary artery disease. In addition, patients may not be compliant with taking prescribed medications or treatments, or following up with scheduled appointments, if they are prevented from doing so by their controlling, abusive partner. Elliott reported that none of the female victims of current IPV presented to the health care providers for routine health maintenance visits, compared with more than half of the non-abused women patients *(47)*.

Among pregnant patients, unwanted pregnancies, requests for pregnancy termination, late entry into prenatal care, miscarriages, placental abruption, preterm labor, substance abuse, low birth weight babies, and impaired bonding should all alert the health care provider to the possibility of underlying IPV.

Mental Status Examination

Health care providers should assess suspected victims of IPV for mental health conditions frequently associated with IPV. Depression scores among victims of IPV have been found to be double the standard norms *(48)*. Abbott found that, among women who had ever attempted suicide, 81% had a lifetime history of IPV, compared with a lifetime history of 19% among women who had not attempted suicide *(49)*. Research has shown that posttraumatic stress disorder was diagnosed in 33 to 84% of victims of IPV, with more severe symptoms among those women experiencing more severe abuse *(50)*. In addition, patients should be assessed for use of alcohol and illegal substances, as these may be used by victims of IPV as a way to "escape" the abuse.

Patients should be assessed for suicidal or homicidal ideation, and the appropriate referrals made, if identified. Health care providers should be aware that if a patient with homicidal ideation specifically names an individual related to that ideation, they have a duty to warn under the Tarasoff vs. University of California decision *(51,52)*.

CHILDREN IN FAMILIES WITH ONGOING IPV

Estimates of numbers of children in IPV homes ranges from 3.3 million to 10 million annually in the United States *(53–56)*. Children who live in IPV homes are at increased risk for child abuse, "caught in the cross-fire" injury, neglect, and emotional trauma through exposure to IPV. Ross *(57)* and McCloskey *(58)* found that children in an IPV home were at significantly heightened risk of physical abuse from the fathers. Appel and Holden *(59)* published a meta-analysis of 31 studies and found a median co-occurrence rate of IPV and child abuse to be 40%. Edelson, in 1999 *(60)*, identified 35 studies that address the overlap of IPV and child abuse and found that rates varied depending on the source of the information. If child protection records were reviewed, the co-occurrence rate was 29%; if adult IPV victims were interviewed, they disclosed 46% rate of abuse by either parent; if child abuse victims were interviewed, they disclosed IPV in 59% of cases. Similar rates of co-occurrence for child sexual abuse and IPV have also been found. Only a few studies have examined the co-occurrence of neglect and IPV.

Studies during the last 20 years have demonstrated the negative impact of IPV on children across all age groups, and the impact seems to extend into adulthood. Abusive relationships impact the health of the pregnancy, with increased rates of miscarriage, prematurity, and increased rates of alcohol, tobacco, and other drugs by abused mothers *(61–63)*. Infants suffer higher rates of attachment disorders, sleep disorders, and failure to thrive *(64)*. Neurobiological studies confirm that violence-exposed children experience an interruption in brain homeostasis that results in persistent fear-associated neurophysiological patterns, similar to PTSD in adults *(65)*. Changes in brain structure, volume, growth, and dominance performance patterns have been documented in children exposed to traumatic events *(66–69)*. School-aged children seem to be the most vulnerable group and experience guilt, self-blame, and diminished levels of self-competency *(70–72)*. Edleson reviewed 31 studies *(60)* that addressed child witness to partner physical violence and found that these children exhibited more aggressive and antisocial behaviors, as well as fearful and inhibited behaviors, and they showed lower social competency than other children. Although the direct impact on adolescents has not been well-studied, childhood exposure to IPV predicted future delinquency *(73)*, and much of this was for dating violence. Adolescents show many of the same PTSD symptoms as younger children *(71,74,75)*, and are often placed in the role of protecting siblings or hiding the violence from neighbors, friends, and teachers *(64)*. Long-term impact studies identify exposure to IPV as an "adverse childhood event" that leads to increased rates of unintended adult pregnancy, lifetime illicit drug use, greater distress, and lower social adjustment *(76)*. Hotaling *(77)* and Freedman *(78)* showed child exposure to IPV to be the single greatest predictor of IPV victimization and perpetration in later life.

Early identification is encouraged. The American Academy of Pediatrics recognizes that IPV is harmful to children and recommends that clinicians attempt to recognize the problem and intervene for the safety of both mother and child victims *(25)*. The Family Violence Prevention Fund, in their national consensus guidelines for child and adolescent health *(79)*, recommends that assessment for partner violence be performed without children, especially those older than age 3 years, in the room because sometimes children may inadvertently disclose the discussion to the abusing parent and endanger both the adult victim and the child. When questions related to inappropriate touching or discipline practices arise with older children, adding a question regarding family conflict resolution or witnessing physical fighting may be appropriate.

Joint intervention for both adult and child victims is the preferred modality, but child protection agencies and domestic violence service providers must jointly arrange protocols for the removal of children thought to be in physical danger and/or suffering health consequences from continued exposure. Once partner violence is identified, the Family Violence Prevention Fund guidelines recommend reassuring the child or adolescent that the problem at home is not their fault, conducting a thorough assessment for signs of physical abuse, sexual abuse, or health sequelae caused by violence exposure, addressing safety needs, and providing resources for both the child and the parent *(79)*. Most IPV victims think that they are doing the best they can to protect the health and welfare of their children, but may also be unaware of how their children are being negatively impacted and unaware of alternatives or resources to assist them.

TEEN DATING VIOLENCE

Although the CDC and most penal codes include dating violence by young couples as IPV, there are some differences in the manifestation of the violence and even greater problems in its identification and intervention. Adolescent dating violence is surprisingly common in the United States. In a national survey of youth health risk behaviors, 9 to 10% of both male and female high school students reported being the victims of physical violence from a dating partner *(80)*. "Mutual combat," in which both partners engage in abusive and violent behavior, may be more common among adolescents than adults *(81)*. Girls are more likely to report severe violence, such as being choked, burned, beaten, threatened with a weapon, or raped. Boys report less severe acts, such as being pinched, slapped, scratched, or kicked *(82–86)*. Whereas boys report strategies to minimize the victimization, such as "laughing or ignoring it," girls report having "fought back" or "obeyed their partner" after experiencing violence *(84)*.

The dynamics of teen dating violence differ somewhat from adult IPV. Adolescents' developmental tasks include separation and individuation as well as experimenting with intimate relationships. Teens distance themselves from parents during the individuation process and become more private regarding relationship issues. Therefore, if they are hurt by a dating partner, they experience a "double whammy" in that they think that they have failed to individuate and failed in their dating efforts. In addition, based on their previous role modeling and inexperience, adolescents can confuse control with devotion, jealousy with love, and violence with passion. Levy *(87)*, in a study of adolescent attitudes toward IPV, found that 25 to 35% of victims of physical dating violence interpreted the behavior as signs of devotion and love, and almost 60% said the violent behavior had "no effect" overall on the relationship. Adults may be just as guilty as children in minimizing teen dating violence because parents and teacher often minimize the importance of romantic attachments in young people and view violence as "fighting" or justify it as "kids will be kids."

Adolescents exposed to IPV as children or teens are at increased risk for victimization and perpetration. In a 5-year study of 1291 8th and 9th graders in North Carolina, Foshee and colleagues found that victimization in boys was predicted by having a friend who was a victim of dating violence, being hit by an adult with intent to harm, lacking maternal supervision, low self-esteem, holding traditional gender stereotypes, having poor conflict resolution skills, and using alcohol. In girls, victimization was predicted by having a friend who had been a victim, being hit by an adult with intention to harm, lacking maternal supervision, having been in a physical fight with a peer, and having been forced to do something sexual by someone other than a date *(88)*.

There seems to be general agreement that health professionals begin anticipatory guidance regarding interpersonal violence at age 11 years, just before patients begin dating relationships. The AMA recommends providers ask about emotional, physical, and sexual abuse regularly through adolescence *(89)*. Practitioners can ask simple questions to open up discussion of the issue, such as *(90)*:

- What happens if you and your boyfriend have a disagreement or a fight?
- Does your girlfriend seem jealous? What does she do when she is feeling this way?

Or, practitioners can raise the issue within the context of health and safety issues, such as:

- Do you own a bicycle helmet? Do you wear it when riding a bike?
- Have you observed kids fight? Have you ever been in a fight?
- Is there a gun in your home? Do you know where it is?
- Have any of your friends hit or hurt their girlfriend? Have you ever hit your girlfriend? Have you ever been hit or hurt physically by your girlfriend?
- Have you ever been forced or pressured to have sexual activity that you did not really want?

Before asking any of these questions, the clinician should know their reporting obligations for child abuse, teen dating violence, and IPV, including unlawful sexual intercourse (intercourse with a minor). Both community agencies and schools have recently become more active in prevention and intervention of teen IPV. In most states, teens can obtain restraining orders against abusive dating partners. The principle problem is that neither teens nor their parents understand that dating violence is a crime and has short- and long-term health consequences. Therefore, anticipatory guidance, routine inquiry, and the early recognition of risk factors for victimization may be the best tools currently available to address this important health risk.

THE BATTERER

No doubt the primary care provider encounters as many patients with violent and abusive tendencies as they do victims. Although some tools and guidelines exist for the identification of female victims of domestic violence, very few guidelines exist for identifying male or female perpetrators of IPV. Oriel and Fleming *(91)* asked whether men in a primary care setting would be willing to discuss acts of partner violence and found that 12% admitted to minor acts of partner violence and 4.2% disclosed severe violence against their partners. The researchers used a direct, verbal inquiry process. Few other guidelines exist.

In the Family Violence Prevention Fund's National Consensus Guidelines *(5)*, the authors extort caution regarding universal screening for victimization, and advocate more research regarding screening for perpetration. Although they postulate that screening females for victimization history can result in more good than harm; they further postulate that screening males for victimization or perpetration could result in more harm than good. Alerting the male perpetrator to health care practices that could undermine his ability to control his partner could lead to decreased access to health care services for his partner or retaliatory behavior. Both of these hypotheses need further study.

Batterer interventions emerged that are based on the preferred etiological theory for IPV. Mental health professionals built cognitive–behavioral and psychodynamic models, whereas feminists, credited with bringing this problem to the forefront, developed sociopolitical models. Unfortunately, whether any of these programs work and whether one approach is better than another remains unclear. Treatment effects seem to be small overall. One study by Gondolf *(92)*, using a quasi-experimental design, showed that program completion by batterers reduced the likelihood of re-assault by 44 to 64%, however, the study design is not fully embraced by the batterer intervention research community. Babcock, Green, and Robie *(93)* conducted a meta-analysis of 68 batterer treatment outcome studies that were classified according to methodology. They examined effect size for various treatment modalities, such as the cognitive–behavioral approach and the Duluth feminist model. They found the effect size to be small, with no statistical difference in effect size between treatment programs.

What does seem to have consensus among researchers is that perpetrators are a heterogeneous group in terms of their psychopathology, means, and severity of violence, and that more targeted interventions may be necessary. Perpetrators with antisocial traits seem to do better with feminist cognitive–behavioral treatment, and those with dependent personalities may have better outcomes with psychodynamic treatment approaches *(94)*. Treatment matching will no doubt result in more costly assessments than the "one size fits all" approach.

Although further research is much needed, primary care providers will identify violence perpetration as an issue with their patients and will need to be informed of assessment and treatment options in their community, and will need to exercise caution in recommending conjoint couples therapy.

DOCUMENTATION

Once considered, IPV should be viewed as an "iceberg" phenomenon, meaning that there is more danger lurking below the surface than what has been revealed. The patient may be disclosing bits and pieces of their story as a way of testing the provider's empathy, trust, and ability to respond appropriately. However, once identified through disclosure or suspected through pattern recognition, the clinician must document and properly diagnosis this health risk. Coker looked at physician documentation of partner violence in a primary care setting *(95)*. Two hundred and ninety-one women were interviewed for IPV using a modified Index of Spouse Abuse and the Women's Experience With Battering tools. The medical records of those women identified as IPV patients were then scrutinized for the next 2 previous years for any documentation, even vague, that suggested that problems existed between intimate partners. On only 21 (14.7%) of 144 charts reviewed had the clinician documented any indication that IPV may be a concern for the patient. Therefore, either the clinicians missed the diagnosis or the clinician failed to document their concerns regarding IPV in approx 85% of cases.

When IPV is identified in the health care setting, the ICD indicates it should be coded to the greatest degree of specificity as Adult Maltreatment and Abuse (995.8_), as shown in Table 7 *(96)*. The ICD-10 coding guidelines now allow modifiers to indicate if the Adult Maltreatment and Abuse is confirmed (T74) or suspected (T76) *(97)*. Adult maltreatment may be suspected by the clinician but denied by the patient. Documentation is dependent on the degree of suspicion; higher degrees may lead to diagnosis, lower degrees to written discussion in the differential diagnosis. Wherever suspected, despite a denial, IPV patients should be offered basic education regarding IPV and referral information for community resources.

Making an accurate diagnosis is a foundation of good patient care, but the process also leads to collecting and reporting accurate public health data and appropriate reimbursement for services. At times, however, making the diagnosis may seem to be in conflict with the patient's need for privacy and protection. Victims' medical records must be scrupulously protected and may have to be sequestered to prevent information regarding IPV from getting into the hands of the perpetrator. For example, the records of the child whose mother discloses that

Table 7
International Classification of Diseases (ICD)-10 Diagnostic Codes for Use in Intimate Partner Violence *(96,97)*

Adult Maltreatment and Abuse (995.8_)
995.81: Physically abused person, battered person, spouse, or woman
995.82: Adult emotional/psychological abuse
995.83: Adult sexual abuse
995.84: Adult neglect (nutritional)
995.85: Other adult abuse and neglect (multiple forms)

IPV is an issue at home may need to be restricted to the father/perpetrator, which the health care provider can do if they think it is in the best interest of the child. Another example is the patient admitted to the hospital after physical abuse who needs to be registered with an alias, with access to medical records severely restricted. According to the Health Insurance Portability and Accountability Act (HIPAA), patients must be given information regarding their privacy rights (Notice of Privacy Practices), but it is up to patients to specify who cannot get the information and how they can best or most safely be contacted (i.e., mail, phone, or email) *(98)*. Many states have taken active legislative steps to protect victims of IPV from additional harm by preventing insurance discrimination *(99)*.

IPV is a crime in all 50 states, therefore, there is increased likelihood that once physical abuse or sexual abuse occurs, the criminal or civil justice system will be involved. Medical records may be subpoenaed and health professionals will be asked to provide testimony. Meticulous documentation of physical injuries will be helpful if trial proceedings occur months or even years later. A US Department of Justice report made recommendations for medical record documentation of IPV by health care providers that may be helpful to victims (Table 8) *(100)*.

Clinical forensic specialists have, for many years, been responsible for the examination and documentation of findings in child abuse and adult sexual assault cases. Recently, standardized forms and protocols for both domestic violence and elder abuse have been advocated. The standardized forms and protocols created in California (OES 502 and 602), are one example, and are readily accessible on the internet *(101)*. These forms and protocols can be used in whole or in part by forensic specialists or individual practitioners to facilitate the thorough and comprehensive documentation that can prove invaluable in court proceedings. In an analysis of domestic violence prosecution outcomes in a large Midwest jurisdiction, photographs of injuries and medical records were found to be two of the five best predictors of a guilty verdict *(102)*.

Table 8
Recommendations for Documentation of Intimate Partner Violence by Health Care Providers That Can Help Victims *(100)*

Take photographs of injuries
Write legibly
Set patient's own words in quotation marks
Use phrase "patient states" and avoid phrases like "patient claims" or "patient alleges"
Identify person who hurt patient in quotation marks and avoid legal terms like "alleged perpetrator"
Domestic violence is a legal finding; use Adult Maltreatment, a medical diagnosis
Record patient demeanor
Record time/day of event and physical examination

Many states have requirements regarding the reporting of violence and abuse to either health or criminal justice agencies *(103)*. Although the ethics and intervention value of reporting mandates have been challenged, the practitioner who fails to comply with state laws risks considerable liability should the patient suffer further harm *(104)*.

Primary care providers may be asked to testify in court regarding their patients. On the rare occasions that this occurs, contact the issuing attorney, get the name of the patient, review the medical record, and arrange a pretrial conference by telephone or in person. During the pretrial conference, the provider should ascertain anticipated questions by both the prosecution and the defense, problems or questions regarding the medical evidence to be introduced, and get clear information regarding the time and location of the trial. It is entirely reasonable to ask for an "on-call" status, because there are many reasons why testimony can be delayed or cancelled at the last minute, most of which are out of control of the attorneys. Most health care providers are considered percipient witnesses (i.e., presenting evidence that is material to the case) and can request very modest witness fees. Expert witnesses are prearranged through a contractual process so that the expert can review the case and render an opinion *(98)*.

In summary, medical records demonstrate the competency of the clinician who has conducted an assessment of violence as a health risk exposure, discussed IPV in the differential diagnosis, or considered Adult Maltreatment as the working diagnosis. Documentation of a care plan demonstrates a good faith effort to help the victim and documentation of patient statements, and physical findings constitute a valuable record that may later be accessed for civil or criminal proceedings.

VICTIM INTERVENTIONS AND REFERRALS

Although "Interventions and Referrals" are addressed as the last section of this chapter, understanding and preparing for intervention is a first step in upgrading your practice to address IPV. Asking patients about IPV without having any available educational resources or interventions to which to refer a victim may further increase their despair. The National Health Resource Center on Domestic Violence can provide information for clinicians to develop a protocol to respond to IPV patients in their practice setting (phone 1-888-Rx-Abuse; www.endabuse.org).

Recommendations regarding intervention are based on expert opinion and a gradually emerging body of outcomes research. When a patient is identified as having been a victim of IPV, the first therapeutic message is to validate the victim's experiences by telling her that she is believed, she does not deserve the abuse, the abuse is not her fault, there are options and alternatives, and that the clinician will provide her with information and resources. The victim's immediate safety needs should be assessed by establishing the location of the perpetrator, keeping in mind that the perpetrator may be in the waiting room. The safety of her children, if any, should also be assessed, as the perpetrator may have kept the children at home to ensure that she would return home. They should also be asked if they have a safe place to go to if needed.

The clinician should assess the patient's situation and needs, to provide her with appropriate interventions and referrals (Fig. 1). In some clinical situations, this assessment may be conducted by a social worker or an advocate from a community-based organization. Assessment includes:

- Determine the nature and severity of the abuse. The Danger Assessment tool developed by Campbell may be used as part of this assessment to determine her current risk for danger (Fig. 2) *(106)*. A positive response to any one question is considered to indicate danger. However, a scoring system has being developed to provide ranges for various degrees of danger.
- Consider the safety of any children in the home. The patient should be asked if her abusive partner has harmed the children. Victims should be questioned regarding whether they have abused the children, as this may occur because of difficulty coping on the part of the victim *(107)*.
- Determine the patient's perception of her situation. She may see the abuse as an isolated incident, or she may already recognize it as a pattern of ongoing, escalating violence. She may think that she has no way out of her situation, or she may be contemplating making a change in her life. In assessing a victim's perception of her situation, it is often helpful for the clinician to think of the Transtheoretical Model's five stages in the process of change *(108)*. This model has been used in assisting patients make changes related to other health risks, such as smoking, obesity, and alcohol abuse. More recently, clinicians have applied it to IPV *(109)*. The five stages are:

Steps	Level I	Level II	Level III	
			Recent or present abuse	
			Without injuries Danger Assessment (-)	With injuries OR Danger Assessment (+)
SCREEN	No history or present threat of abuse	Past history of abuse	↓	↓
INTERVENE	Provide patient education about IPV; give information regarding community resources.	Assess for sequelae of past abuse. Provide patient education about IPV and information regarding community resources.	Comprehensive assessment; individual counseling; assist patient in contacting community IPVS services, safety planning. Arrange follow-up visit.	Crisis intervention; notify police if required by state law; consider protective orders; Contact IPV services and request advocate to see or talk to patient. Arrange follow-up visit.
DOCUMENT	Statement of no abuse or threat of abuse; handouts/educational materials given to patient.	Statement of past abuse and sequelae; education/resources given to patient Add IPV to problem list and address periodically at subsequent visits.	Describe present or recent abuse and any sequelae; counsel patient; resources given, safety planning done Add IPV to problem list and indicate next follow-up visit.	Complete forensic exam and body diagram or photo documentation. If required by law, complete injury report form and forward to law enforcement or designated agency. Describe law enforcement intervention; describe advocacy intervention. Add IPV to problem list.

Adapted from: Lazzaro MV, McFarlane J (105)
Adapted by C. Mitchell, California Medical Training, Center, University of California Davis
Adapted by D. Anglin (to be applicable for all states' legal requirements)

Fig. 1. Intimate Partner Violence Screening and Intervention Guidelines.

DANGER ASSESSMENT

Jacquelyn C. Campbell, PhD, RN, FAAN

Several risk factors have been associated with increased risk of homicides (murders) of men and women in violent relationships. We cannot predict what will happen in your case, but we would like you to be aware of the danger of homicide in situations of abuse and for you to see how many of the risk factors apply to your situation.

Using the calendar, please mark the approximate dates during the past year when you were abused by your partner. Write on that date how bad the incident was according to the following scale:

1. Slapping, pushing; no injuries and/or lasting pain
2. Punching, kicking; bruises, cuts, and/or continuing pain
3. "Beating up"; severe contusions, burns, broken bones
4. Threat to use weapon; head injury, internal injury, permanent injury, miscarriage
5. Use of weapon; wounds from weapon

(If **any** of the descriptions for the higher number apply, use the higher number.)

Mark **Yes** or **No** for each of the following.
("He" refers to your husband, partner, ex-husband, ex-partner, or whoever is currently physically hurting you.)

Yes	No		
____	____	1.	Has the physical violence increased in severity or frequency over the past year?
____	____	2.	Does he own a gun?
____	____	3.	Have you left him after living together during the past year? 3a. (If have *never* lived with him, check here____)
____	____	4.	Is he unemployed?
____	____	5.	Has he ever used a weapon against you or threatened you with a weapon? 5a. (if yes, was the weapon a gun____)
____	____	6.	Does he threaten to kill you?
____	____	7.	Has he avoided being arrested for domestic violence?
____	____	8.	Do you have a child that is not his?
____	____	9.	Has he ever forced you to have sex when you did not wish to do so?
____	____	10.	Does he ever try to choke you?
____	____	11.	Does he use illegal drugs? By drugs, I mean "uppers" or amphetamines, speed, angel dust, cocaine, "crack", street drugs or mixtures.
____	____	12.	Is he an alcoholic or problem drinker?
____	____	13.	Does he control most or all of your daily activities? For instance: does he tell you who you can be friends with, when you can see your family, how much money you can use, or when you can take the car? (If he tries, but you do not let him, check here: _____)
____	____	14.	Is he violently and constantly jealous of you? (For instance, does he say "If I can't have you, no one can.")
____	____	15.	Have you ever been beaten by him while you were pregnant? (If you have never been pregnant by him, check here: _____)
____	____	16.	Has he ever threatened or tried to commit suicide?
____	____	17.	Does he threaten to harm your children?
____	____	18.	Do you believe he is capable of killing you?
____	____	19.	Does he follow or spy on you, leave threatening notes or messages on your answering machine, destroy your property, or call you when you don't want him to?
____	____	20.	Have you ever threatened or tried to commit suicide?

__________ Total "Yes" Answers

Thank you. Please talk to your nurse, advocate or counselor about what the Danger Assessment means in terms of your situation.

Fig. 2. Danger Assessment instrument. (From ref. *105*. Permission to use this instrument in clinical settings has been universally granted by its creator. Dr. Campbell requests notification if the instrument is used in formal research studies).

1. *Precontemplation*—when the patient has not yet thought about change as a possibility.
2. *Contemplation*—when the patient begins to consider that there may be alternatives to her abusive situation.
3. *Preparation*—when the patient has decided to make a change in her situation and is going through the planning stages.
4. *Action*—when the patient actually makes a change, such as obtaining a protective order, leaving her abusive partner.
5. *Maintenance*—the patient goes through healing, but may also have mixed emotions, such as relief, sadness, and happiness.

It is not uncommon for victims of IPV who have made a change to relapse to an earlier stage, much as patients trying to lose weight or stop drinking often do. Interventions that are appropriate to the patient's stage of change may prove to be more successful.

- Patients should be asked what resources, if any, they have tried and which ones they found helpful.
- Patients should be asked about cultural considerations (i.e., race/ethnicity, sex, religion, sexual orientation, age, immigration status, and disability status) that may impact a patient's preference for and use of certain interventions. Health care providers must be aware of and address their own biases and prejudices, because these may compound victimization issues for patients.

IPV patients should be assisted with developing a safety plan for themselves and their children that addresses a variety of situations including leaving temporarily, recurrent violence if she should decide to return to her partner or her partner returns, and workplace violence. Law enforcement may issue an emergency protective order (EPO) 24 hours a day on the request of a patient or her health care provider. If emergency housing is needed, community-based advocacy programs should be contacted. Frequently, the need for shelter exceeds the bed availability. On occasion, a patient may need to be admitted to the hospital to provide for her health or safety. In these instances, she should be admitted as a "Jane Doe."

There are numerous additional resources to which a patient may be referred. Medical centers and clinics may partner with community-based advocacy services to provide immediate crisis intervention for patients. There are also a few hospital-based IPV intervention programs in the country. Clinicians may also contact a local advocacy program's hotline to obtain counseling for a patient over the phone. The National Domestic Violence Hotline may be contacted if local services are not accessible (1-800-799-7233; TTY:1-800-787-3224). The patient should be given a follow-up appointment with her primary care provider. Additional medical consultations may be needed for acute medical problems, or for rehabilitation for chronic medical problems. Referrals should also be made for patient follow-up for counseling for mental health needs. Advocacy programs can also assist IPV victims to obtain protective orders, victim of crime compensation for medical and mental health expenses, long-term counseling for victims of IPV and for children who have witnessed IPV, education, employment assistance, and assistance finding permanent housing.

There is an increasing emphasis on outcomes studies in IPV. In the few studies that have been conducted, there are some hopeful results. McFarlane compared the effect of providing prenatal patients experiencing IPV a pocket card, counseling, or counseling with ongoing mentoring. She found that at follow-up at 6, 12, and 18 months, all groups experienced a decrease in violence *(110)*. Sullivan compared the effect of community-based advocacy after a shelter stay. She found that at 2-year follow-up, IPV victims who had received the advocacy experienced less physical abuse, an increased quality of life, and were using more community resources. In addition, 25% of the intervention group compared with 10% of the controls had experienced no further violence *(111)*. These results should provide clinicians with additional motivation to identify and refer their patients exposed to IPV.

SUMMARY

If you are like most health care providers, you have not previously appreciated how domestic violence harms your patients, complicates your care of them, and impedes their progress to better health. You, like most others, have, no doubt, missed the diagnosis, not even realizing there was a medical diagnosis or a medical issue at hand. Addressing violence and abuse in a health care setting is preferred by many patients, and most professional and academic health organizations now support early identification, documentation, and intervention by health professionals. The research on violence and abuse as a health problem has grown exponentially in the last 20 years, and the research regarding effective intervention is increasing. Addressing the health consequences of violence and abuse for adult and child victims and perpetrators is a knowledge and skill set that every practitioner must gradually acquire because, unfortunately, many patients suffer from exposure to this significant health problem.

REFERENCES

1. McCauley J, Kern DE, Kolodner K, et al. The "Battering Syndrome": Prevalence and clinical characteristics of domestic violence in primary care internal medicine practices. Ann Intern Med 1995;123:737–746.
2. Sharps P, Koziol-McLain J, Campbell J, et al. Health care providers' missed opportunities for preventing femicide. Prev Med 2001;33:373–380.
3. Wisner CL, Gilmer TP, Saltzman LE, et al. Intimate partner violence against women: do victims cost health plans more? J Fam Pract 1999;48:439–443.

4. Max W, Rice DP, Bardwell RA, et al. The economic toll of intimate partner violence against women in the United States. Violence Vict 2004;19:259–272.
5. National Consensus Guidelines on Identifying and Responding to Domestic Violence Victimization in Health Care Settings, 2nd ed. Family Violence Prevention Fund, San Francisco, CA, 2004.
6. Saltzman LE, Fanslow JL, McMahon PM, et al. Intimate Partner Violence Surveillance—Uniform Definitions and Recommended Data Elements Version 1.0. National Center for Injury Prevention and Control, Centers for Disease Control and Prevention, Atlanta, GA, 1999.
7. Rudman WJ. Coding and Documentation of Domestic Violence. Family Violence Prevention Fund, San Francisco, CA, 2000.
8. Waalen J, Goodwin MM, Spitz AM, et al. Screening for intimate partner violence by health care providers. Am J Prev Med 2000;19:230–237.
9. Naumann P, Langford D, Torres S, et al. Women battering in primary care practice. Fam Pract 1999;16:343–352.
10. Rennison CM. US. Department of Justice; Bureau of Justice Statistics Special Report, Intimate Partner Violence and Age of Victim, Washington, DC, 1993–1999, 2001.
11. Gin NE, Rucker L, Frayne S, et al. Prevalence of domestic violence among patients in three ambulatory care internal medicine clinics. J Gen Intern Med 1991;6:317–322.
12. Tjaden P, Thoennes N, Allison CJ. Comparing violence over the life span in samples of same-sex and opposite-sex cohabitants. Violence Vict 1999;14:413–425.
13. Gazmararian JA, Lazorick S, Spitz AM, et al. Prevalence of violence against pregnant women. JAMA 1996;275:1915–1920.
14. Moffitt TE, Caspi A. Findings about Partner Violence from the Dunnedin Multidisciplinary Health and Development Study. National Institute of Justice, Washnigton, DC, 1999.
15. Brandl B, Cook-Daniels L. Domestic abuse in later life: a research review. National Center on Elder Abuse. Available at: www.elderabusecenter.org.
16. Heise LL. Violence against women: an integrated, ecological framework. Violence Against Women 1998;4:262–290.
17. Johnson MP. Patriarchal terrorism and common couple violence: two forms of violence against women. J Marriage Fam 1995;57:283–297.
18. Hamberger LK, Lohr JM, Bonge D, et al. A large sample of empirical typology of male spouse abusers and its relationship to dimensions of abuse. Violence Vict 1996;11: 277–293.
19. Holtzworth-Munroe A, Stuart GL. Typologies of male batterers. Three subtypes and the differences among them. Psychol Bull 1994;116:476–497.
20. Hamberger LK. Risk factors for intimate partner violence perpetrators: typologies and characteristics of batterers. In: Intimate Partner Violence (Mitchell C, Anglin D, eds.). Oxford University Press, New York (in press).
21. American Medical Association. Diagnostic and treatment guidelines on domestic violence. Arch Fam Med 1992;1:39–47.
22. American Academy of Family Practice. Family violence. Am Fam Phys 1994;50:1636–1646.
23. American College of Physicians. Domestic Violence: Position Paper of the American College of Physicians. Philadelphia, 1986.
24. American College of Obstetricians and Gynecologists. Domestic violence: ACOG Bulletin No. 209. Int J Gynaecol Obstet 1995;51:161–170.
25. Committee on Child Abuse and Neglect. The role of the pediatrician in recognizing and intervening on behalf of abused women. Pediatrics 1998;101:1091–1092.
26. Quillian JP. Domestic violence. J Am Acad Nurse Pract 1995;7:351–356.
27. Friedman LS, Samet JG, Roberts MS. Inquiry about victimization experiences: a survey of patient preferences. Arch Int Med 1992;152:1186–1190.

28. Gielen AC, O'Campo PJ, Campbell JC, et al. Women's opinions about domestic violence screening and mandatory reporting. Am J Prev Med 2000;19:279–285.
29. Burge SK, Schneider FD, Ivy L, et al. Patients' advice to physicians about intervening in family conflict. Ann Fam Med 2005;3:248–254.
30. Hamberger LK, Ambuel B, Marbella A, et al. Physicians' interactions with battered women: the women's perspective. Arch Fam Med 1998;7:575–582.
31. Rodriguez MA, Quiroga SS, Bauer HM, et al. Breaking the silence: battered women's perspectives on medical care. Arch Fam Med 1996;5:153–157.
32. Rhodes K, Lauderdale DS, Stocking CB, et al. Better health while you wait: a controlled trial of a computer-based intervention for screening and health promotion in the emergency department. Ann Emerg Med 2001;37:284–291.
33. Soeken KL, McFarlane J, Parker B, et al. The abuse assessment screen. In: Empowering Survivors of Abuse (Campbell JC, ed.). Sage Publications, Thousand Oaks, CA, 1998.
34. Sherin KM, Sinacore JM, Li XQ, et al. HITS: a short domestic violence screening tool for use in a family practice setting. Fam Med 1998;30:508–512.
35. Coker AL, Pope BO, Smith PH, et al. Assessment of clinical partner violence screening tools. J Am Womens Assoc 2001;56:19–23.
36. Brown JB, Lent B, Schmidt G, et al. Application of the Woman Abuse Screening Tool (WAST) and WAST-short in the family practice setting. J Fam Pract 2000;49:896–903.
37. Nelson HD, Nygren P, McInerney Y, et al. Screening women and elderly adults for family and intimate partner violence: a review of the evidence for the US Preventive Services Task Force. Ann Int Med 2004;140:387–396.
38. Campbell JC, Soeken K. Forced sex and intimate partner violence: effects on women's risk and women's health. Violence Against Women 1999;51:1017–1035.
39. Olson L, Anctil C, Fullerton L, et al. Increasing emergency physician recognition of domestic violence. Ann Emerg Med 1996;27:741–746.
40. US Preventive Services Task Force. Screening for family and intimate partner violence: recommendation statement. Ann Int Med 2004;140:382–386.
41. Lachs MS. Screening for family violence: what's an evidence-based doctor to do? Ann Int Med 2004;140:399–400.
42. Muelleman RI, Lenaghan PA, Pakieser RA. Battered women: injury location and types. Ann Emerg Med 1996;28:486–492.
43. McClane GE, Strack GB, Hawley DA. A review of 300 attempted strangulation cases. Part II: clinical evaluation of the surviving victim. J Emerg Med 2001;21:311–315.
44. Hawley DA, McClane GE, Strack GB. A review of 300 attempted strangulation cases. Part III: injuries in fatal cases. J Emerg Med 2001;21:317–322.
45. Smith DJ, Mills T, Taliaferro EH. Frequency and relationship of reported symptomatology in victims of intimate partner violence: the effect of multiple strangulation attacks. J Emerg Med 2001;21:323–329.
46. Diaz-Olavarrieta C, Campbell J, Garcia de la Cadena C, et al. Domestic violence against patients with chronic neurologic disorders. Arch Neurol 1999;56:681–685.
47. Elliott BA, Johnson MMP. Domestic violence in a primary care setting: patterns and prevalence. Arch Fam Med 1995;4:113–119.
48. Walker LE. The Battered Woman Syndrome, 2nd ed. Springer Publishing, New York, 2000.
49. Abbott J, Johnson R, Koziol-McLain J, et al. Domestic violence against women: incidence and prevalence in an emergency department population. JAMA 1995;273:1763–1767.
50. Vitanza S, Vogel LC, Marshall LL, et al. Distress and symptoms of posttraumatic stress disorder in abused women. Violence Vict 1995;10:23–34.
51. Bloom JD, Rogers JL. The duty to protect others from your patients—Tarasoff spreads to the northwest. West J Med 1988;148:231–234.

52. Oppenheimer K, Swanson G. Duty to warn: when should confidentiality be breached? J Fam Pract 1990;30:179–184.
53. Straus MA, Gelles RJ. How violent are American families? Estimates from the National Family Violence Survey and other studies. In: Physical Violence in American Families: Risk factors and Adaptations to Violence in 8,145 Families (Straus MA, Gelles RJ, Smith C, eds.). Transaction Publishers, New Brunswick, NJ, 1990; pp. 95–112.
54. Fantuzzo J, Boruch R, Beriama A. Domestic violence and children: prevalence and risk in five major U.S. cities. J Am Acad Child Adoles Psychiatry 1997;36:116–122.
55. Fantuzzo JW, Mohr WK. Prevalence and effects of child exposure to domestic violence. Future Child 1999;9:21–32.
56. O'Brien M, John RS, Margolin G, et al. Reliability and diagnostic efficacy of parents' reports regarding children's exposure to marital aggression. Violence Vict 1994;9:45–62.
57. Ross SM. Risk of physical abuse to children of spouse abusing parents. Fam Soc 1996;20: 589–598.
58. McCloskey LA. The "Media Complex" among men: the instrumental abuse of children to injure wives. Violence Vict 2001;16:19–37.
59. Appel AE, Holden GW. The co-occurrence of spouse and physical child abuse: a review and appraisal. J Fam Psychol 1998;12:578–599.
60. Edleson JL. The overlap between child maltreatment and woman battering. Violence Against Women 1999;5:134–154.
61. McFarlane J, Parker B, Soeken K. Physical abuse, smoking, and substance use during pregnancy: prevalence, interrelationships, and effects on birth weight. J Obstet Gynecol Neonatal Nurs 1996;25:313–320.
62. Huth-Bocks AC, Levendosky AA, Semel MA. The direct and indirect effects of domestic violence on young children's intellectual functioning. J Fam Violence 2001;16: 269–290.
63. Kearney MH, Haggerty LA, Munro BH, et al. Birth outcomes and maternal morbidity in abused pregnant women with public versus private health insurance. J Nurs Scholarsh 2003;35:345–349.
64. Wolfe DA, Korsch B. Witnessing domestic violence during childhood and adolescence: implication for pediatric practice. Pediatrics 1994;94:594–599.
65. Perry BD, Pollard R. Homeostasis, stress, trauma, and adaptation. A neurodevelopmental view of childhood trauma. Child Adolesc Psychiatr Clin N Am 1998;7:33–51.
66. Glaser D. Child abuse and neglect and the brain—a review. J Child Psychol Psychiatry 2000;41:97–116.
67. Thomas LA, De Bellis MD. Pituitary volumes in pediatric maltreatment-related posttraumatic stress disorder. Biol Psychiatry 2004;55:752–758.
68. De Bellis MD, Keshavan MS, Frustaci K, et al. Superior temporal gyrus volumes in maltreated children and adolescents with PTSD. Biol Psychiatry 2002;51:544–552.
69. De Bellis MD, Keshavan MS, Clark DB, et al. Developmental traumatology. Part II: Brain development. Biol Psychiatry 1999;45:1271–1284.
70. Graham-Bermann SA, Levendosky AA. Traumatic stress symptoms in children of battered women. J Interpers Violence 1998;13:111–118.
71. Osofsky JD. The impact of violence on children. The Future of Children: Domestic Violence and Children 1999;9:33–49.
72. Wolfe DA, Zak L, Wilson S. Child witness to violence between parents: critical issues in behavioral and social adjustment. J Abnorm Child Psychol 1986;14:93–104.
73. Herrera VM, McCloskey LA. Gender differences in the risk for delinquency among youth exposed to family violence. Child Abuse Negl 2001;25:1037–1051.
74. Kilpatrick DG, Ruggiero KJ, Acierno R, et al. Violence and risk of PTSD, major depression, substance abuse/dependence, and comorbidity: results from the National Survey of Adolescents. J Consult Clin Psychol 2003;71:692–700.

75. Li X, Howard D, Stanton B, et al. Distress symptoms among urban African American children and adolescents: a psychometric evaluation of the Checklist of Children's Distress Symptoms. Arch Pediatr Adolesc Med 1998;152:569–577.
76. Felitti VJ, Anda RF, Nordenberg D, et al. Relationship of childhood abuse and household dysfunction to many of the leading causes of death in adults: the Adverse Childhood Experiences (ACE) study. Am J Prev Med 1998;14:245–258.
77. Hotaling GT, Sugarman DB. An analysis of risk markers in husband to wife violence: the current state of knowledge. Violence Vict 1986;1:101–124.
78. Freedman D, Hemenway D. Precursors of lethal violence: a death row sample. Soc Sci Med, 2000;50:1757–1770.
79. Groves BM, Augustyn M, Lee D, et al. Identifying and Responding to Domestic Violence: Consensus Recommendations for Child and Adolescent Health. Family Violence Prevention Fund, San Francisco, CA, 2002.
80. CDC. Youth Risk Behavior Surveillance—United States, 2003. MMWR 2004;53:SS–2.
81. Wekerle C, Wolfe DA. Dating violence in mid-adolescence: theory, significance, and emerging prevention initiatives. Clin Psychol Rev 1999;19:435–456.
82. Gray HM, Foshee V. Adolescent dating violence: differences between one-sided and mutually violent profiles. J Interpers Violence 1997;12:126–141.
83. Makepeace J. Life events stress and courtship violence. Fam Relat 1983;32:101–109.
84. Molidor C, Tolman RM, Kober J. Gender and contextual factors in adolescent dating violence. Prevention Researcher 2000;7:1–4.
85. O'Keefe M, Treister L. Victims of dating violence among high school students. Violence Against Women 1998;4:193–228.
86. Symons PY, Groer MW, Kepler-Youngblood P, et al. Prevalence and predictors of adolescent dating violence. J Child Adolescent Pediatric Nursing 1994;7:14–23.
87. Levy B. In Love and In Danger: A Teen's Guide to Breaking Free of Abusive Relationships. Seal Press, Seattle, 1993.
88. Foshee VA, Bauman KE, Ennett ST, et al. Assessing the long-term effects of the safe dates program and a booster in preventing and reducing adolescent dating violence victimization and perpetration. Am J Public Health 2004;94:619–624.
89. American Medical Association. Guidelines for Adolescent Preventive Services (GAPS): Recommendations Monograph. American Medical Association, Chicago, 1997.
90. Ginsburg KR. Youth violence: if we are not active in prevention efforts, who will be? Arch Pediatr Adolesc Med 1998;152:527–530.
91. Oriel KA, Fleming MF. Screening men for partner violence in a primary care setting: a new strategy for detecting domestic violence. J Fam Pract 1998;46:493–498.
92. Gondolf EW, Jones AS. The program effect of batterer programs in three cities. Violence Vict 2001;16:693–704.
93. Babcock JC, Green CE, Robie C. Does batterers' treatment work? A meta-analytic review of domestic violence treatment. Clin Psychol Rev 2004;23:1023–1053.
94. Saunders D. Feminist-cognitive-behavioral and process-psychodynamic treatment for men who batter: interaction of abuser traits and treatment model. Violence Vict 1996;11: 393–414.
95. Coker AL, Bethea L, Smith PH, et al. Missed opportunities: intimate partner violence in family practice settings. Prev Med 2002;34:445–454.
96. James L, Rudman W, Sawires P, et al. Coding is critical for health care's response to domestic violence. Advance for Health Information Professionals, May 7, 2001.
97. World Health Organization. International Classification of Diseases 10th ed. World Health Organization, 1994-2003. Available at: www.who.int/classifications/icd/en.
98. Mitchell C. Guidelines for the Health Care of Intimate Partner Violence for California Health Professionals. California Office of Emergency Services, California Medical Training Center, Sacramento, CA. 2004.

99. United States Department of Health and Human Services, Office for Civil Rights—HIPAA. Available at: www.hhs.gov/ocr/hipaa.
100. Isaac NE, Enos VP. Documenting Domestic Violence: How Health Care Providers Can Help Victims. National Institute of Justice, 2001.
101. State of California, Governor's Office of Emergency Services. Available at: www.oes.ca.gov (search OES 502 or OES 602).
102. Belknap J, Graham D, Allen GP, et al. Predicting court outcomes in intimate partner violence cases: preliminary findings. Domestic Violence Report 1999;5:1–2, 9–10.
103. Houry D, Sachs CJ, Feldhaus KM, et al. Violence-inflicted injuries: reporting laws in the fifty states. Ann Emerg Med 2002;39:56–60.
104. Brown-Cranstoun J. Kringen v. Boslough and Saint Vincent Hospital: a new trend for healthcare professionals who treat victims of domestic violence? J Health Law 2000;33: 629–655.
105. Lazzaro MV, McFarlane J. Establishing a screening program for abused women. J Nurs Admin 1991;21:24–29.
106. Campbell J. Danger Assessment 2004. Available at: www.dangerassessment.org.
107. Wolfner GD, Gelles RJ. A profile of violence toward children: a national study. Child Abuse Negl 1993;17:197–212.
108. Prochaska JO, DiClemente CC, Norcross JC. In search of how people change: applications to addictive behaviors. Am Psychol 1992;47:1102–1114.
109. Zink T, Elder N, Jacobson J, et al. Medical management of intimate partner violence considering the stages of change: precontemplation and contemplation. Ann Fam Med 2004;2:231–239.
110. McFarlane J, Soeken K, Wiist W. An evaluation of interventions to decrease intimate partner violence to pregnant women. Pub Health Nurs 2000;17:443–451.
111. Sullivan CM, Bybee DI. Reducing violence using community-based advocacy for women with abusive partners. J Consult Clin Psychol 1999;67:43–53.

Index

D

E

J

L

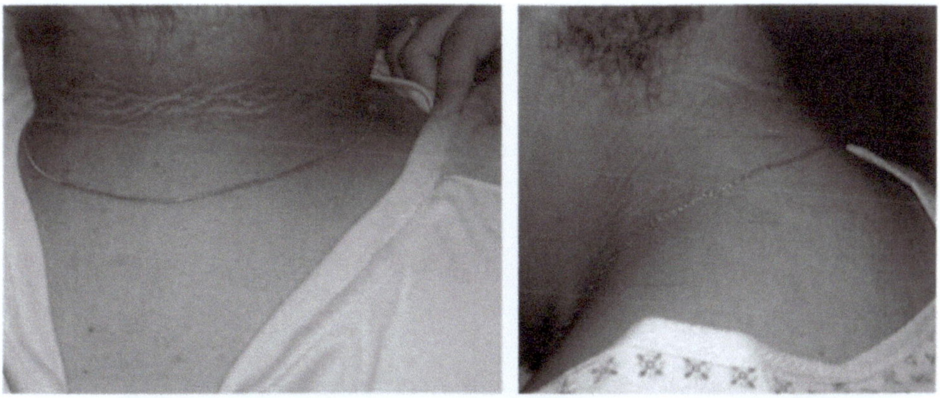

Color Plate 1. Fig. 10.1. *See* legend on p. 188 and discussion on p. 189.

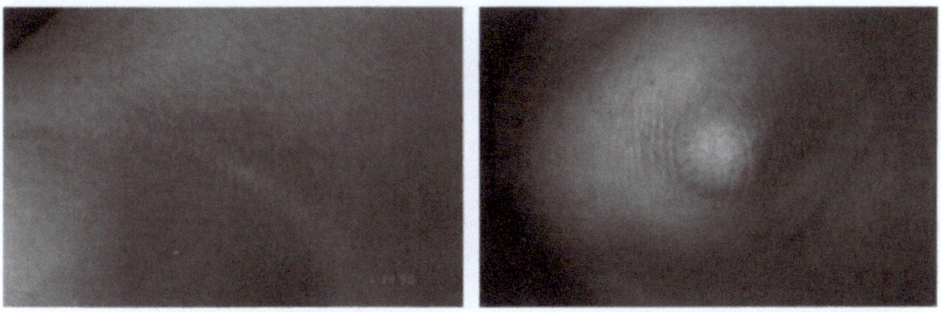

Color Plate 2. Fig. 10.2. *See* legend on p. 189 and discussion on p. 189.

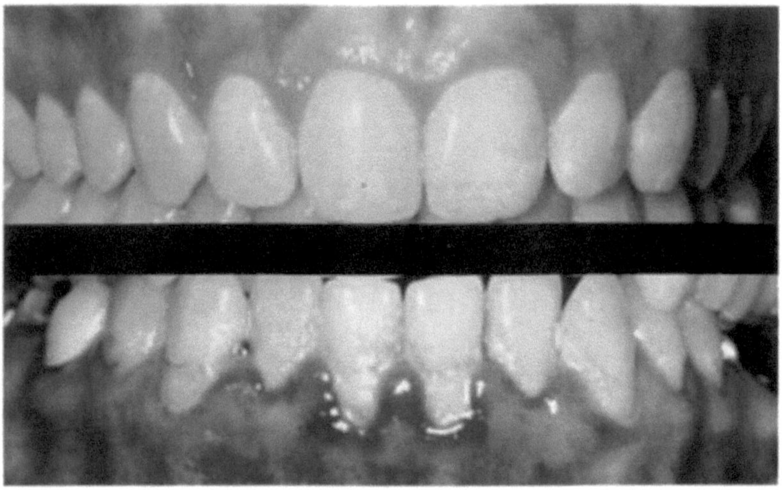

Color Plate 3. Fig. 14.1. *See* legend on p. 275 and discussion on p. 274.

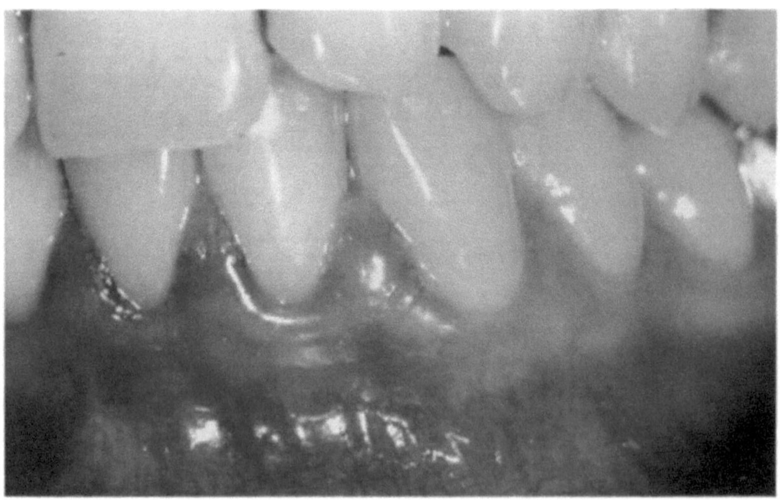

Color Plate 4. Fig. 14.2. *See* legend on p. 277 and discussion on p. 276.

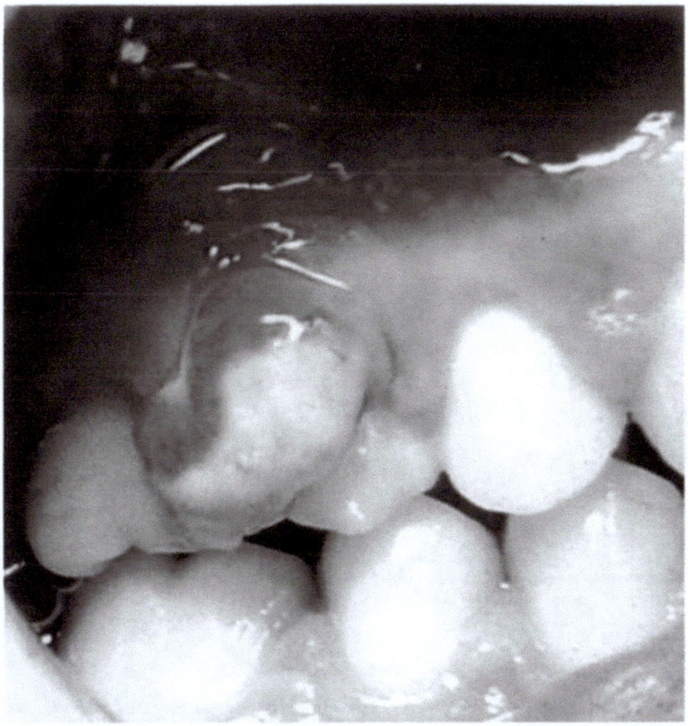

Color Plate 5. Fig. 14.3. *See* legend on p. 278 and discussion on p. 277.

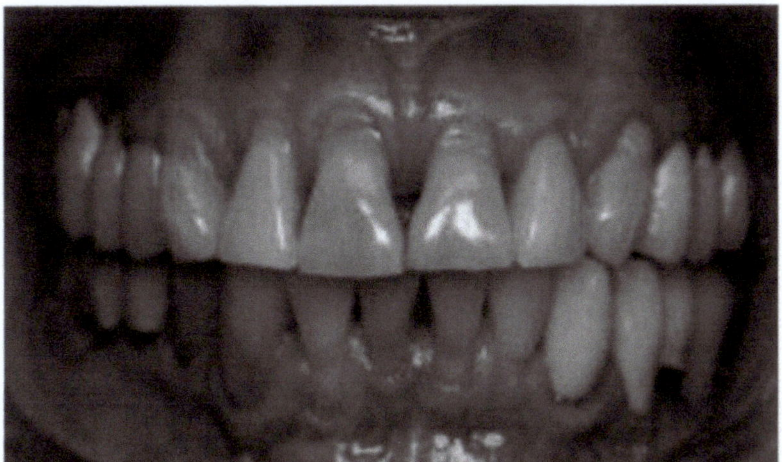

Color Plate 6. Fig. 14.4. *See* legend on p. 287 and discussion on p. 286.

MIX
Papier aus verantwortungsvollen Quellen
Paper from responsible sources
FSC® C105338
FSC
www.fsc.org

If you have any concerns about our products,
you can contact us on
ProductSafety@springernature.com

In case Publisher is established outside the EU,
the EU authorized representative is:
Springer Nature Customer Service Center GmbH
Europaplatz 3, 69115 Heidelberg, Germany

Printed by Libri Plureos GmbH
in Hamburg, Germany